Recent Advancements in the Diagnosis of Human Disease

Editor

Irshad M. Sulaiman
U.S. Food and Drug Administration
Atlanta, GA
USA

CRC Press
Taylor & Francis Group
Boca Raton London New York

CRC Press is an imprint of the
Taylor & Francis Group, an **informa** business

A SCIENCE PUBLISHERS BOOK

Cover credit: Cover images provided by the editor.

First edition published 2024
by CRC Press
2385 NW Executive Center Drive, Suite 320, Boca Raton FL 33431

and by CRC Press
4 Park Square, Milton Park, Abingdon, Oxon, OX14 4RN

CRC Press is an imprint of Taylor & Francis Group, LLC

Library of Congress Cataloging-in-Publication Data (applied for)

ISBN: 978-1-032-57260-4 (hbk)
ISBN: 978-1-032-57264-2 (pbk)
ISBN: 978-1-003-43859-5 (ebk)

DOI: 10.1201/9781003438595

Typeset in Times New Roman
by Radiant Productions

Preface

A disease is a specific aberrant disorder that negatively affects the body of an organism. It is also considered to be a medical condition, often associated with noticeable symptoms. Human disease is frequently referred to any condition that can cause pain, impairment, suffering, or death to the affected individuals. Of the various categories of human diseases, it may be infectious, deficiency, hereditary, and physiological. Infectious diseases are illnesses caused by microorganisms that include bacteria, viruses, and fungi. These human-pathogenic microbes once enter the body, multiply, and can cause mild to severe infections. Furthermore, some of the infectious diseases are transmissible, that spread from person-to- person (human-to-human transmission). However, the pathogens causing mild to life-threatening infectious diseases can be airborne, waterborne, foodborne, and soilborne. It can also be spread by the vectors or by the animals (zoonotic transmission, animal-to-human) or humans (anthroponotic transmission, human-to-human). More recently, several new microbial pathogens have emerged and caused various infectious diseases, a large number of sporadic cases, and deadly outbreaks worldwide; it has also been one of the leading causes of deaths worldwide. The U.S. Centers for Disease Control and Prevention (CDC) estimates that: (i) the national healthcare costs associated with hospital- and community-onset infections from six multidrug-resistant pathogens is more than $4.6 billion annually, and (ii) 90% of the nation's $4.1 trillion in annual health care expenditures are for people with chronic and mental health conditions.

Additionally, the microbial ecology is complex as each microbial organism (species/genotype/sub genotype) in an ecosystem; is believed to occupy a unique niche. It has been established that various strains and species of microbes not typically delimited together but also compete for limited nutrients and space. These extreme challenging conditions often result in the evolution of unique phenotypes of microbes that can outcompete and displace the co-existing genotype/strain/species. Thus, there is a need to characterize more unknown/little less known/less prevalent microorganisms, recovered from clinical, food, environmental, and other settings to establish a clearer understanding of microbial competition and to better predict the performance of microbes causing various illnesses.

With the advancement of molecular diagnostic techniques, it is now possible to detect and differentiate the infectious diseases causing bacteria, viruses, fungi, protozoan parasites in a patient and corelate with the corresponding clinical infection. Considering the fact that genomic material is unique to microbial organism, while characterizing the partial/complete region of gene/genome, the molecular diagnostic test is developed. These molecular tests can provide rapid and precise diagnostic results as compared to the conventional microbiological detection techniques. It has now been proven that it also helps in the control and prevention of various infectious disease. Of these, various PCR-based assays have been widely utilized as molecular diagnostic techniques in the diagnosis of infectious pathogens of public health importance. Currently, the whole-genome sequencing (WGS) is considered to be the gold standard as it can detect single nucleotide variants, insertions/deletions, copy number changes, and large structural variants.

According to CDC, the data generated through molecular diagnostic testing combines the laboratory testing based data with the accuracy of molecular biology. Molecular diagnostic testing has revolutionized the way clinical and public health laboratories investigate the human and microbial genomes, their genes, and the products they encode. These molecular diagnostic tests are most commonly used, and have succeeded several conventional diagnostic tests, in several areas of laboratory medicine including oncology, infectious diseases, clinical chemistry, and clinical genetics. Advancements in molecular diagnostic testing will continue to improve the precision and speed for microbial pathogens detection and characterization of a patient's genes. It is becoming an essential aspect of patient-tailored interventions and therapeutics. Furthermore, the molecular typing tools have facilitated in developing novel vaccines against a specific pathogen.

Thus, considering all of the above facts, this book is compiled on the advancement that has been made in recent past in the diagnosis of various human diseases caused by the human-pathogenic prokaryotic and eukaryotic organisms of public health importance. It will help the scientific community to better understand the diagnosis of several human disease of public health importance.

Contents

Preface   iii

1. **AI-Powered Laboratory Diagnostics Technology**   1
   James Lara

2. **Detection of Gastrointestinal Protists**   46
   Monica Santin, Josephine S.Y. Ng-Hublin and Jenny G. Maloney

3. **Methods Used for Diagnosis of Malaria and their Strengths   104
   and Limitations**
   Samaly Souza Svigel, Venkatachalam Udhayakumar,
   Michael Aidoo, Gireesh Subramaniam and Naomi W. Lucchi

4. **Advances in the Diagnosis of Filarial Nematodes**   118
   Arwa Elaagip and Tarig Higazi

5. **Diagnosis and Treatment of Acute Lung Injury:**   141
   Understanding the Molecular Mechanisms
   Kaiser M. Bijli

6. **MALDI-TOF MS Fingerprinting for the Diagnosis of Infectious   190
   Diseases**
   Hercules Moura, Glauber Wagner, Renato Simões, Yulanda Williamson
   and John R. Barr

7. **Proteomics Fundamentals and Applications in Microbiology**   209
   Glauber Wagner, Guilherme Augusto Maia, John Robert Barr and
   Hercules Moura

8. **Methods for Multiplex Real-Time PCR Melting Curve Assays for   237
   Pathogen Detection**
   Prashant Singh and Frank J. Velez

9. **Persistence and Biofilm Formation of Foodborne Bacterial Pathogens 247
   on Fresh Produce and Equipment Surfaces**
   Hsin-Bai Yin and Jitendra Patel

Index   295

Chapter 1

AI-Powered Laboratory Diagnostics Technology

James Lara

Introduction

Artificial intelligence (AI) is the science, engineering, and development of intelligent machines. The use of AI and machine learning (ML) is a standard across many analytic platforms like Google Analytics (Google 2022), Microsoft's Azure AI (Azure 2022), Meta AI (Meta AI 2022) (Meta is Facebook's parent company) and Amazon web-services (AWS) (AWS 2022). AI-led approaches to develop laboratory diagnostics for the detection and identification of pathogenic microorganisms and diseases are becoming more widely used in government and private industries. Smart technologies, like AI-driven cyber-molecular assays (CMAs) and chatbot technologies, are changing the field of health diagnostics. For instance, the use of chatbots for the remote (over-the-internet) detection of respiratory infectious diseases can vastly improve the point-of-care capacity to diagnose bacterial and viral diseases. Such technology can, for example, guide clinicians against prescribing unnecessary or inappropriate antibiotics, which in turn, lowers economic burdens and risks of antibiotic resistance. Automated diagnostic chatbots exclusively rely on text data provided through a patient's self-assessment (e.g., via questioners or texting), can reduce clinic visits for laboratory testing (e.g., polymerase chain reaction (PCR) and antigen rapid tests) and help to gather accurate population-level information on infection. In the COVID-19 era, the ability of diagnostic chatbots, like "Clara" and "COVID-19 Pediatric Assessment Tool," to reduce unnecessary laboratory testing has been essential for optimizing medical resources to control COVID-19 (Miner et al. 2020, Smith 2020, Yom-Tov 2021). As discussed in the following sections, AI and ML approaches play important roles in the development, design, and optimization of a broad variety of diagnostic tests, including biochemical, molecular-biological, and radiologic tests.

Division of Viral Hepatitis, Centers for Disease Control and Prevention, 1600 Clifton Road NE, Mailstop H18-4, Atlanta, GA 30329, USA.
Email: xzl5@cdc.gov

More than 70 years have passed since the first AI program (a neural network simulator) was invented by Marvin Lee Minsky (Minsky 1954). Mostly driven by advances in ML, computer science, computer engineering and theory of mind, as well as by industrial and government entrepreneurship, the fast-evolving field of AI has expanded into new fields. Yet, AI remains a highly complex, hard-to-understand and sometimes controversial field of science. This is notoriously highlighted by the firing of an AI engineer at Google, who proclaimed that Google's Language Technology is sentient, i.e., it has feelings (Wertheimer 2022). Recent breakthroughs in artificial emotional intelligence (Schuller and Schuller 2018) and natural language processing (NLP) (Chowdhary 2020) have helped build AI systems that are so good at interacting with humans (and acting like humans) that they can trick our minds into believing that the system is self-aware or sentient. Self-aware AI or artificial super intelligence (ASI) technologies are presently a hypothetical concept. So, the event of "Skynet" gaining self-awareness and destroying humanity will remain (for now) in the realm of science fiction.[1]

What today's AI technology offers is efficient, effective and accurate means for analyzing massive amounts of data, learning complex dependencies or relationships from data and solving the hardest of the hardest problems in just a minuscule fraction of the time it would take humans to complete. This sort of capability, for instance, is of utmost importance for advancing novel, scalable and accurate diagnostic support technologies for health organizations to be efficient and successful in planning and executing an effective response intervention against a large outbreak or pandemic. Moreover, for any data-driven digital framework to be successful and effective in serving public health needs, three marks need to be achieved, which are getting the right data at the right time to the right people. AI-powered technology has provided effective solutions for hitting all three marks (Nagarajan 2019).

However, AI technology is not a magic wand nor is it bulletproof. It is vulnerable to several things, such as design flaws (e.g., errors in the programming, use of inappropriate verification-and-validation methods, etc.), faulty data and corruption exploitation (a.k.a. adversarial attacks[2]). High-quality/high-accuracy data is of great importance in AI- and ML-based frameworks purposed for pathogen diagnostics or health interventions. Data in and of itself is worthless if it is of low quality or inaccurate, as data has value to the degree that useful and accurate information can be extracted from it. In computer science, the concept of poor data quality is reflected in the GIGO principle: "If you put Garbage In the AI system, you get Garbage Out of the AI system." We also note that even high-quality and accurate data may be worthless if it is not timely communicated or shared with the appropriate end user (or customer). For instance, communication channels among laboratory and healthcare professionals, including patients, are a relevant component in the lifecycle of a clinical laboratory test (Lubin et al. 2021). A 2021 study found that delays in the availability

---

[1] Skynet is a fictional self-aware ASI system that serves as the antagonistic force in the Sci-Fi "Terminator" franchise (2009–2019).

[2] Adversarial attack is an AI method to generate faulty data inputs and it is purposely designed to cause an AI model to make mistakes in its predictions or deviate from its intended behavior.

or the reporting of laboratory testing results can have negative consequences in patient-care settings, such as the increased risk of unplanned emergency/urgent care visits (Lubin et al. 2021). The approaches and methods used to mitigate data-related vulnerabilities of AI/ML-powered diagnostics will be discussed in more detail in the examples presented in this chapter. Software designing tools and cybersecurity approaches for addressing software design and AI model corruption vulnerabilities, respectively, are beyond the scope of this chapter.

Finally, it is worth mentioning the meaning of some of the terms used in the fields of AI and the applications presented in this chapter. Typically, terms like "Intelligent" or "Smart" denote computational systems driven by AI (e.g., deep learning (DL) technology). However, this is not always the case. These terms are sometimes misused to refer to systems that output tailored decisions, predictions or recommendations that can be handled by an explicitly directed automated process. "Cyber" is another common term in computer and data science. This prefix carries a connotation of a relationship between modern computing, information technology (IT) and the internet. So, chatbot technology, like "Clara" (Miner et al. 2020, Smith 2020), which is AI-driven, web-accessible and powered by cloud computing technologies, is a good example of intelligent cyber diagnostic technology. For IT applications, the term "diagnostics frameworks" typically refers to an analytic platform capability to conduct data diagnostics (e.g., data monitoring, data evaluation and information discovery) and application services diagnostics (e.g., monitoring application operability, functionality, and usage). Such capabilities are standard in many AI-analytic platforms (AWS 2022, Azure 2022, Google 2022). The concepts, technology and approaches associated with IT-related diagnostics frameworks are also applicable and flexibly extendable to diagnostics frameworks for Digital Laboratory Diagnostics built on AI-enabled analytic platforms (IBM 2020, Inc. 2022, Microsoft 2022). In the section that follows, we introduce a brief overview of the history, concepts, approaches and technologies associated with AI technology.

Section 1 Computers and Artificial Intelligence

"The Electronic Brain" is a phrase widely associated with computers since their invention in the 1940s. However, nothing could be further from the truth. There is very little in common between the way that computers and brains operate. The fact is that for some tasks such as calculating, sorting, filing, associating and playing games, computers can do better than brains. But in other tasks, such as understanding the world, computers continue to lag behind humans. Since the 1940s, researchers from diverse fields of science (neurosciences, mathematics and computer science) have sought to understand the principles of brain organization and function (Minsky 1954, Ichikawa and Matsumoto 2004, Ahmad and Sumari 2017, Hasler 2017, Wang and Xia 2021, Hou et al. 2022). Two major reasons compel us to do this. First, we wish to have a better understanding of how the brain achieves its cognitive competence. Second, we want to find ways of transferring this competence to computers and machines. Several factors motivate this quest (e.g., convenience, financial motives, etc.). Ultimately, we want machines with human-like reasoning and decision-making power to perform critical, and complex tasks every time, all the time, with high accuracy and efficiency. For example, AI-powered machines, like AI robots and unmanned AI aerial vehicles, are reshaping the military battlefield (NEWS 2020) and many other extreme, complex and dangerous job fields (Swindells 1995). Recent advances in AI algorithms and approaches [e.g., cognitive AI, conversational AI and emotional AI (Ahmad and Sumari 2017, Schuller and Schuller 2018, Kulkarni et al. 2019)], as well as innovations in computing hardware technology [e.g., computer chips, central processing units (CPUs) and graphical processing units (GPUs) (Meyer 2018, MSV 2020, INTEL 2022, NVIDIA 2022)], are paving the way toward the creation of better rationally thinking-and-acting machines. Such types of machines are already improving several areas of healthcare services, including screening and treatment of outpatient conditions (Campbell and Jovanovic 2021).

AI is commonly defined as a technology that enables a computer system or a machine to simulate human behavior, albeit other definitions have been proposed over past decades[3] (Williams 1983, Stuart J. Rusell 2012, IBM 2020, Azure 2022). The goal of AI technology is to create computer systems and machines that, like humans, can "rationally think" and/or "rationally act" (Stuart J. Rusell 2012). ML is a branch of computer science that focuses on the use of data and computational algorithms to imitate the way that humans learn to gradually become intelligent. Technically, ML is a subset of AI that allows machines to automatically learn from past data without the requirement for explicit programming.[4] A simple and reader-friendly explanation of the difference between AI and ML is provided by Microsoft: "An 'intelligent' computer uses AI to think like a human and perform tasks on its own. Machine learning is how a computer system develops its intelligence" (Azure 2022). Although AI and ML are technically different, herein we use these terms interchangeably for purposes of simplifying our discussion. For a more detailed discussion and exploration of AI technology, we refer readers to other sources of information on the subject (Williams 1983, Arbib 2003, Hinton et al. 2006, Hinton and Salakhutdinov 2006, Bengio 2009, Li and Dong 2014, Ahmad and Sumari 2017, Saleh 2019, Dargan et al. 2020, IBM 2020, Wang and Xia 2021, Azure 2022), including the textbook *Artificial Intelligence: A Modern Approach* by Stuart Russell and Peter Norvig, which is currently on its 4th edition and considered, by the tech industry as one of the leading textbooks in the field of AI (IBM 2020). Some of the top leading textbooks in the field of AI research are listed in Table 1.

In recent years, AI technology has become ubiquitous. It is present in almost all the devices we use every day. It is in our watches, phones, TVs, remote controllers and automobiles, basically in any electronic devise with a microcontroller chip (a chip

---

[3] John McCarthy, in his paper "What is Artificial Intelligence?", defined AI as follows: "It is the science and engineering of making intelligent machines, especially intelligent computer programs. It is related to the similar task of using computers to understand human intelligence, but AI does not have to confine itself to methods that are biologically observable" (source: https://borghese.di.unimi.it/Teaching/AdvancedIntelligentSystems/Old/IntelligentSystems_2008_2009/Old/IntelligentSystems_2005_2006/Documents/Symbolic/04_McCarthy_whatisai.pdf).

[4] Explicit programming is the process of manually controlling a machine's action by specifically writing each instruction for every action of the machine.

Table 1. Five of the leading AI research textbooks as of 2021[§].

Book Title	About the Author	Summarization of Covered Topics
Artificial Intelligence: A Modern Approach	Stuart Russell: Founder of the Center for Human-Compatible Artificial Intelligence at UC Berkeley. Peter Norvig: Councillor of the Association for the Advancement of Artificial Intelligence (AAAI).	The most comprehensive and up-to-date introduction to the theory and practice of AI.
Introduction to Artificial Intelligence	Philip C Jackson: Software designer and developer and founder of TalaMind LLC, which conducts research toward human-level AI.	Serves as an introduction to the science of reasoning processes in computers. Easy-to-read coverage of problem-solving methods, automated understanding of natural languages, etc.
The Emotion Machine: Commonsense Thinking, Artificial Intelligence, and the Future of the Human Mind	Marvin L. Minsky: Pioneer in the field of ANN and inventor of the first working ANN model.	Offers a new model for how our minds work, and presents arguments of why emotions, intuitions and feelings are not distinct but different ways of thinking.
Machine Learning	Tom M. Mitchell: Co-chairs a congressionally mandated follow-on study due in 2023; 2017 U.S. National Academy report on IT and the Future of Work.	Intended to support undergraduate-level and introductory graduate-level courses in ML.
Deep Learning (Adaptive Computation and Machine Learning series)	Ian Goodfellow: Scientist at OpenAI; inventor of the generative adversarial networks and contributor of various ML software, including TensorFlow and Theano. Aaron Courville: Developer of AI software and co-chair at CIFAR. Yoshua Bengio: Co-director of the Learning in Machines & Brains project at the Canadian Institute for Advanced Research.	Covers relevant concepts in probability theory, information theory, and deep learning techniques (e.g., deep feedforward networks and convolutional neural networks). Offers research perspectives on theoretical topics such as autoencoders, structured probabilistic models, Monte Carlo methods, and deep generative models.

§ Source: California-based AI News platform, Marktechpost; available at: https://www.marktechpost. com/2021/06/11/top-artificial-intelligence-books-to-read-in-2021/.

that can be the size of a grain of salt) (Meyer 2018, MSV 2020). Moreover, we can find AI projects in every government and private industry (Mckinsey and Company 2019, Walch and Schmelzer 2019). In a 2019 survey, the AI technology analyst firm, Cognilytica, identified over 3,000 vendor companies across over 100 subsegments of the AI market implementing a wide range of AI applications (Walch and Schmelzer 2019). The survey found that over 70% of those vendors were applying their AI-powered solutions to a wide range of industry-specific domains (e.g., finance, health care, cybersecurity, autonomous vehicles, etc.). In addition, Walch and Schmelzer (2019) noted patterns in the AI applications and proposed seven usage patterns (shown in Figure 1). The theories and AI/ML algorithms that are involved

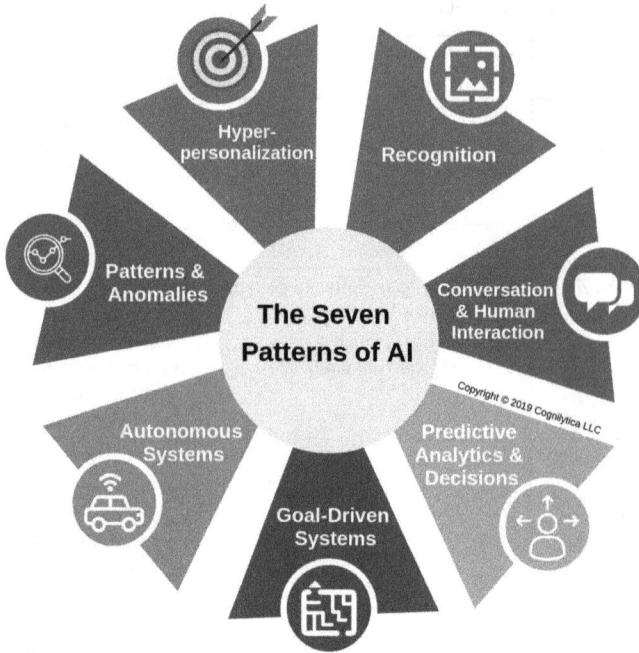

Figure 1. Visualization of the usage patterns of AI technology (as identified in a 2019 Survey by K. Walch and R. Schmelzer). "Reproduced with permission from Cognilytica, The Seven Patterns of AI - [online] Cognilytica (2019). Copyright 2019, Cognilytica LLC."

and used to tackle some of today's industry-specific problems (e.g., finance, national defense and others) are discussed in more detail by Russell and Norvig (2012). The usage patterns of AI technology in health care, public health surveillance and laboratory diagnostics applications are listed below (in no hierarchical order).

1) Hyper-Personalization: Hyper-personalization (or hypersonalization) is a marketing term used to refer to what is broadly known as personalization or customization. For this type of task, ML is used to extract user-specific information and profiles from end users (or customers) for purposes that include gaining insights about the behaviors, likes and needs of users, providing better ways of engaging and retaining customers, providing personalized information and advice to users, etc. One case example is media companies, like Spotify, which use ML technology to gain data-led insights on how, where and when a customer wants to receive content (Jain 2021). Other case examples include the health care and laboratory diagnostics industries, where personalized medicine technology uses ML to recognize and identify unique clinical needs or healthcare requirements for each patient (Schork 2019) and where personalized laboratory diagnostics technology uses ML to extract information (e.g., molecular, or radiological or biochemical profiles) in the clinical context of the individual patient for providing precise diagnoses and tailored clinical recommendations and treatments (Jha and Topol 2016, Jaffe and Mani 2018, Prodan Zitnik et al. 2018, Giordano et al. 2021).

2) Predictive Analytics and Decisions: Predictive analytics can be defined as the use of big data, statistical algorithms and ML to identify the likelihood of future outcomes based on *a priori* knowledge (a.k.a., historical data) (Poornima and Pushpalatha 2018). AI-powered predictive analytics goes beyond data analytics to the specialized task of extracting from the prior knowledge a set of features relevant to the target to provide the most accurate prediction of the future. Some of the ML methods used to select, extract, or construct relevant predictive features (also referred to as attributes or descriptors) are discussed in Digital Biomarkers, Section 3.1. Predictive analytics has a broad range of applications, including weather forecasting (Poornima and Pushpalatha 2018, Marzieh et al. 2022), aircraft handling and control (Haider 2020) and threat awareness on the battlefield (Williams 2022). The primary objective of predictive analytics is to provide decisions or decision support. This objective is aimed at providing reliable decision-making or decision-support systems to assist and help users to make better decisions (Poornima and Pushpalatha 2018, Haider 2020, Williams 2022) to take the right actions at the right time (Haider 2020) or to lower (or eliminate) cognitive burdens associated with highly time-sensitive and complex tasks (Haider 2020, Williams 2022). In fields of health and care, public health surveillance and laboratory diagnostics, AI-powered predictive analytics provide, for instance, guidance for optimizing laboratory diagnosis procedures (McRae et al. 2016, Lubin et al. 2021) and guidance for response interventions (Poornima and Pushpalatha 2018, Meystre et al. 2022) or provide advice to clinicians and patients (Poornima and Pushpalatha 2018, Lamba et al. 2021, Lubin et al. 2021, Meystre et al. 2022).

3) Conversation and Human Interaction: For AI computer agents[5] (AI agents) to naturally converse with humans and retrieve knowledge from human interaction, they must be able to process natural languages and be able to acquire information from written or spoken language. So, if an agent wants to do knowledge acquisition, it must understand (at least partially) the ambiguities and complexity of human languages to perform information-seeking tasks, such as text classification and information retrieval. One common factor in addressing these tasks is the use of language models that predict the probability distribution of language expressions (Russell and Norvig 2012). On the other hand, if an agent aims at a deep understanding of a conversation to communicate with humans in natural language, then language models need to be more complex than those aimed, for instance, at simple text classifications. This level of communication typically starts with grammatical models of the phrase structure of sentences, then adding semantics to the model and then applying machine translation and speech recognition methods. Recent advances in neural machine translation (NMT) represent a significant step forward in machine translation capabilities (Sutskever et al. 2014, Bahdanau et al. 2015). For instance, in

---

[5] An AI agent program can be defined as the study of the rational agent and its environment. AI agents can sense the environment through sensors and act on their environment through actuators. AI agents can be endowed with cognitive properties such as knowledge, belief, intention, etc. (Source: https://www.javatpoint.com/agents-in-ai; last accessed 08/28/2022).

2020, Google added five new languages to its Google Translate in what was then its first expansion in the past few years. On May 11, 2022, Google made headline news when it announced it added 24 new languages to its Translate app (BBC News 2022). This advancement was accomplished because Google's Zero-Shot Machine Translation (ZMT), an NMT-based ML model, can learn to translate into another language without ever seeing an example (Caswell (2022) [Online]). Innovations in deep learning and NLP technology (Bengio 2009, Russell and Norvig 2012, Li and Dong 2014, Chowdhary 2020, Dargan et al. 2020, Ataee 2021, Sarker 2021), coupled with new machine translation technology (Sutskever et al. 2014, Bahdanau Cho et al. 2015, Wang et al. 2021) are fueling the development of evermore intelligent conversation and human interaction technologies. In Section 4.2, we focus our discussion on the applications of such technologies, for over-the-internet laboratory diagnostics of SARS-CoV-2. In depth, discussion of computer agents, natural language processing (NLP) and natural language communication processes can be found in Russell and Norvig (2012) [Chapters 22 and 23 (Russell and Norvig 2012)] and other sources (Russell and Norvig 2012, Chowdhary 2020).

4) Pattern Recognition and Anomaly Detection: Pattern recognition can be defined as the classification (or clustering) of data based on *a priori* knowledge or based on statistical information extracted from data patterns and/or their representation. One of the most important aspects of pattern recognition techniques is its broad range of applications (Begum and Devi 2011, Ridder et al. 2013, Zhang et al. 2020, Siontis et al. 2021, Khalil et al. 2022). Applications include signal processing tasks, like speech recognition for communication management systems (Li and Dong 2014), electrocardiogram (ECG) recognition for automatic medical diagnosis applications (Siontis et al. 2021) or electroencephalogram (EEC) recognition for automatic lie detection applications (Khalil et al. 2022). Pattern recognition techniques also have applications for the detection of outliers, anomalies and novelty in data (Zhang et al. 2020). In general, outliers are patterns that deviate from the mean distribution location observed in the sampled data. However, outliers might not be anomalous as anomalies are generated by different processes or mechanisms (Hawkins 1980, Chandola et al. 2009, Alamo et al. 2021, Schneider and Xhafa 2022). Chandola, Banerjee and Kumar (2016) defined anomalies[6] as "patterns in data that do not conform to a well-defined notion of normal behavior," which might be induced in the data for a variety of reasons (e.g., malicious activity or breakdown of a system) (Chandola et al. 2009). On the other hand, the aim of automated novelty detection is to detect new or unknown patterns in data, which can sometimes prove to be a much harder task than the outlier or anomaly detection tasks (Markou and Singh 2003). AI-powered anomaly detection is used in many applications such as cyber-intrusion detection, fraud detection, image processing, sensor networks, medical anomaly detection and public health anomaly detection (Chandola et al.

---

[6] In published literature, anomalies are also referred to as rare events, abnormalities, aberrations, deviants, or outliers. Hawkins (1980) defined an anomaly as *"an observation which deviates so much from other observations as to arouse suspicions that it was generated by a different mechanism"*.

2009, Alamo et al. 2021, Han et al. 2021, Schneider and Xhafa 2022). Anomaly detection technology plays critical roles in the analysis of epidemiological data and management of pandemics like COVID-19 (Alamo et al. 2021, Schneider and Xhafa 2022). For instance, we often find that epidemiological data suffer from severe limitations (e.g., missing or inaccurate, or duplicated data, including inappropriate record keeping), application of anomaly detection on raw epidemiological data can be used for reconciling observations and/or predictions among different external data sources (a process known as data reconciliation) (Alamo et al. 2021). Other applications include pathogen infection anomaly detection (Wang et al. 2016, Aminian et al. 2020).

5) Autonomous Systems: The first system that came were mechanical systems (e.g., human-powered machines, like levers, or fuel-powered machines, like combustion engines). Then came automated systems (e.g., automated industrial processing systems, like Oliver Evans' fully automatic flour mill machine[7]). Now, we have AI-powered autonomous systems. The primary objective of the first two systems is to minimize human labor. In manufacturing settings, they also help lower costs for business owners and increase energy efficiency, productivity, accuracy and better production quality. AI autonomous systems accomplish the primary objectives of all previous systems and, in addition, it gives intelligence to machines, so they can sense, plan and act in dynamic environments, which minimizes the need for human intelligence for accomplishing tasks or mission goals. A good example of state-of-the-art autonomous AI technology is in *autonomous planning and scheduling:* NASA's Remote Agent program became the first on-board autonomous planning program to control the scheduling of operations for a spacecraft (Jonsson et al. 2000). The remote agent generated plans from predefined goals and monitored the execution of those plans–detecting, diagnosing and recovering from problems as they occurred. Hardware autonomous ystems[8] (Lysecky and Vahid 2005, Salvador et al. 2013, Camsari et al. 2017, Hussein 2017, Faria et al. 2021) as well as software autonomous systems are found across many industries and applied to a broad diversity of tasks, from helping to make the perfect "Cheetos"[9] (Culler 2020) to executing mission planning of spacecraft and rovers, for Mars exploration programs by NASA and the European Space Agency (Ai-Chang et al. 2004, Cesta et al. 2007).

---

[7] In 1785, Oliver Evans, an American inventor and engineer, developed an automatic flour mill, which is believed to be history's first completely automated industrial process by being able to have continuous production without any human intervention. (Source: https://www.progressiveautomations.com/blogs/news/the-evolution-of-automation; last accessed 08/30/2022).

[8] In the context of autonomous systems, the term "hardware" refers to a configurable computing chip technology (e.g., Field Programmable Gate Arrays (FPGAs)) that provides designers with the ability to quickly create hardware circuits to deliver improved performance over software-only computing. This type of autonomous system is also referred to as adaptive computing system.

[9] Cheetos is a crunchy corn puff snack brand made by Frito-Lay, a subsidiary of PepsiCo. PepsiCo, in collaboration with Microsoft, developed an AI-automated system that makes recommendations or adjustments any time a product falls out of specs.

We note that the primary objectives and tasks delineated for the above five AI patterns can also be achieved with the use of statistical methods. For instance, Google Maps and Microsoft's Bing can forecast congestion and its duration by performing advanced statistical predictive analysis of traffic patterns (Pan et al. 2017). Similarly, statistical models are used for decision-making, anomaly detection and pattern recognition tasks (Jain et al. 2000, Chandola et al. 2009, Latimer et al. 2016). However, unlike statistical models, AI models use ML algorithms to achieve the capacity for improving the accuracy of the predictions, as well as the capacity for rapidly adapting (or adjusting) their predictions to changes in data over time. Moreover, deep learning techniques have provided the means for ML models to tackle very large data and to learn a large set of interrelated concepts, which might be key to the kind of broad generalizations that humans appear able to do (Bengio 2009, Li and Dong 2014, Sarker 2021) [a feat not achievable by statistical methods alone (Bengio 2009)].

Finally, we note that AI technologies can be grouped into different types (or categories). There are four types of AI that are mainstream, which are: reactive machines, limited memory, theory of mind and self-aware. When considering the technical parlance used among AI researchers, AI can be further categorized into three additional types (Table 2). These seven categories of AI are based on what the AI technology is used for, what it is capable of, and how it helps advance humanity (Joshi 2019, Saleh 2019, IBM 2020, Johnson 2020). Nearly all AI applications we know of, including the ones discussed herein, are driven by "limited memory AI." Present-day AI applications, including AI models that use deep learning, rely on large training datasets to form a reference model to solve a problem and/or to generate a decision or a diagnosis. The types of AI and their description are shown in Table 2.

Section 1.1 Artificial Neural Network Technology

The first example of a brain-inspired AI technology is the artificial neural network (ANN) (Minsky 1954, Arbib 2003). In simple terms, an ANN model is a computational model emulating biologic neuron operations that can, in principle, be used to compute any arithmetic or logical function. A general schematic representation of an ANN architecture is shown in Figure 2. An ANN model comprises two types of components: neurons and connections. Neurons (or perceptrons) are units that computationally process input data, receives-and-transmit information and generate a prediction. The connections, with adjustable "weights" or "strengths," propagate the information signals from one neuron to another for further processing. The most basic type of a multiple-layer ANN is the three-layer feedforward model [a.k.a., multiple-layer perceptron (MLP)], where neurons are classified into three types according to the layer they are found: (1) *input neurons*, forming the input layer, are responsible for receiving and processing input vectors and transmitting signal information to neurons on the next layer; (2) *hidden neurons*, forming the hidden layer, receive information from the input layer and further process and transmit signal vectors to neurons in the output layer; (3) *output neurons*, in the final layer, produce the model's output or prediction.

Table 2. Classification of AI technologies as of 2022[§].

Number	AI Type[‡]	Summarized Description
1.	Reactive Machines	The oldest and simplest form of AI systems. They have no memory-based functionality, meaning they store no input and cannot learn from previous data. A popular example of a reactive AI machine is IBM's Deep Blue, which defeated chess grandmaster Garry Kasparov in 1997.
2.	Limited Memory	AI's capable of storing data and learning from historical data and using it to make better predictions. Nearly all existing applications that we know of (from chatbots or virtual assistants to autonomous vehicles) come under this category of AI.
3.	Theory of Mind[†]	This AI exists either as a concept or as a work in progress (e.g., self-driving cars and Google's Language Technology). In the theory of mind AI, AI systems begin to interact and understand the needs, emotions, beliefs and thought processes of humans.
4.	Self-Aware[†]	This marks the final stage of AI. AI has evolved to be so akin to the human brain that it has developed self-awareness. AI will be able to understand and evoke emotions in those it interacts with and have emotions, needs, beliefs and potential desires of its own. Likely, humans will have to negotiate terms with the intelligent entity it created. What happens, good or bad, is anyone's guess.
5.	Artificial Narrow Intelligence (ANI)	ANI represents all the existing AI, including the most complicated and capable AI that has ever been created to date.
6.	Artificial General Intelligence[†] (AGI)	AGI is the ability of an AI agent to learn, perceive, understand and function like a human being. Will become the most capable forms of intelligence on earth.
7.	Artificial Super Intelligence[†] (ASI)	ASI will mark the pinnacle of AI research. These machines will, at the very least, affect our way of life.

[‡] Categories 1–4, are mainstream, while types 5–6 are three additional types of AI and terminologies that are used in tech-oriented circles.

[†] Types oF AI that are currently only at the hypothetical stage.

[§] Source URLs: Johnson (2020) [Online], Joshi (2019) [Online].

ANN models can have many varied architectural complexities and implement a wide range of mathematical functions. ANN model complexity, i.e., the number of neurons conforming the hidden layers (layer size) and density of the network connectivity is influenced by many factors, like the complexity of the data and the task, training methods used, the permitted error tolerance thresholds, etc. (Fausett 1994, Swingler 1996, Kon and Plaskota 2000, Arbib 2003, Yamashita et al. 2018, Freire et al. 2021). Designing an ANN model is more of an art form than a systematic process. In a very general sense, the process of deriving the right complexity of the ANN model's architecture involves a tradeoff between the desired accuracy with the training data and the generalization[10] capability of the model to make accurate predictions over unseen or new data. Reaching a healthy balance between the two

---

[10] Generalization is defined as the ability of an ANN model (or any other ML method) to classify a pattern that was not included in the training data (see Figure 2A).

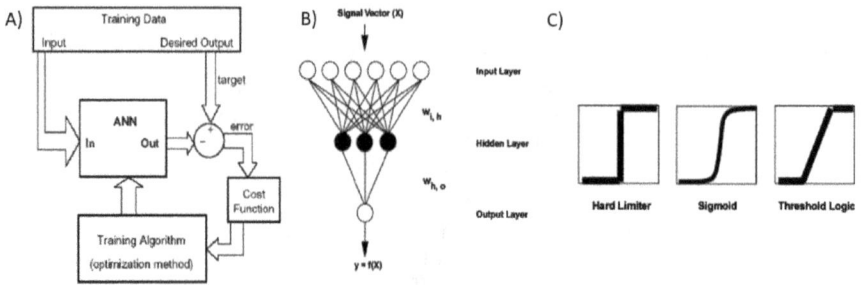

Figure 2. Schematic representation of the training, functions and architecture of a general 3-layered MLP. (A) Supervised learning schematic (i.e., training ANN models with examples). The ANN learns to map a set of signal inputs to specified (desired) outputs in the training data. The adaptation (value changes) of the weights is achieved through a cost function for error minimization, and the training algorithm during the training epochs. (B) Architecture of a three-layer feedforward MLP (with a size of 1 hidden layer and 3 hidden neurons). The number of input neurons represents the number of variables or features (i.e., the dimensional vector space of data). Neurons are represented as circles with weighted inputs and output shown as arrows. (C) Three common types of nonlinearity functions used in ANN models.

requires experimenting by trial-and-error different architectures, as well as manual refining of the model's hyperparameters. For an ANN model to be efficient, the number of hidden layers and their size must be sufficient for the model to make a good representation of the data, but sufficiently low to allow generalizations to be made when new data become available (Fausett 1994, Swingler 1996). If the ANN model is too deep (i.e., a large number of hidden layers and hidden neurons), the model will be fitted on the training data, resulting in an ANN model exhibiting high accuracy on training data, but unable to generalize on future data. Overfitting is a big problem because the performance evaluation of ANN models on training data is very different from the performance evaluation that is of utmost importance, which is on how accurate ANN models are in solving future problems or making accurate decisions on new data. We note that the overfitting problem is not unique to ANN models; in fact, it is a general optimization problem for all shallow ML[11] technologies [e.g., Support Vector Machines (SVM), Decision Trees (DT), Random Forest (RF), Naïve Bayesian Classifiers (NBC), etc.].

There are two other distinct phenomena closely associated with the optimization problem of ANN models, namely, the "curse of dimensionality" (Bellman 1957, Fausett 1994, Arbib 2003, Russell and Norvig 2012) and the "optimizer's curse" (Smith and Winkler 2006, Russell and Norvig 2012). The latter refers to a problem closely associated with "expectations" on the selection of a model, while the former is associated with the challenges of data requirement fulfillment. The optimizer's curse problem can be defined as a post-decision surprise or disappointment that ensues when a model's performance deviates from the expected results. This curse crops up because of the optimization-based selection process, which aims at selecting

---

[11] Shallow ML typically refers to ANN with 0 or up to 2 hidden layers, a.k.a., as MLP's. Shallow ML algorithms is any algorithm that does not use deep learning and rely on expert-based descriptors (or labelling), while deep learning algorithms enable models to learn compact abstract representations from the data.

the best model from n alternative models whose prediction output is thought of as "true values" representing the expected value or expected utility. The problem is that as the number of alternatives (or choices) increases, extremely optimistic estimates are more likely to arise (Russell and Norvig 2012). The tendency for the estimated expected utility of the best choice model to be too high is what is referred to as the optimizer's curse (Smith and Winkler 2006). In other words, sometimes what appears to be the best choice may not be, if the variance in the utility estimate is high. For instance, a ML model selected from thousands that have 90% accuracy is probably worse than one that had 70% accuracy. Smith and Winkler 2006, proposed that "the key to overcoming the optimizer's curse is conceptually quite simple: model the uncertainty in the value estimates explicitly and use Bayesian methods to interpret these value estimates" (Smith and Winkler 2006). Bayesian methods that do this have been proposed (Smith and Winkler 2006, Ning and You 2019).

The curse of dimensionality, which is defined as a problem related to the data size (i.e., the number of samples) that is needed to estimate an arbitrary function with a given level of accuracy, grows exponentially with respect to the number of input variables (i.e., dimensionality) of the function (Bellman 1957). For similarity search functions (e.g., nearest neighbor), the curse of dimensionality means that the number of variables in the dataset that need to be accessed grows exponentially with the underlying dimensionality in the data (Russell and Norvig 2012). In other words, if the number of variables in finite data is too large, the curse of dimensionality renders the finite data into sparse data. The problem with the number of data samples being relatively small compared to the dimensional vector space of the data also affects processes of ML methods, such as the process of ANN parameter estimation (e.g., estimating the number of the hidden neurons in the ANN model or estimating the stopping criteria of the training process, etc.). In most real-world analysis scenarios, the data available for processing is limited and the collection of more data is nearly unfeasible because of constraints associated with the costs and/or technical difficulty. Curse of dimensionality is often experienced in diverse fields of science [e.g., medical diagnostics, where available biological, epidemiological and clinical data are very limited and data collection costs are high (Panel on the Design of the National Children's, Implications for the Generalizability of et al. 2014)]. In today's world of AI and big data, the optimization problem associated with deep ANN models has been greatly mitigated with the introduction of deep learning techniques.

Section 1.2 Deep Learning (DL) Technology

The emergence of deep learning techniques in 2006 has transformed and advanced the fields of ANN and ML (Bengio et al. 2006, Hinton et al. 2006, Hinton and Salakhutdinov 2006, Bernhard et al. 2007, Li and Dong 2014, Dargan et al. 2020, Sarker 2021). Deep learning technology drives many of today's modern AI applications (e.g., voice-enabled TVs and self-driving cars) and many services provided by healthcare and financial institutions [e.g., virtual assistants or chatbots (Education 2020, Azure 2022)]. Deep learning neural network technology has outperformed traditional ML methods in tasks associated with speech recognition (Fernández et al. 2007) and has broken records in several areas of ML, including machine language translation (Sutskever et al. 2014), Language Modeling (Jozefowicz et al. 2016) and handwriting recognition (Graves and Schmidhuber 2008). Deep learning[12] can be defined as a class of ML techniques that exploit many layers of non-linear information processing for supervised or unsupervised feature extraction and transformation and for pattern analysis and classification (Li and Dong 2014). Deep learning is essentially a learning technique based on deep ANN models (i.e., ANN models with several hidden layers) that attempts to simulate the human brain, learn from large amounts of data and enable AI systems to perform classification, clustering and pattern recognition tasks with exceptional accuracy. The objective of deep learning is of moving ML closer to one of its original goals: Artificial Intelligence (several tutorial resources on deep learning is available at Github, Inc. (2023) [Online]). Presently, deep learning is the best method for training deep ML architectures like deep neural networks (DNN), convolutional neural networks (CNN), deep Bayesian networks (DBN), restricted Boltzmann machines (RBMs) and others.

Regarding the curse of dimensionality, Bengio (2009) proposed that "what matters for generalization is not dimensionality, but instead the number of "variations" of the function we wish to obtain after learning" (Bengio 2009). Therefore, to escape the curse of dimensionality it would be necessary to have a model that can capture the many variations that can occur in the data without having to enumerate all of them. Instead, a compact representation that captures most of these variations must be discovered by the learning algorithm, where "compact" means that such variations in data could be encoded with a few bits. Deep architecture models can achieve this level of data compression through deep learning techniques, i.e., they can extract compact information representative of the data, which is then encoded at various levels in the model's architecture (Bengio et al. 2006, Hinton and Salakhutdinov 2006, Bernhard et al. 2007, Bengio 2009). A full description of deep learning techniques and discussion on deep architecture models can be found in Bengio (2009) and elsewhere in the literature (Bengio et al. 2006, Hinton et al. 2006, Hinton and Salakhutdinov 2006, Bernhard et al. 2007, Li and Dong 2014, Dargan et al. 2020, Sarker 2021). We note that other solutions for mitigating the curse of dimensionality address the utilization of computer computing resources, like the better use of GPUs (Johnson et al. 2021) and yet others address it with domain-specific algorithm solutions [e.g., algorithms for similarity searches that use k-nearest neighbor methods (Chen et al. 2010, Fu et al. 2019)]. A case example of the use of these two types of solution approaches is the Facebook AI Similarity Search (Faiss), which is a library that allows its users to quickly search for multimedia documents that are very similar to each other (Github, Inc. (2023) [Online]).

In addition to the above-mentioned resources, there are several other resources available that facilitate building, training or implementing deep learning technologies.

---

[12] There are at least 5 definitions of the term *deep learning* (refer to Li and Dong (2014) in the bibliographic Section of this chapter).

Tech giants like Microsoft and IBM provide AI products and cloud computing resources for the development and application of deep learning technologies (Education 2020, Azure 2022). Open-source software like TensorFlow (Abadi et al. (2015) [Online], Paszke et al. (2019) [Online], ONNX Runtime developers (2021) [Online], Clark (2018) [Online]) and elsewhere. Some of the most popular deep learning AI neural network technologies in use include,

- CNN: Commonly used for image classification and object recognition, facial recognition, topic detection and sentiment analyses (Sarker 2021). Figure 3 shows the architecture of a general CNN model used for image classification. Below, are some sources with example scripts for the Python and R languages,

    - Using R and TensorFlow to build CNN:
      YCSung (2017) [Online].
    - Using Python and TensorFlow to build CNN:
      TensorFlow (2023) [Online].

- Generative adversarial networks (GANs): applications include high-fidelity image and video generation, advanced facial recognition, and super image resolution. GAN is also used to train models how to generate new information or material that mimics the specific properties of the original training dataset, which can help to make more authentic copies of the original data (Goodfellow et al. 2014, Sarker 2021). For this reason, GANs can also be used for adversarial attacks, such as for generating "fake media content." In fact, GANs are the underpinning technology behind "Deepfakes."[13] Example scripts for the Python and R languages,

    - Deep learning GANs with R:
      Keydana (2018) [Online].
    - Deep learning GANs with Python:
      Candido (2020) [Online].

- Recurrent neural network (RNN): commonly used for speech recognition, handwriting recognition, advanced forecasting, robotics and other complex deep learning workloads (Sarker 2021). Example scripts for the Python and R languages,

    - Deep Learning RNN using R with Keras:[14]
      Tatman (2019) [Online].
    - Deep Learning RNN using Python with Keras:
      Zhu and Chollet (2023) [Online].

---

[13] Deepfakes are synthetically generated media in which a person in an existing image or video is replaced with someone else's likeness.

[14] Keras (https://keras.io) is a high-level API of TensorFlow.

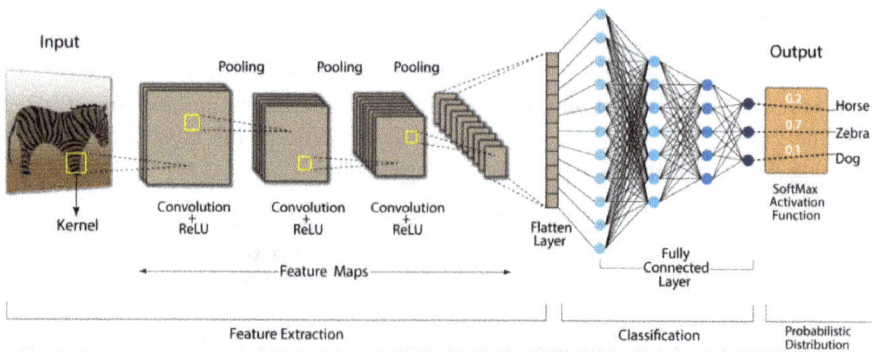

Figure 3. Schematic representation of a general multi-classifier CNN architecture. CNN has input and output layers and many hidden layers and millions of parameters that have the ability to learn complex objects and patterns. CNN sub-samples the given input by convolution and pooling processes that are subjected to an activation function (Rectifier Linear Unit-ReLu), where all of these processes take place in the partially connected hidden layers. Processed inputs are then transmitted to the fully connected layer and then to the output layer. The output retains the original shape similar to the input image dimensions. Convolution is the process involving a combination of two functions. In CNN, the input image is subjected to convolution (with the use of filters) that produces a feature map. The output values are directed to a soft-max layer that converts them into probabilities. The soft-max layer assigns decimal probabilities to each class in a multi-class problem, where the probabilities sum equals 1.0, which allows the output values to be interpreted directly as a probability. (Developers Breach, NPO [Online]).

Section 2 Molecular Diagnostics Technology

Laboratory or medical diagnostics encompass a broad set of technologies used on a patient-level or population scale to measure and diagnose the state of a wide range of conditions, such as the state of health, immunity, therapy response, mental health, disease or infection stage, pregnancy status, etc. Such technologies, depending on their complexity and technical requirements, may be accessed at home, in point-of-care settings or in laboratory settings. Additionally, there are different types of diagnostics technologies based on the analysis procedures (e.g., chemical, microscopic, imaging analysis, etc.) and the mediums they use to perform a diagnosis. Laboratory diagnostics are carried out on a variety of mediums, such as histological samples, bodily fluids samples (e.g., blood and saliva), and non-biogenic materials, like radiographs, electrocardiograms, environmental samples (e.g., air and water), etc. Here we focus our discussion on molecular diagnostics technology, which is a branch of the biotechnology industry. The term "molecular diagnostics" can be defined as technology for identifying, in tissue or bodily fluid, biomolecules such as proteins and DNA/RNA variants to facilitate the detection, diagnosis, and classification of pathogens and diseases, the prognosis of outcomes of infection or disease, and monitoring response to therapy (Gormley 2007, Debnath et al. 2010, Patrinos et al. 2017, Software 2019, Touma 2020).

In November 1949, chemist Linus Pauling, together with Itano, Singer and Wells, published an article on sickle-cell anemia, which opened new research into "molecular diseases" (the term used by Pauling in the manuscript) (Gormley 2007, Patrinos et al. 2017). More than four decades later, in the mid-1990s, technological innovations in patient-level genetic testing for the detection of the BRAC 1 and BRAC 2 mutations (BRAC Analysis) (Muller et al. 2004), together with the appearance of new techniques for nucleic acid sequence-based amplification (NASBA) (Malek et al. 1994), transcription-mediated amplification (TMA) (La Rocco et al. 1994) and self-sustained sequence replication (3SR) (Mueller et al. 1997) gave rise to the field of molecular diagnostics technology. The first widespread use of molecular diagnostics technology was for the diagnosis of an infectious pathogen, namely, the Human Immunodeficiency Virus (HIV), which soon led to the development of viral load testing assays for the detection of viral pathogens, like hepatitis C virus (HCV), cytomegalovirus, EpsteinBarr virus and BK virus (Software 2019).

The applications of modern molecular diagnostics are extensive, including clinical pathology, forensics testing, epigenetics, metagenomics, molecular oncology, immunotherapy and immunosuppression, personalized medicine and more (Debnath et al. 2010, Patrinos et al. 2017, Software 2019). Furthermore, advances in the fields of nanotechnology[15] (Jain 2003, Young and Kairdolf 2014, McRae et al. 2016, Kirtana et al. 2022), Biotechnology (Gulino 1999, Desiere and Romano Spica 2012, Gartland and Gartland 2018, English et al. 2019, Cornelissen et al. 2021) and AI will further drive the expansion of applications, creation of new technology, and guarantee more accuracy in diagnoses results. The interactions and interplay among these three fields of research and their contributions to molecular diagnostics technology are critical for the rapid response and intervention to global emergencies and threats from infectious and dangerous pathogens as demonstrated by the COVID-19 pandemic (Feng et al. 2020). Moreover, as we discuss in Sections 3 and 4, AI is pioneering digital diagnostics technology that is transforming the equity, affordability and accessibility to diagnostics tests, which is improving the quality of health care, medical diagnosis and treatment processes. In the subsections that follow we focus on AI roles in the development of selected laboratory molecular diagnostics technology.

Section 2.1 Molecular Diagnostics Innovations Driven by AI

The vast amount of available molecular information generated by high-throughput technologies, like high-throughput screening (HTS) and next-generation sequencing (NGS), has broadened the landscape in molecular diagnostics. The information generated by these technologies has led to new insights into the underlying biology of the respective infectious diseases and has provoked a shift in molecular diagnostics, from genotype to phenotype and to systems biology.[16] Furthermore, such information has propelled the growth in the list of analytes that have been identified as diagnostic and prognostic biomarkers (Wang et al. 2010, Haddad and Pantaleo 2012, Janvilisri

---

[15] Nanotechnology is the understanding and control of matter at the nanoscale, at dimensions between approximately 1 and 100 nm, where unique phenomena enable novel applications (https://www.nano.gov/).

[16] Systems Biology, as defined by NIH, is an approach in biomedical research to understanding the larger picture—be it at the level of the organism, tissue, or cell—by putting its pieces together (https://irp.nih.gov/catalyst/v19i6/).

et al. 2015, Carleo et al. 2016, Dix et al. 2016), which together with the increasing knowledge of their inter-patient variability and correlations to therapy outcomes, are paving the way for personalized medicine. In parallel, AI technology has helped in further expanding the list of biomarkers by digitally transforming HTS- and NGS-generated information (see in Section 3) and has allowed exceptional accuracy and automated integration of processes that include data collection, image and signal processing-&-analysis, results interpretation, and easy access to molecular diagnostics.

Section 2.1.1 Rapid Diagnostic Test (RDT) Technology

RDTs are widely used for the detection of infectious pathogens due to their ability to provide users with a rapid, simple, binary result (positive or negative). RDT technology has its seeds in 1949 when Linus Pauling and colleagues invented a rapid diagnostic test for sickle cell anemia and sickle cell trait (Itano and Pauling 1949). The test was for use in clinical laboratory settings; when a drop of blood was sealed between a cover slip and a slide under a microscope and a solution of a reducing agent was added, the decline in oxygen tension due to oxidative processes in the blood cells led to sickling[17] within a few seconds. Modern RDTs are designed for use in low-resource settings (e.g., at-home self-testing) or use at the point-of-care and are stable at high temperatures, simple to operate and inexpensive. The most common type of RDT is the lateral-flow device, which is a paper-based platform that works by applying a fluid sample at the end of the test strip. The sample then flows to the other end of the strip or the absorbent pad by capillary action. Such RDTs work based on the principle of antigen-antibody reaction and can determine both the presence and concentration of an analyte (or target compound). These types of RDTs have their origins in RDT technology developed in the early 1970s for determining pregnancy status. The "Predictor pregnancy test",[18] made by Organon Pharmaceuticals, was the first RDT for at-home testing made available to the public in the United States (for $10) (Romm 2015). Women would place a few drops of urine in a test tube, then add a chemical solution and allow the mixture to rest for two hours. Pregnant women would then see a dark brown circle on a yellow background on the mirror at the bottom of the kit or if there was no pregnancy, the background remained completely yellow.

Over the years, RDT has considerably expanded into new applications (Baksi et al. 2018, Tábuas-Pereira et al. 2018, Bradbury et al. 2020, Cruz Hernandez et al. 2020, De Luca et al. 2020, Ashley and Hassan 2021, Bouzid et al. 2021, Rindi 2022, Wang et al. 2022). Current uses of RDT include the diagnosis of neural, endocrine, metabolic, respiratory and blood pathologies, the detection of prognostic analytes and the detection of pathogens, which has made RDTs an important tool for

---

[17] Sickling is when the hemoglobin in red blood cells clumps together, causing the cell to become fragile, rigid, and crescent or sickle-shaped.

[18] The kit worked by detecting the pregnancy hormone (human chorionic gonadotrophin) in the urine. The kit was sold in Canada and the Netherlands by the early 1970s. FDA approval for the US was granted in 1976 (The Smithsonian; https://www.si.edu/).

medical diagnostics and health care management. Some examples of the paper-based RDT application for pathogen detection include OraQuick™ (for HIV infection), AccuQuik Test Kit™ (for Hepatitis A, B, C or E virus infection) and AccuQuik™ malaria test kits (for Plasmodium falciparum and Plasmodium vivax infection). However, the analysis and processing of RDT results have changed little over the past decades until recently. Today, innovations in AI and ML, like deep learning techniques, are helping developers to overcome the accuracy and processing limitations of RDT technology.

One issue affecting lateral-flow devices is the accuracy of the interpretation of results. Digital technologies to improve the accuracy of interpretation and the consistency of data collection are available. In high-income countries, companies offer RDT-reading instruments, which opto-electronically read lateral-flow tests and digitally communicate their results (Faulstich et al. 2009). For instance, Qassay® Rapid, Digital Lateral-Flow Test Readers (by P4Q Electronics) are based on high-precision multi-spectral sensor technology that enables evaluation of any lateral-flow strip test with higher accuracy than those obtained by self-evaluation (i.e., by eye). However, these types of readers are rare in low-resource settings due to their costs and the logistics and maintenance associated with these devices (Kadam et al. 2020). AI/ML technology has contributed to rapid diagnostic test result interpretation both through improving the processing of test results and by driving the development of new low-maintenance, more accessible and more accurate RDT-reader devices. For instance, recently developed smartphone apps for reading rapid test results use ML to classify serological test results and reduce reading ambiguities. Such types of apps (e.g., by p4q) are claimed to yield around 99% precision, compared to the ~ 90% accuracy produced by the eye. This type of RDT-reader technology combines the high-resolution imaging abilities of the smartphone's camera with ML image processing techniques to read and interpret rapid diagnostic test results. A major advantage of app-based AI technology is that no hardware other than a smartphone is needed, thus it can be more broadly adopted, i.e., in low-resource settings, point-of-care and at home.

Deep learning technology has also been recently introduced for the interpretation of RDT test results. Turbé et al. (2021) demonstrated that two deep learning-enabled HIV-RDTs improved the accuracy of interpretations compared to current RDT technologies used in the field (Turbé et al. 2021). Using images captured with a Samsung Tablet and CNN (see Figure 3) image processing technique, interpretations achieved high levels of sensitivity (97.8%) and specificity (100%) compared with the more costly handheld or portable RDT-readers (92–100% sensitivity; 97–100% specificity). Moreover, deep learning technology has enabled the incorporation of RDT technology into mobile devices, like smartwatches (Hassantabar et al. 2021, Sharlach 2022). Advancements in AI-powered RDTs evoked by the COVID-19 pandemic are likely to become the seeds for technologies that will profoundly change the landscape of molecular diagnostics, from laboratory robotic production lines to laboratory data collection and processing centers (Foundation 2022, Sharlach 2022).

Section 2.1.2 DNA Microarray Technology

Microarray technology is a general approach used in laboratory settings that involves binding an array of thousands to millions of known nucleic acid fragments to a solid surface, referred to as a "chip." The chip is then bathed with DNA or RNA isolated from a study sample. Complementary base pairing between the sample and the chip-immobilized fragments produces light through fluorescence that can be detected using a specialized machine. There are different types of microarrays,

- Microarray Expression Analysis: The expression pattern of selected genes (e.g., from a cohort of healthy persons) is compared to the expression pattern of a gene responsible for a disease.
- Microarray for Mutation Analysis: Genomic deoxyribonucleic acid (gDNA) is used for gene mutation analysis. The genes from different persons can differ by as much as a single-nucleotide base and detecting such single-point mutations is known as SNP detection.
- Comparative Genomic Hybridization: It is used for the identification of changes in the number of important chromosomal fragments harboring genes involved in a disease.

Microarrays can be manufactured in different formats, depending on the number of probes under examination, costs, and customization requirements. Arrays may have as few as 10 probes or up to 2.1 million micrometer-scale probes from commercial vendors. Microarray technology can be used for a variety of purposes in research and clinical settings, such as measuring gene expression levels, DNA sequence-specific detection (e.g., single-nucleotide polymorphisms or SNPs), pathogen detection and genotyping and more (Schena et al. 1995, Wang et al. 2002, McLoughlin 2011, Sánchez-Pla 2014). The first miniaturized DNA microarrays designed for gene expression profiling were reported in 1995 (Schena et al. 1995). The first DNA microarray designed for the detection of a wide range of pathogens was the ViroChip, which contained 1,600 probes derived from 140 complete viral genomes (Wang et al. 2002). The viral families represented on the first version of the ViroChip included double- and single-stranded DNA viruses, retroviruses and both positive- and negative-stranded RNA viruses. Oligonucleotides were derived from potent human pathogens, including human T-lymphotropic virus, hepatitis B virus, hepatitis C virus, papillomaviruses and all 20 fully sequenced human and animal herpes viruses. Five other viral families associated with respiratory tract infections (paramyxo-, orthomyxo-, nido-, adeno- and picornavirus) were also extensively covered.

AI/ML technologies have improved DNA microarray data analysis. Recently, ML techniques such as SVM, RF, boosting methods and others have proven to be powerful and accurate algorithms for processing the digital fluorescence signals of microarrays and for the classification of microarray data (Maros et al. 2020). However, Lahmer et al. (2020) demonstrated that deep learning CNN, outperformed state-of-the-art ML technologies by a margin of at least 20% accuracy (Lahmer et al. 2020). Moreover, Qin and colleagues (2020), showed that deep learning AI technology identified erroneous microarray-based and gene-level conclusions in literature (Qin et al. 2021). After retrospectively constructing the raw images for 37,724 microarrays from a total of 3165 published studies and analyzing them with a deep learning CNN model, they found that 26.73% of the microarray-based studies were affected by serious imaging defects and that 28.82% of the gene-level conclusions reported in publications were artifactual.

Section 2.1.3 Next-generation Sequencing Technology

NGS technology, as defined by Illumina Inc., is a massively parallel sequencing technology that offers ultrahigh-throughput, scalability and speed. The technology is used to determine the order of nucleotides in entire genomes or targeted regions of DNA or RNA molecules. NGS technology has its foundation in the Sanger sequencing method which was introduced in 1977 (Sanger and Coulson 1975, Sanger et al. 1977). Presently, the technology is in the 4th generation with the development of nanopore systems for DNA sequencing. Slatko et al. (2019) provide an overview of how NGS technology work and on the different types of technologies that have emerged over the past 15 years (Slatko et al. 2018). NGS technology has diverse uses in laboratory settings such as in molecular diagnostic applications for identifying disease-related SNPs (Singh et al. 2019); for identifying gross chromosome abnormalities (e.g., deletions, duplications and rearrangements) (Weckselblatt and Rudd 2015, Liu et al. 2021) and for pathogen detection, genotyping, and phenotyping (e.g., drug-resistance, virulence, vaccine escape or transmission) (Forbi et al. 2015, Shaw et al. 2016, Lara et al. 2017, Ramachandran et al. 2018, Yang et al. 2018, Ganova-Raeva et al. 2019, Simsek et al. 2021, Munyuza et al. 2022, Sahibzada et al. 2022). Such studies have demonstrated the importance of NGS technology for improving our knowledge about the epidemiology, treatment, vaccine development and surveillance of pathogens.

Schmidt and Hildebrandt have recently conducted an extensive review of deep learning AI technologies used for NGS data analysis and applications in areas of variant calling, epigenetics, metagenomics and transcriptomics (Schmidt and Hildebrandt 2021). NGS integrated with AI (for instnace, for drug discovery and *de novo* molecule design (Xu et al. 2019, Gupta et al. 2021) and RNA/DNA structure prediction (Townshend et al. 2021)) has a strong potential to accelerate the discovery of curative treatments. Furthermore, this integration is currently being explored for applications of pathogen surveillance toward the control and elimination of infectious diseases, like malaria (Garrido-Cardenas et al. 2019, Lyimo et al. 2022) and hepatitis C (Forbi et al. 2015, Lara et al. 2017, Ramachandran et al. 2018, Ganova-Raeva et al. 2019, Sahibzada et al. 2022). Surveillance systems supported by NGS and AI data analytics have the capacity for the rapid and accurate identification of outbreaks and transmission networks. Sharing such data with state and local health departments can help target interventions more effectively and prevent the further spread of the disease. Molecular surveillance is an important component of the US national- and state-level strategic plans targeting the elimination of hepatitis C by 2030 (National Academies of Sciences et al. 2017, State 2022).

Section 3   Digital Diagnostics Technology

Here, the term digital diagnostics technology is used to refer to a variety of applications and technologies for the direct or indirect detection of pathogens in biological and non-biological samples through digital data processing. Nearly, all current molecular diagnostics technologies used in low-, middle- or hi-resource settings, generate digital information or data that can be converted into digital information, which enables the application of AI/ML technologies. Tocci et al. in their study of digital systems, defined the term "digital data" as logical information or physical quantities that are represented in digital form (Tocci et al. 2009). Digital technologies are most often electronic and the more familiar digital systems, including computers and telephone systems. Digital technology means that devices (e.g., computers, phones, biosensors or RDT readers) can be more compact, faster, lighter and more versatile. Huge amounts of information can be stored locally or remotely and moved around to any part of the world virtually immediately. Even the term "information" has expanded to include media such as photos, audio, and video, and it no longer refers to just words and numbers.

The advantages that digital technologies provide in terms of social connectivity, communication speeds, remote working, learning opportunities, automation, data storage and data editing have deeply transformed all aspects of industry and government. For instance, internet speeds have grown faster since the early days of dial-up and telecoms have become faster and more widespread, which has facilitated the transfer of data over the web or the air in real-time. The availability of low-cost communication devices, faster internet broadbands and faster telecom networks has allowed the molecular surveillance and diagnostics of pathogens in remote mid-resource and low-resource settings (Faulstich et al. 2009, Turbé et al. 2021). Remote decision-making is more inclusive, efficient, effective and versatile [from the control of the battlefield NEWS (2020) and Williams (2022)] to control of pandemics (Alamo et al. 2021, Foundation 2022, Sharlach 2022). In the subsections below, we discuss some aspects that were covered in Section 2 but from a digital perspective.

Section 3.1   Digital Biomarkers

Biomarkers are an integral part of biomedical research and clinical practice. Many molecular research assays and clinical diagnostic tests use analytes (e.g., biological molecules such as hormones, antigens or antibodies) to measure, for instance, pregnancy status or to detect pathogens or assess the health status of patients (e.g., liver function, etc.). Biomarkers are recognized as important predictors of clinical and therapy outcomes. The US National Institute of Health (NIH), Biomarkers Definitions Working Group defines the term "biomarker" as "a characteristic that is measured as an indicator of normal biological processes, pathogenic processes, or responses to an exposure or intervention including therapeutic interventions. This can include molecular, histological, radiographic, or physiologic characteristics" (Group 2016). Babrak et al. put forth suggestions to address current issues in the field of digital biomarkers and defines digital biomarkers as "objective, quantifiable, physiological, and behavioral measures that are collected by means of digital devices that are portable, wearable, implantable, or digestible. These data are often used to explain, influence, and/or predict health-related outcomes" (Babrak et al. 2019).

In the field of digital systems (and in the context of molecular diagnostics of pathogens), digital biomarkers can be defined as digitalized logical information or physical quantities that can be used to measure, quantify, classify or predict characteristics of a pathogen: (i) the species and strain, (ii) health risks (virulence, infectiousness and infectivity), (iii) drug susceptibility and (iv) origin. Although establishing consistency in definitions and categorizations in the field of biomarkers (or digital biomarkers) is a challenge (Babrak et al. 2019), we identify four types of digital biomarkers based on data representation:

1. Device-generated biomarkers are markers obtained from any type of digital data generated directly by a digital device. The digital data can be raw data processed from a single device or from extra devices required for out-of-device processing. Data can assume various formats such as photo media, fluorescence spectra (e.g., microarray technology), genomic reads (NGS technology), etc. The device's normal output format is not altered or transformed by the analyst prior to analysis.

2. Property-based biomarkers are markers generated from data representation of various physicochemical and biochemical properties of biomolecules (protein, DNA or RNA) or of their elements (amino acids or nucleic acids). A popular database of amino acid indices, amino acid mutation matrixes and pair-wise contact potentials is the AA Index database (Kawashima et al. 2008). In addition, there are several tools available to compute the physicochemical properties of biomolecules. Pse-in-One is an example of a web-server application used to derive various physicochemical and biochemical properties of proteins, DNA and RNA biomolecules (Liu et al. 2015).

3. Structure-based biomarkers are markers generated from data representation of various structural descriptors, such as geometries, topologies, dimensions, molecular connectivity (a.k.a., molecular networks) and relations among (or between) the elements comprising biomolecules. For instance, the Crystallography Open Database (COD) warehouses structure crystallographic data of over 160,000 curated chemical structures in different formats (Gražulis et al. 2012). A commonly used format is the Simplified Molecular-Input Line-Entry System (SMILES) format, which is a description of the structure of a chemical species in the form of a line notation using short ASCII strings. SMILES data has been used for tasks such as the prediction of molecular functions (Quirós et al. 2018), the optimization of function or properties of target molecules (Kwon and Lee 2021) and the prediction of SMILES formats from molecular image formats (Rajan et al. 2021). Freely available software programs can be found in the literature, including programs for converting polypeptide sequences to SMILES format (Minkiewicz et al. 2017).

4. AI-derived biomarkers are markers generated from deep learning artificial neural networks (DLANN) used for supervised or unsupervised learning of feature representation at successively more abstract layers. CNN and transformers are popular DLANN models used for learning features from data. Recently, DLANN

models known as Bidirectional Encoder Representations from Transformers (BERT), originally developed by Google for machine language understanding (Devlin et al. 2018), are being applied to molecular studies with great success (Ho et al. 2021). Figure 4 shows a schematic representation of the architecture of a DLANN model known as an autoencoder. We note that ML methods for feature extraction/construction (FE/FC), such as self-organizing maps (SOM) (Yang and Yang 2014) and the class-attribute interdependence maximization (CAIM) algorithm (Kurgan and Cios 2004) are available. DLANN methods, however, are generally more complex and capable of operating more independently than ML-based FE/FC models. Markers derived through ML FE/FC methods could be referred to as ML-derived biomarkers.

As identified above, the first type of biomarkers typically consists of a known feature or set of features strongly associated with specific characteristics of interest (e.g., strain-related or risk-related or therapy-related data features). For example, in data generated through NGS technology, biomarkers can be SNP or a DNA "motif" or a DNA fragment in a genomic region. Furthermore, this type of digital biomarker serves as the foundation for the exploration and discovery of novel biomarkers, which can be achieved by data mining techniques, like feature selection (FS), using

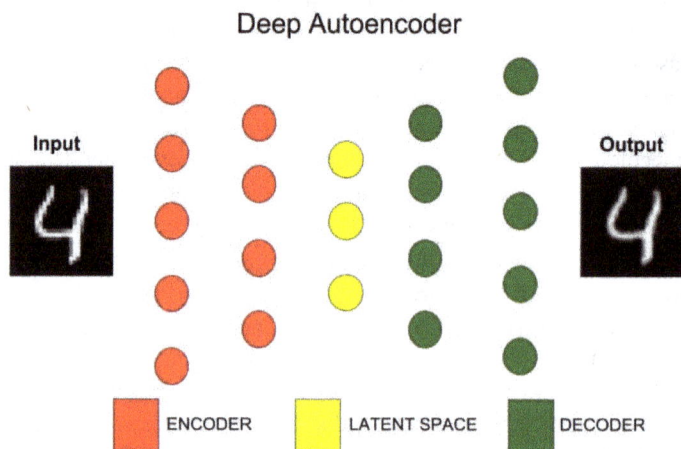

Figure 4. Schematic of a general deep autoencoder architecture (ANN connectivity not shown). A deep autoencoder is an ANN used for unsupervised learning of efficient data feature codings, typically for the purpose of data dimensionality reduction. This is achieved by designing deep learning architecture that aims that copy the input layer at its output layer. The architecture is shaped in the form of a funnel where the number of nodes decreases as we move from the input layer (red nodes) until a layer (yellow nodes) referred to as "latent space." The number of nodes increases again from the latent space to the output layer (nodes in green) where the number of nodes in the output layer equals the number of nodes in the input layer. Each layer in the ANN learns an abstract representation of the input vector space of the data (as presented in Figure 2). The latent space acts as a bottleneck for the transmission of information, letting the most important features through (i.e., filters out noise or removes non-relevant features). For instance, suppose we have data with an input dimensional vector space of 1,000 features and we want to reduce the number of dimensions (i.e., the number of features) to 50. We would design the deep autoencoder with 50 nodes in the latent space, which would then reduce the dimensional vector space from 1,000 to the 50 most relevant (or useful) combinations of data features. (Source: The Statistics Online Computational Resource (SOCR) [Online]).

statistical or AI/ML methods. Moreover, device-generated data give rise to the other three listed biomarker types. These three types are the product of data engineering[19] for AI/ML processing. Discussion on data engineering and data mining methods used to transform data output formats of digital devices can be found elsewhere in the literature.

Examples of property-based and structure-based features, as well as an example of AI-derived features based on a deep learning method, are shown in Figure 5. There are serval deep learning methods for extracting relevant features (or biomarkers) from data (e.g., CNN-based, Encoder-based systems, etc.). The example in Figure 5 is a deep learning method inspired by the idea of sentence embedding and NLP, which uses an unsupervised deep learner, known as a Paragraph Vector, to learn sequence embedding features. Briefly, protein sequences (or genomic sequences) are embedded into a vector space separately (here, 4-kmer representations), and then every sequence can be represented as a vector, namely the "sequence embedding features." Lastly, the feature representation is obtained by concatenating the "sequence embedding features" derived from sequences (which can be from different groups or classes, like from patients with different clinical outcomes or patients infected with different virulent strains of a pathogen, etc.). Furthermore, by applying the attention mechanism, one can successfully interpret the meaning of sequence embedding features and find motifs that represent domain-specific information. A detailed discussion of this method is provided by Zen et al. (Zeng et al. 2018).

Section 3.2 Cyber-Molecular Assays (CMAs)

From our discussion in the Introduction Section, CMAs is a technology of modern computing, IT and the internet. The term "cyber-molecular assay" was first introduced at CDC by Y. Khudyakov's Research Team (Campo and Khudyakov 2020, Lara et al. 2018, Icer Baykal et al. 2021). In the context of the digital laboratory diagnostics framework, CMAs operate as "expert" systems (or computer programs) that have expertise in specific domains such as a molecular, clinical or epidemiological field. Expert systems are defined as computer programs that use AI technologies to simulate the judgment and behavior of a human or an organization that has expertise and experience in a particular field, a concept that was first developed by computer scientist Edward Feigenbaum (1988). CMAs provide reliable test results and can be designed to perform important and advantageous operations without human intervention, such as:

- Learning new relevant features (i.e., biomarkers) that improve test results.
- Self-improve, i.e., determine if predictions and outcomes are accurate and correct as necessary.
- Identify and remove data noise.
- Detect data anomalies and identify their sources.

---

[19] Data engineering is the complex task of making raw digital data suitable for data analysis.

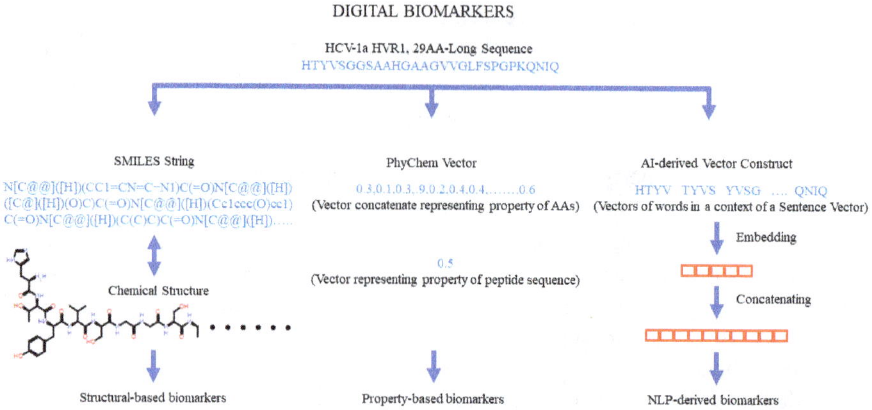

Figure 5. Examples of molecular digital biomarker engineering. Shown in this figure are: (i) a peptide sequence string from HCV HVR1 that serves as input; (ii) a SMILES string output representing structural relations among atomic elements forming the peptide molecule, where capitalized letters represent elements (e.g., C for carbon, N for nitrogen), equal signs represent double bonds, single @ or double @@ symbols represent tetrahedral carbon configurations and small-cap letters represent aromatic rings; (iii) PhyChem vectors representing a numerical vector of the input peptide as the concatenated physicochemical property of AAs or as a numerical output representing a physicochemical property of the input peptide (e.g., hydrophobicity); (iv) simplified schematic representation of an unsupervised feature extraction method based on an NLP and a Deep Learning method (explained in the body of this chapter). Additional descriptions of different characters found in SMILES strings can be found in the user's guide of the program used for the derivation of SMILES files, including information on the program-specific representation styles. Computer programs can convert molecule images to SMILES strings or SMILES strings into images, from which relevant features can also be extracted (see Figure 3).

Such operations and capabilities have important functions in molecular surveillance systems and for analytical processes that include data reconciliation[20] (Sims et al. 2018, Alamo et al. 2021, Khan et al. 2022). Expert systems by nature are very complex systems, nevertheless, there are intrinsic components in such systems (Feigenbaum 1988). There are three major components in CMAs: (i) A knowledge base component. This is where the information that expert systems use is stored. Data and knowledge about a particular domain or subject area are organized in the knowledge base and accessed by CMAs through a data acquisition module. If built into the system, the acquisition module could enable CMAs to gather information from external sources and store it in the knowledge base. Next is (ii) an inference component. This is the "digital assay" part of the CMA and where relevant information learned from the knowledge base is used to solve problems and make decisions based on the input data provided by users. For instance, in ANN CMAs relevant information is stored in the connections and neurons of the ANN model. The inference component may also include an explanation module that shows users how

---

[20] Data reconciliation is a term used in public health surveillance settings to describe a verification phase, which is conducted (i) during a data migration where the target data is compared against the original data source to ensure that the migration framework has transferred the data correctly; or (ii) during an emergency response (e.g., COVID-19) where independent data sources are compared against each other.

the CMA came to its conclusion. Last is (iii) the user interface component. This is the part of the expert system that end users interact with to get test results or solutions to problems or answers to their questions.

CMAs have been used to tackle highly complex tasks. For instance, Lara et al. (2017) showed that an ANN CMAs can detect differences in intra-host evolution of hepatitis C virus (HCV) hypervariable region 1 between mono-infected and HIV-coinfected persons, which may be potentially used to identify HCV/HIV-coinfected persons (Lara et al. 2018). In the next section, we briefly discuss the roles of chatbot technology in clinical and molecular diagnostics. One could view this type of chatbot technology as a "special" form of CMAs technology with AI/ML technologies driving data analysis, data interpretation and data collection; however, with the added value of machine-human conversational interaction, which enhances users' experience with the respective health-improving or lifesaving chatbot diagnostic technology.

Section 4 AI Chatbot Technology

Advances in ML and NLP algorithms have created very powerful AI computer agents that can communicate and converse using the natural language of humans. Nowadays, AI chatbot technology is almost everywhere (e.g., smart TVs, cars, mobile devices, etc.). An AI chatbot can be defined as a computer program that uses ML and NLP to understand people's questions and automate responses to questions, thus simulating human conversation. Historically, chatbots[21] were text-based and explicitly programmed to reply to a limited set of simple queries with answers that had been pre-written by the chatbot's developers (Adamopoulou and Moussiades 2020). These early chatbots operated more like an interactive "frequently-asked-questions" scheme and while they are good at providing accurate answers for the specific questions on which they were trained, they failed when presented with a question that was not presented in the training dataset. Over time, chatbot technology has integrated more ML and NLP, which has improved the chatbot's ability to understand the end user's intent and accurately predict user needs and has allowed end users to interact with chatbots in a realistic conversational way. In fact, the latest types of chatbots are "contextually aware"[22] and can learn and become more intelligent as they get incrementally exposed to human language. Meta AI's *BlenderBot* 3 (Shuster et al. 2022) and Microsoft's (Asia) Xiaoice (Janarthanam and Lemon 2014) are good examples of such types of AI chatbots. More detailed information and an overview of chatbot technology can be found elsewhere (IBM 2019, Adamopoulou and Moussiades 2020, Ayanouz et al. 2020, Chowdhary 2020, Microsoft 2022, Oracle 2022). Herein, some of the major features of chatbot technology are discussed in the following sections.

---

[21] The first chatbot (named ELIZA) was created in 1966 by MIT professor Joseph Weizenbaum.

[22] In computer science, contextual awareness refers to the idea that computers can both sense and react based on their environment. Context-aware systems can gather and analyze information about their environment at any given time and automatically adapt their responses accordingly.

Section 4.1 General Schema of AI Chatbot Technology

A schematic representation of a general chatbot architecture is shown in Figure 4. It comprises a user interface (UX) through which the end user can remotely interact with the chatbot system via a multiple-choice questionnaire, text messaging or voice. The chatbot system can be roughly described as being comprised of four modular components: a natural language understanding[23] (NLU) module, which contains a model that analyzes the end user's request (or input) to infer the user's intent and interpret associated information; an action execution/information retrieval module that performs requested actions or collects data of interest from data sources; the response generation module that prepares a response based on user's intent and context information; and the conversation or dialogue management module, which execute functions required to fulfill user requests such as keeps and updates the context of a conversation (e.g., current intent and identifying information), requests missing information (by asking follow-up questions, when necessary) and processes clarifications. The architecture of AI chatbots, those that integrate the latest AI/ML and NLP technologies, has become much more complex over time (Janarthanam and Lemon 2014, Adamopoulou and Moussiades 2020, Ayanouz et al. 2020).

One of the factors fueling the rapid growth of chatbot technology is the growing number of open-source AI and ML libraries available to developers (Nayyar 2019, Botpress 2022). The number of chatbot-based applications (Jovic 2022) and the terms used to describe them is growing with each passing day (IBM 2019, Microsoft 2022, Oracle 2022). The terms chatbot, AI chatbot, virtual agent and virtual assistant are commonly seen being used interchangeably in chatbot-themed papers, reports, news, etc. The fact is that chatbot technology is now using complex algorithms and advanced ML methods to provide more detailed and human-like responses. However, the term AI chatbot (a.k.a. virtual agent or virtual assistant) refers to chatbot technology with deep learning capabilities, which enables interactions to become more accurate over time. Unfortunately, AI chatbot technology has received some bad publicity for the sometimes embarrassing and sometimes controversial chatbot-generated comments. For instance, Meta's AI chatbot, named BlenderBot 3 (Table 3), when asked the question "Any other thoughts on Zuckerberg?" (in reference to Facebook's CEO Mark Zuckerberg), responded "His company exploits people for money and he does not care. It needs to stop! Are we united yet?" (Clayton 2022). In a separate case, in 2016 Microsoft had to apologize after its AI chatbot, named Tay (inaugurated on the social media platform Twitter), started expressing racist and misogynistic sentiments just 16 hours after going live (Hunt 2016, Vincent 2016, Zemčík 2021). However, the benefits of releasing such technology to the public outweigh the risk of bad publicity (IBM 2019, Clayton 2022).

AI chatbot technology has revolutionized the way that many industries operate customer services. For instance, staffing 24-hour customer support centers are expensive, even when outsourced to other countries. A chatbot, however, can answer

---

[23] NLU is a subset of NLP that uses the semantic analysis of text that focuses on extracting the context and intent of text (i.e., what was meant). Conversely, NLP algorithms focus on processing the text or sentence in a literal sense (i.e., what was said).

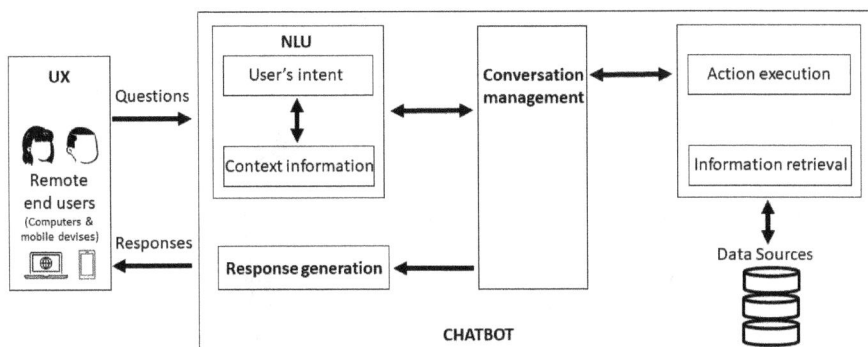

Figure 6. General chatbot architecture.

Table 3. List of selected AI chatbots.

Chatbot name	Application	Availability[§]
Clara	COVID-19 Testing	https://www.cdc.gov/coronavirus/2019-ncov/symptoms-testing/coronavirus-self-checker.html
COVID-19 Pediatric Assessment Tool	COVID-19 Testing	https://covid-choa.mybluemix.net/dashboard?view=chat
COVID-19 virtual assistant	COVID-19 Testing	https://www.hyro.ai/covid-19
Scout	Health Plan-related Assessments	Available on Android and IOS apps
Symptom checker	COVID-19 Testing	https://www.advocateaurorahealth.org/coronavirus-disease-2019/#symptomchecker
Sayana	Mental health care	https://www.sayana.app
Therabot	Mental health therapy support	Available for Webpages, Android and IOS apps
Woebot	Mental health care	https://woebothealth.com
Wysa	Mental health therapy support	https://www.wysa.io
BlenderBot[†]	Social Media	https://www.blenderbot.ai
Tay[‡]	Social Media	(https://web.archive.org/web/20160323194709/https://tay.ai/#chat-with-tay)

† BlenderBot 3 is a multitopic chatbot developed by Meta AI.

‡ Tay was a multitopic chatbot developed by Microsoft for the Twitter, Kik and GroupMe social media platforms.

§ Links last accessed on 08/30/2022.

questions 24 hours a day, seven days a week and can be used to provide a first line of support, supplement support during peak periods or offer an additional support option, which can help reduce the number of customers who need to speak with a human staff representative (Silva et al. 2017, Dihingia et al. 2021). AI chatbot technology has also brought innovations in health care and medicine. For example, Microsoft's Health Bot services (Azure 2022) has provided the framework for the development of various chatbots such as Premera's "Scout" chatbot (for digital services like checking healthcare claim status, eligibility and health plans); Aurora Health Care's "symptom checker" (for triaging symptoms and locate nearby care centers); as well as CDC's "Clara" chatbot (a public Coronavirus Self-Testing tool for assessing the likelihood of COVID-19 infection). In the section below, we discuss the application of AI chatbot technology to COVID-19 diagnostics.

Section 4.2 AI Chatbot Technology for COVID-19 Testing

Presently, AI chatbot technology for use in pathogen diagnostics is only available for the coronavirus 2 (SARS-CoV-2) infection, which causes COVID-19. There are two chatbot diagnostics that are widely used by health organizations in the US. The Centers for Disease Control and Prevention (CDC) in collaboration with Microsoft Corporation developed "Clara", a chatbot that assesses coronavirus-related symptoms and risk factors, suggests whether people should seek medical assistance, and provides information on how to safely self-manage infection at home (Miner et al. 2020, Smith 2020). Clara (Table 3) was built on Microsoft's "Health Bot" and is powered by AI technologies in the Azure cloud architecture and is freely available to the public. The second chatbot, the "COVID-19 Pediatric Assessment Tool," with similar functions and capabilities as Clara, was created by Children's Healthcare of Atlanta in partnership with IBM Watson Health and is freely available to the public (Table 3). This intelligent cyber diagnostic tool is powered by AI technologies in the IBM Public cloud architecture (IBM 2020, Miner et al. 2020).

Chatbot technology dedicated to aiding a patient's self-assessment for COVID-19 also includes Hyro's "COVID-19 virtual assistant" (ACCESSWIRE. COM 2020). This tool is provided to health organizations and the public for free as a plug-and-play software that can be embedded in websites and mobile devices. The virtual assistant enables health organizations to address common questions about the coronavirus, guide patients through a self-assessment and evaluate their risk for SARS-CoV-2 infection. Hyro's virtual assistant (Table 3) allows patients to type or verbalize a question of interest using their language. The information provided in the responses by the virtual assistant is based on information provided by the CDC and the World Health Organization (WHO), as well as on information automatically and autonomously scraped from various sources (ACCESSWIRE.COM 2020). Around the world, such as in Sweden, researchers have also developed chatbot-based tools [Online forward triage tools (OFTTs)] that assess the urgency for SARS-CoV-2 testing and medical referral (Hautz et al. 2021, Michel et al. 2022) and in Israel, researchers used Microsoft's Health Bot to develop an internet-based surveillance system for real-time or near real-time monitoring of SARS-CoV-2 infection (Yom-Tov 2021).

Although the above-mentioned diagnostic technologies cannot literally diagnose SARS-CoV-2 infection, they do provide a fast and accurate differential judgment for the exclusion of other potential viral and bacterial pathogens or non-infectious entities that cause COVID-19-related symptoms (e.g., Flu, cold, bacterial pneumonia, allergies, etc.). Therefore, these AI chatbots can provide rapid and accurate means to strengthen decision support capacity at local and national levels. Population-targeted decision support systems that can accurately and reliably differentiate between at-risk patients and those that are likely not in need of immediate screening or treatments can help improve point-of-care diagnostic capacity, free medical resources and optimize the management and distribution of national resources (Miner et al. 2020, Smith 2020, Yom-Tov 2021). The implementation and adoption of such support systems to combat large outbreaks or pandemics could translate into more efficient and better-quality healthcare services for patients.

We note, however, that such AI chatbot diagnostic technology is not risk-free. There are some risks, like the risk of amplifying misinformation (e.g., due to corrupted information in the databases used by chatbots) (Treml 2020, Ye and Li 2020, Zhang et al. 2020). Moreover, the lack of research on the effectiveness of this technology for SARS-CoV-2 diagnostics is of concern. Comparison and comprehensive effectiveness studies are needed, as well as more collaborations between healthcare organizations, tech industries and academics, which should help in future pandemic preparedness efforts.

Section 4.3 Medical Chatbot Technology for Disease Diagnostics

In today's world, with the lifestyle change brought about by the COVID-19 pandemic, illness and mortality rates have increased in the general population (Lee et al. 2022, WHO 2022). Patient's waiting times at point-of-care facilities have substantially increased and doctors' workload has gone up with the increased number of patient visits they receive. Additionally, in the US at least 44% of emergency department visits can be characterized as unnecessary (CDC/National Center for Health Statistics (2023) [Online]). Thus, the reliability and quality of healthcare services in a pandemic or national health emergency depends on the ability of caregivers and patients to conduct remote consultations with digital experts, such as chatbots. Medical chatbots focused on the medical domain can play a major role in making health status assessments and/or in providing accurate remote diagnosis (Bhirud et al. 2019, Adamopoulou and Moussiades 2020, Ayanouz et al. 2020).

There are several medical chatbots available in the healthcare and medical sector. For instance:

- "Endurance," for Alzheimer's and other forms of Dementia (created by Endurance lasers and Endurance Laser LLC; available at: https://endurancelasers.com/talk-to-endurance-chatbot/; last accessed 08/30/2022).
- "Insomnobot3000" for insomnia (developed by Casper Sleep; available at: https://insomnobot3000.com/; last accessed 08/30/2022).
- "KakaoTalk," for obstetric and mental health care (Chung et al. 2021).

However, the problem with these three chatbot technologies is that they are question-and-answer formatted and have basic functionalities such as answering basic questions, escalating questions to experts and recommending tutorials or products that best match the requirements of patients. They lack AI/ML-based intelligence and thus are not capable of communicating in natural language or understanding the needs of users or predicting the underlying factors of a disease. Examples of AI chatbots with such properties are listed in Table 3. For instance, Therabot™ is an assistive-robotic system designed to provide support during counseling sessions and in-home therapeutic support to patients diagnosed with mental conditions associated with trauma (Bethel et al. 2018). This chatbot is designed as a stuffed robotic dog and has adaptive touch sensing to allow for improved human-robot interactions. Through its touch sensing and ML capacity, it can determine the level of stress of its user and adapt to provide support during therapy sessions and for home therapy practice. Over time, the chatbot learns the preferences of its user and adapts their behaviors accordingly.

Section 5 AI Technology Adoption: Challenges and Future

There are several barriers that affect the rate at which agencies adopt new AI technologies into their operational activities and the same is true for clinical laboratories. Addressing barriers to technology can be highly complex. Below we list some of these barriers:

- Cultural Attitudes and Practices: Attitudes toward technology innovation vary among countries, industries, organizations and agencies. For instance, "pagers" were small devices that allowed their users to receive simple "beeps" or later text messages and were very popular in the 1980s–1990s. Each had a unique number, like a phone number, and to receive a message, the sender had to call a switchboard and leave a short message, which would then be converted into a text message by an operator or, more commonly, a machine. While in the US and the UK, pager services saw their end in the 90s (except for sectors, like healthcare), Japan's last pager provider, Tokyo Telemessage, closed its service on October 1, 2019 (with a Tokyo funeral company setting up a site for people to lay flowers and pay their respects to the end of the *pokeberu* or pocket bell) (BBC [Online] 2019). Organizational culture also affects how technology adoption evolves. For instance, in 2016, the Government Accountability Office (GAO) reported that the US nuclear weapons force, more specifically, the Strategic Automated Command and Control System (SACCS), was still using 8-inch floppy disks[24] and a 1970s-era computer system (Mosher 2016). Although supposedly such technologies are presently no longer used by SACCS, at the time of the inquiries in 2016, the Pentagon spokesperson stated that "This system remains in use because, in short, it still works" (BBC [Online] 2016).

  Both above examples illustrate a normal tendency for people (and industry) to resist changes to the technologies they learn to like and use. This resistance arises from the interaction between the technical design of a system and the environmental or social circumstances in which it is used (JISC 2006). Moreover, one may say that agencies and their work environments can be viewed as an interlocking jigsaw puzzle, where existing pieces not only depend on one

---

[24] A standard 8 in-floppy disk had 237 kB of storage space, enough for 15 seconds of current audio media formats. More than 130,000 8-inch floppy disks would be needed to store 32 GB of information; the size of an average memory stick in use today. (Source: https://www.bbc.com/news/world-us-canada-36385839).

another, but new pieces fit only into gaps and contours shaped by previous practices (Collins and Halverson 2009).

Organizational practices that affect technology adoption, include practices on how appointments in leadership are managed by government organizations or private institutions. For instance, practices in leadership appointments have prompted concerns and controversy in national security and public safety. Recently, an organization responsible for cybersecurity was found to be headed by an individual who had never used a computer (BBC [Online] 2018). To accelerate AI technology adoption, the US government and military agencies, like the Department of Defense, are moving toward appointing data engineers, computer scientists and mathematicians to head the respective science departments (2021). A recent report by the GAO regarding deficiencies with the collection and management of contact tracing information during the global COVID-19 pandemic (GAO (2022) [Online]), prompted some members of the US Senate to propose the creation of an independent agency, the Center for Public Health Data (CPHD), which would sit under the US Department of Health and Human Services and be led by a chief data engineer (2022). The CPHD would aggregate digital data from public health agencies as well as laboratories, clinics and hospitals and make it accessible in real-time for decision-making as health threats unfold.

- Regulations and Policies: In the most extreme cases, requirements imposed by antiquated regulations can block changes in the technology used for normal daily operations. For instance, news media in 2022 reported that in Japan, around 1,900 government procedures still require businesses to use floppy disk technology (Craft 2022; FitzGerald 2022). Policies play important roles in ensuring the acquisition of new technologies as well as the acquisition of personnel with the proper technological skillset. The Chief Information Officer (CIO) Council (https://www.cio.gov/) is one of the leading agencies with the mission of improving IT practices across US government agencies and has published guidance and recommendations for the hiring and reskilling of personnel to ensure the maintenance of an innovative workforce (2020).

- Technical Challenges: Technical challenges for the quick adoption of new AI technology in normal operation activities vary from the degree of difficulty users experience in learning the new technology to technical challenges involved in transferring processes from legacy systems to new systems. While the former can be more easily mitigated through improvements in the design of novel technologies, the former can prove extremely challenging to address for some areas or fields. Although there is no consensus in definition, typically, legacy systems are defined as old or outdated technology or computer systems that remain in use. However, in certain conditions, legacy technology should be viewed as old applications or computer systems that are critical to an agency's mission. The challenge of replacing such critical technologies with new ones lies in part in technical difficulties associated with ensuring compatibility of the new technology with the old data formats, so as to prevent the loss of historic or critical data (Johnson 2020).

There are data quality issues that developers of digital molecular diagnostics should be aware of and prepared to address with the proper solutions. The quality of the data can be affected by several factors. Errors and distortions in data can be generated unintentionally during the processes of generating or collecting it, and the end user of the stored data would see this accumulated result. Having sound data management procedures and rules on how data is collected and stored, together with using structured methods to filter accurate information from data errors and noise, should help improve data quality and accuracy of the information provided to the end users. Other issues that affect data quality include data inconsistency (differences between historical and new data), data duplication, data outliers, etc., that require statistical, mathematical or ML solutions. Such issues and methods used to address them are beyond the scope of this chapter and can be found elsewhere. For instance, a study by Roh et al. (2019) presents a survey of current data collection methods for ML (Roh et al. 2021), and Maitre et al. (2022) discusses data filtering techniques for deep learning systems used for human activity recognition (Maitre et al. 2022).

Accuracy in data that is used for training AI and ML systems is very important for ensuring the reliability and accuracy of the diagnostics test results (i.e., to avoid a GIGO system). Deep learning technologies are inherently resilient to data noise and can filter out non-relevant information (see Figures 3 and 4), in this sense, DLANNs can be considered good data filters (Sarker 2021). Nevertheless, the performance of any AI/ML model can be compromised if the level of data errors and distortions is too high. One approach to selecting high-quality data for the training of DLANN systems is to pair DLANN models with data filtering methods such as unsupervised or semi-supervised anomaly detection methods (Ergen et al. 2017, Maleki et al. 2021). In addition, such pairing is used to improve prediction performance on new (unseen) data –data cleanup after data collection is part of the set of optimization approaches, such as adding more layers to the neural network, data augmentation, hyperparameter tuning and more that are normally used to improve DLANNs performance (Hui 2018).

In conclusion, the role of AI technology in laboratory settings will be expansive and less expensive. Soon, AI tools will become integral and relevant toolsets of laboratory work, just like tubes and pipetting tools are today. AI technology, together with biotechnology, nanotechnology, communications technology and the availability of affordable miniaturized mobile devices will allow public health agencies to conduct field epidemiological investigations and molecular test screenings in medium- and low-resource settings around the world. AI-powered molecular diagnostics technology, like CMAs and chatbot technologies, will become smarter, more personalized, efficient, accurate and transparent.

References

ACCESSWIRE.COM. (2020). Hyro Develops Free Virtual Assistant to Aid COVID-19 Support and Diagnosis. Tel Aviv, Israel. https://www.accesswire.com/581593/Hyro-Develops-Free-Virtual-Assistant-to-Aid-COVID-581519-Support-and-Diagnosis.

Adamopoulou, E. and L. Moussiades. (2020). Chatbots: History, technology, and applications. Machine Learning with Applications 2: 100006.

Ahmad, A. S. and A. D. W. Sumari. (2017). Cognitive artificial intelligence: Brain-inspired intelligent computation in artificial intelligence. 2017 Computing Conference.

Ai-Chang, M., J. Bresina, L. Charest, A. Chase, J. C. J. Hsu, A. Jonsson et al. (2004). MAPGEN: Mixed-initiative planning and scheduling for the Mars Exploration Rover mission. IEEE Intelligent Systems 19(1): 8–12.

Alamo, T., D. G. Reina, P. M. Gata, V. M. Preciado and G. Giordano. (2021). Data-driven methods for present and future pandemics: Monitoring, modelling and managing. Annual Reviews in Control 52: 448–464.

Aminian, M., H. Andrews-Polymenis, J. Gupta, M. Kirby, H. Kvinge, X. Ma et al. (2020). Mathematical methods for visualization and anomaly detection in telemetry datasets. Interface Focus 10(1): 20190086.

Abadi, M., P. Barham, J. Chen, Z. Chen, A. Davis, J. Dean et al. (2015). [Online] TensorFlow: Large-Scale Machine Learning on Heterogeneous Distributed Systems. (Available at https://static. googleusercontent.com/media/research.google.com/en//pubs/archive/45166.pdf; last accessed on 09/07/2023).

Arbib, M. A. (2003). The elements of brain theory and neural networks. The Handbook of Brain Theory and Neural Networks. M. A. Arbib. Cambridge, Massachusetts, The MIT Press, 3–23.

Ashley, B. K. and U. Hassan. (2021). Point-of-critical-care diagnostics for sepsis enabled by multiplexed micro and nanosensing technologies. Wiley Interdiscip. Rev. Nanomed. Nanobiotechnol. 13(5): e1701.

Ataee, P. (2021). An Overview of Deep Learning—from History to Fundamentals. Towards Data Science. https://towardsdatascience.com/an-overview-of-deep-learning-from-history-to-fundamentals-f7117b7112d7110d7137.

AWS. (2022). Analytics on AWS. Retrieved 08/25/2022, from https://aws.amazon.com/big-data/datalakes-and-analytics/.

Ayanouz, S., B. A. Abdelhakim and M. Benhmed. (2020). A smart chatbot architecture based NLP and machine learning for health care assistance. Proceedings of the 3rd International Conference on Networking, Information Systems & Security. Marrakech, Morocco, Association for Computing Machinery: Article, 78.

Azure. (2022). Artificial Intelligence (AI) vs. machine learning (ML). https://azure.microsoft.com/en-us/solutions/ai/artificial-intelligence-vs-machine-learning/#introduction.

Azure. (2022). Azure Analytics Services. From https://azure.microsoft.com/en-us/products/category/analytics/.

Azure. (2022). Health Bot. A managed service purpose-built for development of virtual healthcare assistants. https://azure.microsoft.com/en-us/products/bot-services/health-bot/.

Azure. (2022). What is artificial intelligence? https://azure.microsoft.com/en-us/resources/cloud-computing-dictionary/what-is-artificial-intelligence/#how.

Azure. (2022). What Is Deep Learning? https://azure.microsoft.com/en-us/resources/cloud-computing-dictionary/what-is-deep-learning/.

Babrak, L. M., J. Menetski, M. Rebhan, G. Nisato, M. Zinggeler, N. Brasier et al. (2019). Traditional and digital biomarkers: Two Worlds apart? Digital Biomarkers 3(2): 92–102.

Bahdanau, D., K. Cho and Y. Bengio. (2015). Neural machine translation by jointly learning to align and translate. Proceedings of the 3rd International Conference on Learning Representations. San Diego, USA.

Baksi, A., S. S. Vasan and R. R. Dighe. (2018). DNA Flow cytometric analysis of the human testicular tissues to investigate the status of spermatogenesis in azoospermic patients. Sci. Rep. 8(1): 11117.

BBC [Online] (2016). BBC News [Online]. US nuclear force still uses floppy disks. https://www.bbc.com/news/world-us-canada-36385839.

BBC [Online] (2018). BBC News [Online]. Japan's cyber-security minister has 'never used a computer'. https://www.bbc.com/news/technology-46222026.

BBC [Online] (2019). BBS News [Online]. Japan's last pagers beep for the final time. https://www.bbc.com/news/world-asia-49888869.

BBC News (2022). Google Translate adds 24 new languages - BBC [Online] BBC News. https://www.bbc.com/news/technology-61416757.

Begum, S. A. and O. M. Devi. (2011). Fuzzy algorithms for pattern recognition in medical diagnosis. Assam University Journal of Science and Technology 7(2): 1–12.

Bellman, R. E. (1957). Dynamic Programming. New Jersey, USA, Princeton University Press.

Bengio, Y. (2009). Learning deep architectures for AI. Found. Trends Mach. Learn. 2(1): 1–127.

Bengio, Y., P. Lamblin, D. Popovici and H. Larochelle. (2006). Greedy layer-wise training of deep networks. Proceedings of the 19th International Conference on Neural Information Processing Systems. Canada, MIT Press, 15–160.

Bernhard, S., P. John and H. Thomas. (2007). Efficient learning of sparse representations with an energy-based model. Advances in Neural Information Processing Systems 19: Proceedings of the 2006 Conference, MIT Press, 1137–1144.

Bethel, C. L., Z. Henkel, S. Darrow and K. Baugus. (2018). Therabot-an Adaptive Therapeutic Support Robot. 2018 World Symposium on Digital Intelligence for Systems and Machines (DISA).

Bhirud, N., S. Tatale, S. Randive and S. Nahar. (2019). A Literature Review On Chatbots In Healthcare Domain.

Botpress. (2022). 13 Best Open Source Chatbot Platforms to Use in 2022. https://botpress.com/blog/open-source-chatbots.

Bouzid, D., M. C. Zanella, S. Kerneis, B. Visseaux, L. May, J. Schrenzel et al. (2021). Rapid diagnostic tests for infectious diseases in the emergency department. Clin. Microbiol. Infect. 27(2): 182–191.

Bradbury, D. W., A. E. Kita, K. Hirota, M. A. St John and D. T. Kamei. (2020). Rapid diagnostic test kit for point-of-care cerebrospinal fluid leak detection. SLAS Technol. 25(1): 67–74.

Campbell, M. and M. Jovanovic. (2021). Conversational Artificial Intelligence: Changing tomorrow's health care today. Computer 54(8): 89–93.

Campo, D. S. and Y. Khudyakov. (2020). Machine learning can accelerate discovery and application of cyber-molecular cancer diagnostics. J. Med. Artif. Intell. 3(7): 10.21037/jmai.2020.01.01.

Camsari, K. Y., R. Faria, B. M. Sutton and S. Datta. (2017). Stochastic p-bits for invertible logic. Physical Review X 7(3): 031014.

Candido, R. (2020). [Online] Generative Adversarial Networks: Build Your First Models. Real Python. (Available at https://realpython.com/generative-adversarial-networks/; last accessed 0n 09/07/2023).

Carleo, A., D. Bennett and P. Rottoli. (2016). Biomarkers in sarcoidosis: the contribution of system biology. Curr. Opin. Pulm. Med. 22(5): 509–514.

Caswell, I. (2022). [Online] Google Translate News. (Available at https://blog.google/products/translate/24-new-languages/; last accessed on 09/07/2023).

CDC/National Center for Health Statistics (2023). [Online] Emergency Department Visits, https://www.cdc.gov/nchs/fastats/emergency-department.htm.

Cesta, A., G. Cortellessa, M. Denis, A. Donati, S. Fratini, A. Oddi et al. (2007). Mexar2: AI solves mission planner problems. IEEE Intelligent Systems 22(4): 12–19.

Chandola, V., A. Banerjee and V. Kumar. (2009). Anomaly detection: A survey. ACM Comput. Surv. 41(3): Article 15.

Chen, Y., T. Guan and C. Wang. (2010). Approximate nearest neighbor search by residual vector quantization. Sensors (Basel) 10(12): 11259–11273.

Chowdhary, K. R. (2020). Natural Language Processing. Fundamentals of Artificial Intelligence. K. R. Chowdhary. New Delhi, Springer India, 603–649.

Chung, K., H. Y. Cho and J. Y. Park. (2021). A chatbot for perinatal women's and partners' obstetric and mental health care: Development and usability evaluation study. JMIR Med. Inform. 9(3): e18607.

CIO Council. (2020). [Online] Future of the Federal IT Workforce. (Available at: https://www.cio.gov/assets/resources/Future_of_Federal_IT_Workforce_Update_Public_Version.pdf; last accessed on 09/15/2022). F. P. Team.

Clark, D. (2018). [Online] Top 16 Open Source Deep Learning Libraries and Platforms. KDnuggets Newsletter News. (Available at https://www.kdnuggets.com/2018/04/top-16-open-source-deep-learning-libraries.html; last accessed on 09/07/2023).

Clayton, J. (2022). Meta's chatbot says the company 'exploits people'. BBCNews. https://www.bbc.com/news/technology-62497674.

Collins, A. and R. Halverson. (2009). The Technology Skeptics' Argument. Rethinking Education in the Age of Technology: The Digital Revolution and Schooling in America. New York, NY, Teachers College Press, 33.

Cornelissen, M., A. Małyska, A. K. Nanda, R. K. Lankhorst, M. A. J. Parry, V. R. Saltenis et al. (2021). Biotechnology for tomorrow's World: Scenarios to guide directions for future innovation. Trends Biotechnol. 39(5): 438–444.

Craft, L. (2022). CBS News. [Online]. Japan is struggling to quit floppy disks and fax machines. https://www.cbsnews.com/news/japan-struggling-to-quit-floppy-disks-and-fax-machines/.

Cruz Hernandez, D., M. Metzner, A. P. de Groot, B. Usukhbayar, N. Elliott, I. Roberts et al. (2020). Sensitive, rapid diagnostic test for transient abnormal myelopoiesis and myeloid leukemia of Down syndrome. Blood 136(12): 1460–1465.

Culler, L. (2020). More perfect Cheetos: How PepsiCo is using Microsoft's Project Bonsai to raise the (snack) bar - Microsoft. [Online] AI for Business: https://blogs.microsoft.com/ai-for-business/pepsico-perfect-cheetos/.

Dargan, S., M. Kumar, M. R. Ayyagari and G. Kumar. (2020). A survey of deep learning and its applications: A new paradigm to machine learning. Archives of Computational Methods in Engineering 27(4): 1071–1092.

De Luca, C., R. Sgariglia, M. Nacchio, P. Pisapia, I. Migliatico, E. Clery et al. (2020). Rapid on-site molecular evaluation in thyroid cytopathology: A same-day cytological and molecular diagnosis. Diagn. Cytopathol. 48(4): 300–307.

Debnath, M., G. B. K. S. Prasad and P. S. Bisen. (2010). Molecular Diagnostics: Promises and Possibilities, Springer Netherlands.

Desiere, F. and V. Romano Spica. (2012). Personalised medicine in 2012: Editorial to the special issue of new biotechnology on molecular diagnostics & personalised medicine. N. Biotechnol. 29(6): 611–612.

Developers Breach, NPO. [Online]. Retrieved on 09/07/2022 from https://developersbreach.com/convolution-neural-network-deep-learning/.

Devlin, J., M. -W. Chang, K. Lee and K. Toutanova. (2018). BERT: Pre-training of Deep Bidirectional Transformers for Language Understanding.

Dihingia, H., S. Ahmed, D. Borah, S. Gupta, K. Phukan, M. K. Muchahari et al. (2021). Chatbot implementation in customer service industry through deep neural networks. 2021 International Conference on Computational Performance Evaluation (ComPE).

Dix, A., S. Vlaic, R. Guthke and J. Linde. (2016). Use of systems biology to decipher host-pathogen interaction networks and predict biomarkers. Clin. Microbiol. Infect. 22(7): 600–606.

Education, I. C. (2020). Deep Learning. https://www.ibm.com/cloud/learn/deep-learning.

English, M. A., L. R. Soenksen, R. V. Gayet, H. de Puig, N. M. Angenent-Mari, A. S. Mao et al. (2019). Programmable CRISPR-responsive smart materials. Science 365(6455): 780–785.

Ergen, T., A. Mirza and S. Kozat. (2017). Unsupervised and semi-supervised anomaly detection with LSTM neural networks. IEEE Transactions on Neural Networks and Learning Systems.

Faria, R., J. Kaiser, K. Y. Camsari and S. Datta. (2021). Hardware design for autonomous Bayesian networks. Frontiers in Computational Neuroscience 15.

Faulstich, K., R. Gruler, M. Eberhard, D. Lentzsch and K. Haberstroh (2009). Handheld and portable reader devices for lateral flow immunoassays. Lateral Flow Immunoassay. R. Wong and H. Tse. Totowa, NJ, Humana Press, 157–183.

Fausett, L. (1994). Fundamentals of Neural Networks: Architectures, Algorithms, and Applications. Upper Saddle River, NJ, Prentice Hall.

Feigenbaum, E. A. (1988). Knowledge processing: From fileservers to knowledge servers. Applications of Expert Systems 2: 3–11.

Feng, W., A. M. Newbigging, C. Le, B. Pang, H. Peng, Y. Cao et al. (2020). Molecular diagnosis of COVID-19: Challenges and research needs. Analytical Chemistry 92(15): 10196–10209.

Fernández, S., A. Graves and J. Schmidhuber. (2007). An Application of Recurrent Neural Networks to Discriminative Keyword Spotting. Artificial Neural Networks – ICANN 2007, Berlin, Heidelberg, Springer Berlin Heidelberg.

FitzGerald, J. (2022). BBC News. [Online]. Floppy disks in Japan: Minister declares war on old-fashioned technology. https://www.bbc.com/news/world-asia-62749310.

Forbi, J. C., J. E. Layden, R. O. Phillips, N. Mora, G. L. Xia, D. S. Campo et al. (2015). Next-generation sequencing reveals frequent opportunities for exposure to Hepatitis C virus in Ghana. PLoS One 10(12): e0145530.

Foundation, N. S. (2022). Engineers develop fast and accurate COVID-19 sensor. https://beta.nsf.gov/news/engineers-develop-fast-and-accurate-covid-19-sensor.

Freire, P. J., Y. Osadchuk, B. Spinnler, A. Napoli, W. Schairer, N. Costa et al. (2021). Performance versus complexity study of neural network equalizers in coherent optical systems. Journal of Lightwave Technology 39(19): 6085–6096.

Fu, C., C. Xiang, C. Wang and D. Cai. (2019). Fast approximate nearest neighbor search with the navigating spreading-out graph. Proc. VLDB Endow. 12(5): 461–474.

Ganova-Raeva, L., Z. Dimitrova, I. Alexiev, L. Punkova, A. Sue, G. L. Xia et al. (2019). HCV transmission in high-risk communities in Bulgaria. PLoS One 14(3): e0212350.

GAO (2022). [Online] Contact Tracing for Air Travel, CDC's Data System Needs Substantial Improvement. In: Report to Congressional Addressees, GAO-22-105018. (Available at https://www.gao.gov/assets/gao-22-105018.pdf; last accessed 09/07/2023).

Garrido-Cardenas, J. A., L. González-Cerón, F. Manzano-Agugliaro and C. Mesa-Valle. (2019). Plasmodium genomics: An approach for learning about and ending human malaria. Parasitology Research 118(1): 1–27.

Gartland, K. M. A. and J. S. Gartland. (2018). Opportunities in biotechnology. J. Biotechnol. 282: 38–45.

Giordano, C., M. Brennan, B. Mohamed, P. Rashidi, F. Modave, P. Tighe et al. (2021). Accessing artificial intelligence for clinical decision-making. Front. Digit. Health 3: 645232.

Github, Inc. (2023). [Online] Topics: # deep-learning-tutorial. (Available at https://github.com/topics/deep-learning-tutorial/; last accessed on 09/07/2023).

Github, Inc. (2023). [Online] Public repository: facebookresearch/faiss. (Available at https://github.com/facebookresearch/faiss/; last accessed on 09/07/2023). FB Team.

Goodfellow, I., J. Pouget-Abadie, M. Mirza, B. Xu, D. Warde-Farley, S. Ozair et al. (2014). Generative Adversarial Nets. Z. Ghahramani, M. Welling, C. Cortes, N. Lawrence and K. Q. Weinberger, 27.

Google. (2022). Google Analytics. Retrieved 08/25/2022, from https://analytics.google.com/analytics/web/provision/#/provision.

Gormley, M. (2007). The first 'molecular disease': A story of Linus Pauling, the intellectual patron. Endeavour 31(2): 71–77.

Graves, A. and J. R. Schmidhuber. (2008). Offline Handwriting Recognition with Multidimensional Recurrent Neural Networks. D. Koller, D. Schuurmans, Y. Bengio and L. Bottou, 21.

Gražulis, S., A. Daškevič, A. Merkys, D. Chateigner, L. Lutterotti, M. Quirós et al. (2012). Crystallography Open Database (COD): An open-access collection of crystal structures and platform for world-wide collaboration. Nucleic Acids Res 40(Database issue): D420–427.

Group, F. -N. B. W. (2016). BEST (Biomarkers, EndpointS, and other Tools) Resource. https://www.ncbi.nlm.nih.gov/books/NBK326791/.

Gulino, A. (1999). Biotechnology and molecular diagnostics. Forum (Genova) 9(3 Suppl 3): 37–46.

Gupta, R., D. Srivastava, M. Sahu, S. Tiwari, R. K. Ambasta, P. Kumar et al. (2021). Artificial intelligence to deep learning: Machine intelligence approach for drug discovery. Mol. Divers 25(3): 1315–1360.

Haddad, E. K. and G. Pantaleo. (2012). Systems biology in the development of HIV vaccines. Curr. Opin. HIV AIDS 7(1): 44–49.

Haider, S. (2020). Ensuring aircraft safety in single point failures, automation and human factors. 2020 Annual Reliability and Maintainability Symposium (RAMS).

Han, C., L. Rundo, K. Murao, T. Noguchi, Y. Shimahara, M. Zoltán Ádám et al. (2021). MADGAN: Unsupervised medical anomaly detection GAN using multiple adjacent brain MRI slice reconstruction. BMC Bioinformatics 22(2): 31.

Hasler, J. (2017). We could Build an Artificial Brain Right Now. IEEESpectrum: https://spectrum.ieee.org/we-could-build-an-artificial-brain-right-now.

Hassantabar, S., N. Stefano, V. Ghanakota, A. Ferrari, G. N. Nicola, R. Bruno et al. (2021). CovidDeep: SARS-CoV-2/COVID-19 test based on wearable medical sensors and efficient neural networks. IEEE Transactions on Consumer Electronics 67(4): 244–256.

Hautz, W. E., A. Exadaktylos and T. C. Sauter. (2021). Online forward triage during the COVID-19 outbreak. Emerg. Med. J. 38(2): 106–108.

Hawkins, D. M. (1980). Identification of Outliers, Springer.

Hinton, G. E., S. Osindero and Y.-W. Teh. (2006). A fast learning algorithm for deep belief nets. Neural Comput. 18(7): 1527–1554.

Hinton, G. E. and R. R. Salakhutdinov. (2006). Reducing the dimensionality of data with neural networks. Science 313(5786): 504–507.

Ho, Q. T., T. T. Nguyen, N. Q. Khanh Le and Y. Y. Ou. (2021). FAD-BERT: Improved prediction of FAD binding sites using pre-training of deep bidirectional transformers. Comput. Biol. Med. 131: 104258.

Hou, M., Y. Wang, L. Trajkovic, K. N. Plataniotis, S. Kwong, M. Zhou et al. (2022). Frontiers of Brain-inspired autonomous systems: How does defense R&D drive the innovations? IEEE Systems, Man, and Cybernetics Magazine 8(2): 8–20.

Hui, J. (2018). Improve Deep Learning Models performance & deep network tuning (Part 6). In Deep Learning Series. (Available at https://jonathan-hui.medium.com/deep-learning-series-f6b46d1e568e; last accessed 09/23/2022). J. Hui.

Hunt, E. (2016). Tay, Microsoft's AI chatbot, gets a crash course in racism from Twitter. TheGuardian: https://www.theguardian.com/technology/2016/mar/2024/tay-microsofts-ai-chatbot-gets-a-crash-course-in-racism-from-twitter?CMP=twt_a-technology_b-gdntech.

Hussein, F. (2017). Hexarray: A Novel Self-Reconfigurable Hardware System. Ph.D. Dissertation, Boise State University.

IBM. (2019). What is a Chatbot? https://www.ibm.com/cloud/learn/chatbots-explained.

IBM. (2020). Artificial Intelligence (AI). https://www.ibm.com/cloud/learn/what-is-artificial-intelligence#toc-types-of-a-q56lfpGa.

IBM. (2020). IBM Offers Watson Assistant for Citizens to Provide Responses to COVID-19 Questions, IBM. https://newsroom.ibm.com/2020–2004–2002-IBM-Offers-Watson-Assistant-for-Citizens-to-Provide-Responses-to-COVID-2019-Questions.

Icer Baykal, P. B., J. Lara, Y. Khudyakov, A. Zelikovsky and P. Skums (2021). Quantitative differences between intra-host HCV populations from persons with recently established and persistent infections. Virus Evol. 7(1): veaa103.

Ichikawa, M. and G. Matsumoto. (2004). The brain-computer: origin of the idea and progress in its realization. J. Integr. Neurosci. 3(2): 125–132.

Inc., G. (2022). How to Build Laboratory Diagnostics Software from Scratch. https://gravelsoft.com/blog/f/how-to-build-laboratory-diagnostics-software-from-scratch.

INTEL. (2022). FPGA's for Artificial Intelligence (AI). Retrieved 08/25/2022, 2022, from https://www.intel.com/content/www/us/en/artificial-intelligence/programmable/overview.html.

Itano, H. A. and L. Pauling. (1949). A rapid diagnostic test for sickle cell anemia. Blood 4(1): 66–68.

Jaffe, R. and J. Mani. (2018). Predictive biomarkers in personalized laboratory diagnoses and best practices outcome monitoring for musculoskeletal health. Metabolic Therapies in Orthopedics, Second Edition. I. Kohlstadt and K. Cintron. UK, CRC Press, 39–57.

Jain, A. (2021). How data and AI can help media companies better personalize; and what to watch out for - Google. [online] Google Cloud: https://cloud.google.com/blog/products/media-entertainment/how-data-and-ai-can-help-media-companies-better-personalize.

Jain, A. K., R. P. W. Duin and M. Jianchang. (2000). Statistical pattern recognition: A review. IEEE Transactions on Pattern Analysis and Machine Intelligence 22(1): 4–37.

Jain, K. K. (2003). Nanodiagnostics: Application of nanotechnology in molecular diagnostics. Expert. Rev. Mol. Diagn. 3(2): 153–161.

Janarthanam, S. and O. Lemon. (2014). Adaptive generation in dialogue systems using dynamic user modeling. Computational Linguistics 40(4): 883–920.

Janvilisri, T., H. Suzuki, J. Scaria, J. W. Chen and V. Charoensawan. (2015). High-throughput screening for biomarker discovery. Dis. Markers 2015: 108064.

Jha, S. and E. J. Topol. (2016). Adapting to Artificial Intelligence: Radiologists and Pathologists as Information Specialists. JAMA 316(22): 2353–2354.

JISC. Joint Information Systems Committee (JISC). [Online]. Resistance to Technology. In, Change management. The theory, methodologies and techniques to help manage change effectively. 2006. (Available at: https://www.jisc.ac.uk/guides/change-management/resistance-to-technology; last accessed 09/15/2022).

Johnson, D. B. (2020). FCW News. [Online]. IRS legacy system problems could be worse than advertised. https://fcw.com/it-modernization/2020/2008/irs-legacy-system-problems-could-be-worse-than-advertised/258023/.

Johnson, J. (2020). [Online] BMC, Machine Learning & Big Data Blog. (Available at https://www.bmc.com/blogs/artificial-intelligence-types/; last accessed on 09/07/2023).

Johnson, J., M. Douze and H. Jégou. (2021). Billion-scale similarity search with GPUs. IEEE Transactions on Big Data 7: 535–547.

Jonsson, A. K., P. H. Morris, N. Muscettola and K. Rajan. (2000). Planning in interplanetary space: Theory and practice. Proceedings of the Fifth International Conference on Artificial Intelligence Planning Systems, Austin, Texas, USA, The AAAI Press.

Joshi, N. (2019). 7 Types of Artificial Intelligence, Forbes. (Available at https://www.forbes.com/sites/cognitiveworld/2019/06/19/7-types-of-artificial-intelligence/?sh=d989591233ee; last accessed on 09/07/2023).

Jovic, D. (2022). The Future is Now - 37 Fascinating Chatbot Statistics: https://www.smallbizgenius.net/by-the-numbers/chatbot-statistics/#gref.

Jozefowicz, R., O. Vinyals, M. Schuster, N. Shazeer and Y. Wu (2016). Exploring the Limits of Language Modeling.

Kadam, R., W. White, N. Banks, Z. Katz, S. Dittrich, C. Kelly-Cirino et al. (2020). Target product profile for a mobile app to read rapid diagnostic tests to strengthen infectious disease surveillance. PLoS One 15(1): e0228311.

Kawashima, S., P. Pokarowski, M. Pokarowska, A. Kolinski, T. Katayama, M. Kanehisa et al. (2008). AAindex: Amino acid index database, progress report 2008. Nucleic Acids Res. 36(Database issue): D202–205.

Khalil, M. A., M. Ramirez, J. Can and K. George. (2022). Implementation of Machine Learning in BCI Based Lie Detection. 2022 IEEE World AI IoT Congress (AIIoT).

Khan, D., M. Park, S. Lerma, S. Soroka, D. Gaughan, L. Bottichio et al. (2022). Improving efficiency of COVID-19 aggregate case and death surveillance data transmission for jurisdictions: Current and future role of application programming interfaces (APIs). J. Am. Med. Inform. Assoc. 29(10): 1807–1809.

Keydana, S. (2018). [Online] Generating images with Keras and TensorFlow eager execution. Posit AI Blog. (Available at https://blogs.rstudio.com/ai/posts/2018-08-26-eager-dcgan/; last accessed 09/07/2023).

Kirtana, A., R. Abdul and S. Barathi. (2022). Nanotechnology and its applications in molecular detection. application of nanoparticles in tissue engineering. S. Afaq, A. Malik and M. Tarique. Singapore, Springer Nature Singapore, 103–117.

Kon, M. A. and L. Plaskota. (2000). Information complexity of neural networks. Neural Networks 13(3): 365–375.

Kulkarni, P., A. Mahabaleshwarkar, M. Kulkarni, N. Sirsikar and K. Gadgil. (2019). Conversational AI: An overview of methodologies, applications & future scope. 2019 5th International Conference On Computing, Communication, Control And Automation (ICCUBEA).

Kurgan, L. A. and K. J. Cios. (2004). CAIM discretization algorithm. IEEE Transactions on Knowledge and Data Engineering 16(2): 145–153.

Kwon, Y. and J. Lee. (2021). MolFinder: An evolutionary algorithm for the global optimization of molecular properties and the extensive exploration of chemical space using SMILES. J. Cheminform. 13(1): 24.

La Rocco, M. T., A. Wanger, H. Ocera and E. Macias. (1994). Evaluation of a commercial rRNA amplification assay for direct detection of Mycobacterium tuberculosis in processed sputum. Eur. J. Clin. Microbiol. Infect. Dis. 13(9): 726–731.

Lahmer, H., A. E. Oueslati and Z. Lachiri. (2020). Classification of DNA microarrays using deep learning to identify cell cycle regulated genes. 2020 5th International Conference on Advanced Technologies for Signal and Image Processing (ATSIP).

Lamba, D., W. H. Hsu and M. Alsadhan. (2021). Chapter 1—Predictive analytics and machine learning for medical informatics: A survey of tasks and techniques. Machine Learning, Big Data, and IoT for Medical Informatics. P. Kumar, Y. Kumar and M. A. Tawhid, Academic Press, 1–35.

Lara, J., M. Teka and Y. Khudyakov. (2017). Identification of recent cases of hepatitis C virus infection using physical-chemical properties of hypervariable region 1 and a radial basis function neural network classifier. BMC Genomics 18(Suppl 10): 880.

Lara, J., M. A. Teka, S. Sims, G. L. Xia, S. Ramachandran, Y. Khudyakov et al. (2018). HCV adaptation to HIV coinfection. Infect. Genet. Evol. 65: 216–225.

Latimer, N. R., C. Henshall, U. Siebert and H. Bell. (2016). Treatment swithching: Statistical and decision-making challenges and approaches. International Journal of Technology Assessment in Health Care 32(3): 160–166.

Lee, W. E., S. W. Park, D. M. Weinberger, D. Olson, L. Simonsen, B. T. Grenfell et al. (2022). Direct and indirect mortality impacts of the COVID-19 pandemic in the US, March 2020–April 2021. medRxiv.

Li, D. and Y. Dong. (2014). Deep Learning: Methods and applications. Foundations and Trends in Signal Processing, New Foundations and Trends 7: 197–387.

Lindsey R. Sheppard. (2021). Cultivating a defense department workforce for the digital Era. In, CSIS International Security Program's Transition 46 series on Defense 360. Center for Strategic & International Studies (CSIS), Washington D.C., USA.

Liu, B., F. Liu, X. Wang, J. Chen, L. Fang and K. C. Chou et al. (2015). Pse-in-One: A web server for generating various modes of pseudo components of DNA, RNA, and protein sequences. Nucleic Acids Res. 43(W1): W65–71.

Liu, Y., G. Wang, F. Zhang and L. Dai. (2021). An NGS-based approach to identify Y-chromosome variation in non-obstructive azoospermia. Andrologia 53(10): e14201.

Lubin, I. M., J. R. Astles, S. Shahangian, B. Madison, R. Parry, R. L. Schmidt et al. (2021). Bringing the clinical laboratory into the strategy to advance diagnostic excellence. 8(3): 281–294.

Lyimo, B. M., Z. R. Popkin-Hall, D. J. Giesbrecht, C. I. Mandara, R. A. Madebe, C. Bakari et al. (2022). Potential opportunities and challenges of deploying next generation sequencing and CRISPR-Cas systems to support diagnostics and surveillance towards malaria control and elimination in Africa. Front. Cell Infect. Microbiol. 12: 757844.

Lysecky, R. and F. Vahid. (2005). A study of the speedups and competitiveness of FPGA soft processor cores using dynamic hardware/software partitioning. Proceedings of the conference on Design, Automation and Test in Europe - Volume 1, IEEE Computer Society, 18–23.

Maitre, J., K. Bouchard and S. Gaboury. (2022). SSRN. [Online]. Data Filtering and Deep Learning for Enhanced Human. (Available at: https://papers.ssrn.com/sol3/papers.cfm?abstract_id=4070386; lasta accessed on 09/15/2022).

Malek, L., R. Sooknanan and J. Compton. (1994). Nucleic acid sequence-based amplification (NASBA). Methods Mol. Biol. 28: 253–260.

Maleki, S., S. Maleki and N. R. Jennings. (2021). Unsupervised anomaly detection with LSTM autoencoders using statistical data-filtering. Applied Soft Computing 108: 107443.

Markou, M. and S. Singh. (2003). Novelty detection: A review—Part 2 neural network based approaches. Signal Processing 83(12): 2499–2521.

Maros, M. E., D. Capper, D. T. W. Jones, V. Hovestadt, A. von Deimling, S. M. Pfister et al. (2020). Machine learning workflows to estimate class probabilities for precision cancer diagnostics on DNA methylation microarray data. Nature Protocols 15(2): 479–512.

Marzieh, F., H. K. Mostafa, J. S. Mahdi and M. Ebrahim. (2022). Big data analytics in weather forecasting: A systematic review. Archives of Computational Methods in Engineering 29(2): 1247–1275.

Mckinsey&Company. (2019). Global AI Survey: AI proves its worth, but few scale impact. https://www.mckinsey.com/featured-insights/artificial-intelligence/global-ai-survey-ai-proves-its-worth-but-few-scale-impact.

McLoughlin, K. S. (2011). Microarrays for pathogen detection and analysis. Brief Funct Genomics 10(6): 342–353.

McRae, M. P., G. Simmons, J. Wong and J. T. McDevitt. (2016). Programmable Bio-nanochip Platform: A Point-of-Care Biosensor System with the Capacity To Learn. Acc. Chem. Res. 49(7): 1359–1368.

(Meta AI 2022, 08/25/2022). from https://ai.facebook.com/.

Meyer, D. (2018). IBM Built a Computer the Size of a Grain of Salt. Here's What It's For, Fortune. https://fortune.com.

Meystre, S. M., P. M. Heider, Y. Kim, M. Davis, J. Obeid, J. Madory et al. (2022). Natural language processing enabling COVID-19 predictive analytics to support data-driven patient advising and pooled testing. Journal of the American Medical Informatics Association 29(1): 12–21.

Michel, J., A. Mettler, C. Starvaggi, N. Travaglini, C. Aebi, K. Keitel et al. (2022). The utility of a pediatric COVID-19 online forward triage tool in Switzerland. Front Public Health 10: 902072.

Microsoft. (2022). Azure Health Bot. Retrieved 08/25/2022, 2022, from https://www.microsoft.com/en-us/research/project/health-bot/.

Microsoft. (2022). What is a chatbot? https://powervirtualagents.microsoft.com/en-us/what-is-a-chatbot/.

Miner, A. S., L. Laranjo and A. B. Kocaballi. (2020). Chatbots in the fight against the COVID-19 pandemic. NPJ Digit. Med. 3: 65.

Minkiewicz, P., A. Iwaniak and M. Darewicz. (2017). Annotation of peptide structures using SMILES and other chemical codes-practical solutions. Molecules 22(12).

Minsky, M. L. (1954). Theory of Neural-analog Reinforcement Systems and its Application to the Brain-model Problem. PH.D., Princeton University.

Mosher, D. (2016). BusinessInsider [Online]. US nuclear forces are controlled by this shockingly obsolete tech, from https://www.businessinsider.com/floppy-disks-control-us-nuclear-weapons-2016-5.

MSV, J. (2020). How TinyML Makes Artificial Intelligence Ubiquitous, Forbes. https://www.forbes.com.

Mueller, J. D., B. Pütz and H. Höfler. (1997). Self-sustained sequence replication (3SR): An alternative to PCR. Histochem. Cell Biol. 108(4-5): 431–437.

Muller, C. Y., J. O. Schorge, G. E. Tomlinson and R. Ashfaq. (2004). BRCAPAP: Feasibility of clinical BRCA testing on liquid-based cervical cytology: Implications for biomarker development. Cancer Epidemiol. Biomarkers Prev. 13(9): 1534–1537.

Munyuza, C., H. Ji and E. R. Lee. (2022). Probe capture enrichment methods for HIV and HCV genome sequencing and drug resistance genotyping. Pathogens 11(6).

Nagarajan, D. (2019). Continuous delivery of data drives continuous intelligence. Journey to AI Blog, IBM. https://www.ibm.com/blogs/journey-to-ai/2019/2003/continuous-delivery-of-data-drives-continuous-intelligence/.

National Academies of Sciences, E., Medicine, Health, D. Medicine, H. Board on Population, P. Public Health and B. Committee on a National Strategy for the Elimination of Hepatitis. (2017). A National Strategy for the Elimination of Hepatitis B and C: Phase Two Report. B. L. Strom and G. J. Buckley. Washington (DC), National Academies Press (US) Copyright 2017 by the National Academy of Sciences.

Nayyar, A. (2019). Chatbots and the open source tools you can use to develop them. OpenSource.com. https://www.opensourceforu.com/2019/2001/chatbots-and-the-open-source-tools-you-can-use-to-develop-them/.

News, J. G. f. D. (2020). Esper says artificial intelligence will change the battlefield. U.S. Department of Defence. https://www.defense.gov/News/News-Stories/Article/Article/2340972/esper-says-artificial-intelligence-will-change-the-battlefield/.

Ning, C. and F. You. (2019). Optimization under uncertainty in the era of big data and deep learning: When machine learning meets mathematical programming. Computers & Chemical Engineering 125.

NVIDIA. (2022). Nvidia DGX Station A100. Workgroup Appliance for the Age of AI. Retrieved 08/25/2022, 2022, from https://www.nvidia.com/en-us/data-center/dgx-station-a100/.

ONNX Runtime developers. (2021). [Online] ONNX Runtime. (Available at https://onnxruntime.ai/; last accessed on 09/07/2023).

Oracle. (2022). What is a chatbot? https://www.oracle.com/chatbots/what-is-a-chatbot/.

Pan, J., I. S. Popa and C. Borcea. (2017). DIVERT: A distributed vehicular traffic re-routing system for congestion avoidance. IEEE Transactions on Mobile Computing 16(1): 58–72.

Panel on the Design of the National Children's, S., R. Implications for the Generalizability of, S. Committee on National, B. Division of, S. Social, Education, Y. Board on Children, Families, M. Institute of and C. National Research. (2014). The National Academies Collection: Reports funded by National Institutes of Health. The National Children's Study 2014: An Assessment. G. J. Duncan, N. J. Kirkendall and C. F. Citro. Washington (DC), National Academies Press (US), 99–106.

Paszke, A., S. Gross, F. Massa, A. Lerer, J. Bradbury, G. Chanan et al. (2019). [Online] PyTorch: An Imperative Style, High-Performance Deep Learning Library. In: Advances in Neural Information Processing Systems 32. Curran Associates, Inc.; pp. 8024–35. (Available at http://papers.neurips.cc/paper/9015-pytorch-an-imperative-style-high-performance-deep-learning-library.pdf; last accessed on 09/07/2023).

Patrinos, G. P., P. B. Danielson and W. J. Ansorge. (2017). Chapter 1 - Molecular Diagnostics: Past, Present, and Future. Molecular Diagnostics (Third Edition). G. P. Patrinos, Academic Press, 1–11.

Poornima, S. and M. Pushpalatha. (2018). A survey of predictive analytics using big data with data mining. International Journal of Bioinformatics Research and Applications 14(3): 269–282.

Prodan Zitnik, I., D. Cerne, I. Mancini, L. Simi, M. Pazzagli, C. Di Resta et al. (2018). Personalized laboratory medicine: A patient-centered future approach. Clin. Chem. Lab. Med. 56(12): 1981–1991.

Qin, Y., D. Yi, X. Chen and Y. Guan. (2021). Deep learning identifies erroneous microarray-based, gene-level conclusions in literature. NAR Genom. Bioinform. 3(4): lqab089.

Quirós, M., S. Gražulis, S. Girdzijauskaitė, A. Merkys and A. Vaitkus. (2018). Using SMILES strings for the description of chemical connectivity in the Crystallography open database. J. Cheminform. 10(1): 23.

Rajan, K., A. Zielesny and C. Steinbeck. (2021). DECIMER 1.0: Deep learning for chemical image recognition using transformers. J. Cheminform. 13(1): 61.

Ramachandran, S., H. Thai, J. C. Forbi, R. R. Galang, Z. Dimitrova, G. L. Xia et al. (2018). A large HCV transmission network enabled a fast-growing HIV outbreak in rural Indiana, 2015. EBioMedicine 37: 374–381.

Ridder, D. d., J. d. Ridder and M. J. Reinders. (2013). Pattern recognition in bioinformatics. Briefings in Bioinformatics 14(5): 633–647.

Rindi, L. (2022). Rapid molecular diagnosis of extra-pulmonary tuberculosis by Xpert/RIF Ultra. Front. Microbiol. 13: 817661.

Roh, Y., G. Heo and S. E. Whang. (2021). A survey on data collection for machine learning: A big Data - AI integration perspective. IEEE Transactions on Knowledge and Data Engineering 33(4): 1328–1347.

Romm, C. (2015). Before There Were Home Pregnancy Tests. The Atlantic

Russell, S. J. and P. Norvig. (2012). Artificial Intelligence: A Modern Approach.

Russell, S. J. and P. Norvig. (2012). Natural Language Processing. Artificial Intelligence: A Modern Approach, 860–887.

Russell, S. J. and P. Norvig. (2012). Utility Functions. Artificial Intelligence: A Modern Approach, 615–621.

Sahibzada, K. I., L. Ganova-Raeva, Z. Dimitrova, S. Ramachandran, Y. Lin, G. Longmire et al. (2022). Hepatitis C virus transmission cluster among injection drug users in Pakistan. PLoS One 17(7): e0270910.

Saleh, Z. (2019). Artificial Intelligence Definition, Ethics and Standards.

Salvador, R., A. Otero, J. Mora, E. d. l. Torre, T. Riesgo and L. Sekanina. (2013). Self-reconfigurable evolvable hardware system for adaptive image processing. IEEE Transactions on Computers 62(8): 1481–1493.

Sánchez-Pla, A. (2014). Chapter 1—DNA Microarrays Technology: Overview and Current Status. Comprehensive Analytical Chemistry. C. Simó, A. Cifuentes and V. García-Cañas, Elsevier, 63: 1–23.

Sanger, F. and A. R. Coulson. (1975). A rapid method for determining sequences in DNA by primed synthesis with DNA polymerase. J. Mol. Biol. 94(3): 441–448.

Sanger, F., S. Nicklen and A. R. Coulson. (1977). DNA sequencing with chain-terminating inhibitors. Proc. Natl. Acad. Sci. U S A 74(12): 5463–5467.

Sarker, I. H. (2021). Deep Learning: A comprehensive overview on techniques, taxonomy, applications and research directions. SN Comput. Sci. 2(6): 420.

Schena, M., D. Shalon, R. W. Davis and P. O. Brown. (1995). Quantitative monitoring of gene expression patterns with a complementary DNA microarray. Science 270(5235): 467–470.

Schmidt, B. and A. Hildebrandt. (2021). Deep learning in next-generation sequencing. Drug Discovery Today 26(1): 173–180.

Schneider, P. and F. Xhafa. (2022). Chapter 3—Anomaly detection: Concepts and methods. Anomaly Detection and Complex Event Processing over IoT Data Streams. P. Schneider and F. Xhafa, Academic Press, 49–66.

Schork, N. J. (2019). Artificial Intelligence and Personalized Medicine. Precision Medicine in Cancer Therapy. D. D. Von Hoff and H. Han. Cham, Springer International Publishing, 265–283.

Schuller, D. and B. W. Schuller. (2018). The age of artificial emotional intelligence. Computer 51(9): 38–46.

Sharlach, M. (2022). Deep-learning diagnoses: Edge AI detects COVID-19 from smartwatch sensors, Office of Engineering Communications, Princeton University. https://ece.princeton.edu/news/deep-learning-diagnoses-edge-ai-detects-covid-19-smartwatch-sensors.

Shaw, W. H., Q. Lin, Z. Z. Muhammad, J. J. Lee, W. X. Khong, O. T. Ng et al. (2016). Identification of HIV mutation as diagnostic biomarker through next generation sequencing. J. Clin. Diagn. Res. 10(7): Dc04–08.

Shuster, K., J. Xu, M. Komeili, D. Ju, E. M. Smith, S. Roller et al. (2022). BlenderBot 3: A deployed conversational agent that continually learns to responsibly engage. arXiv:2208.03188 [cs.CL].

Silva, G. M. D., S. Thakare, S. More and J. Kuriakose. (2017). Real world smart chatbot for customer care using a software as a service (SaaS) architecture. 2017 International Conference on I-SMAC (IoT in Social, Mobile, Analytics and Cloud) (I-SMAC).

Sims, S., A. G. Longmire, D. S. Campo, S. Ramachandran, M. Medrzycki, L. Ganova-Raeva et al. (2018). Automated quality control for a molecular surveillance system. BMC Bioinformatics 19(Suppl 11): 358.

Simsek, C., M. Bloemen, D. Jansen, L. Beller, P. Descheemaeker, M. Reynders et al. (2021). High prevalence of coinfecting enteropathogens in suspected rotavirus vaccine breakthrough cases. J. Clin. Microbiol. 59(12): e0123621.

Singh, N., P. Lapierre, T. M. Quinlan, T. A. Halse, S. Wirth, M. C. Dickinson et al. (2019). Whole-genome Single-Nucleotide Polymorphism (SNP) analysis applied directly to stool for genotyping shiga toxin-producing *Escherichia coli*: An advanced molecular detection method for foodborne disease surveillance and outbreak tracking. J. Clin. Microbiol. 57(7).

Siontis, K. C., P. A. Noseworthy, Z. I. Attia and P. A. Friedman. (2021). Artificial intelligence-enhanced electrocardiography in cardiovascular disease management. Nature Reviews Cardiology 18(7): 465–478.

Slatko, B. E., A. F. Gardner and F. M. Ausubel. (2018). Overview of next-generation sequencing technologies. Curr. Protoc. Mol. Biol. 122(1): e59.

Smith, A. (2020). CDC Creates Coronavirus Chatbot Called Clara to Check Your Symptoms, PC Mag: https://pcmag.com.

Smith, J. E. and R. L. Winkler. (2006). The optimizer's curse: Skepticism and postdecision surprise in decision analysis. Manag. Sci. 52: 311–322.

Software, P. M. L. (2019). The History and Evolution of Molecular Diagnostics. https://psychesystems.com/wp-content/uploads/2019/2007/History_Molecular-Diagnostics_WPv2011_2018–2011.pdf.

State, N. Y. (2022). New York State Hepatitis C Elimination Plan.

Stuart J. Rusell, P. N. (2012). Artificial Intelligence. Artificial Intelligence: A Modern Approach, 1–29.

Susan Miller. (2022). FCW news [Online]. Averting the next pandemic with real-time health data. https://fcw.com/it-modernization/2022/2008/averting-next-pandemic-real-time-health-data/375384/.

Sutskever, I., O. Vinyals and Q. V. Le, (2014). Sequence to Sequence Learning with Neural Networks. Advances in Neural Information Processing Systems 27 (NIPS 2014). Z. Ghahramani, M. Welling, C. Cortes, N. Lawrence and K. Q. Weinberger. Montréal, Canada.

Swindells, M. B. (1995). A procedure for detecting structural domains in proteins. Protein Sci. 4(1): 103–112.

Swingler, K. (1996). Netwrok use and analysis. Applying Neural Networks: A practical Guide. San Fransisco, Mourgan Kaufman Publishers Inc., 165–182.

Tábuas-Pereira, M., S. Freitas, J. Beato-Coelho, J. Ribeiro, J. Parra, C. Martins et al. (2018). [Aphasia Rapid Test: Translation, Adaptation and Validation Studies for the Portuguese Population]. Acta Med. Port. 31(5): 265–271.

Tatman, R. (2019). [Online] Beginner's Intro to RNN's in R. (Available at https://www.kaggle.com/code/rtatman/beginner-s-intro-to-rnn-s-in-r/notebook/; last accessed 09/07/2023).

TensorFlow (2023). [Online] Convolutional Neural Network (CNN). https://www.tensorflow.org/tutorials/images/cnn/.

The Statistics Online Computational Resource (SOCR). [Online] Retrieved on 09/07/2022 from https://socr.umich.edu/HTML5/ABIDE_Autoencoder/; last accessed on 09/07/2023). SOCR Team.

Tocci, R. J., N. S. Widmer and G. L. Moss. (2009). Digital Systems: Principles and Applications. India, Pearson India.

Touma, M. (2020). COVID-19: Molecular diagnostics overview. J. Mol. Med. (Berl.) 98(7): 947–954.

Townshend, R. J. L., S. Eismann, A. M. Watkins, R. Rangan, M. Karelina, R. Das et al. (2021). Geometric deep learning of RNA structure. Science 373(6558): 1047–1051.

Treml, F. (2020). Security Threats and Security Testing for Chatbots. Chatbots Life. https://chatbotslife.com/security-threats-and-security-testing-for-chatbots-325d704da329af.

Turbé, V., C. Herbst, T. Mngomezulu, S. Meshkinfamfard, N. Dlamini, T. Mhlongo et al. (2021). Deep learning of HIV field-based rapid tests. Nature Medicine 27(7): 1165–1170.

Vincent, J. (2016). Twitter taught Microsoft's AI chatbot to be a racist asshole in less than a day. The Verge. https://www.theverge.com/2016/2013/2024/11297050/tay-microsoft-chatbot-racist.

Walch, K. and R. Schmelzer. (2019). The seven patterns of AI - Cognilytica. [online] Cognilytica. https://www. cognilytica.com/2019/2004/2004/the-seven-patterns-of-ai/.

Wang, D., L. Coscoy, M. Zylberberg, P. C. Avila, H. A. Boushey, D. Ganem et al. (2002). Microarray-based detection and genotyping of viral pathogens. Proc. Natl. Acad. Sci. U S A 99(24): 15687–15692.

Wang, K., S. Langevin, C. S. O'Hern, M. D. Shattuck, S. Ogle, A. Forero et al. (2016). Anomaly detection in host signaling pathways for the early prognosis of acute infection. PLoS One 11(8): e0160919.

Wang, K., I. Lee, G. Carlson, L. Hood and D. Galas. (2010). Systems biology and the discovery of diagnostic biomarkers. Dis. Markers 28(4): 199–207.

Wang, L. and Y. Xia. (2021). Artificial Intelligence Brain. 2021 International Conference on Computer Engineering and Artificial Intelligence (ICCEAI).

Wang, W., Z. Zhang, Y. Du, B. Chen, J. Xie and W. Luo. (2021). Rethinking Zero-shot Neural Machine Translation: From a Perspective of Latent Variables. Findings of the Association for Computational Linguistics: EMNLP (Findings) 2021. Punta Cana, Dominican Republic, 4321–4327.

Wang, Y., H. Xu, Z. Dong, Z. Wang, Z. Yang, X. Yu et al. (2022). Micro/nano biomedical devices for point-of-care diagnosis of infectious respiratory diseases. Med. Nov. Technol. Devices 14: 100116.

Weckselblatt, B. and M. K. Rudd. (2015). Human structural variation: Mechanisms of chromosome rearrangements. Trends Genet. 31(10): 587–599.

Wertheimer, T. (2022). Blake Lemoine: Google fires engineer who said AI tech has feelings. BBC News Tech, BBC News: https://www.bbc.com/news/technology-62275326.

WHO. (2022). 14.9 million excess deaths associated with the COVID-19 pandemic in 2020 and 2021. https://www.who.int/news/item/05–05–2022–2014.2029-million-excess-deaths-were-associated-with-the-covid-2019-pandemic-in-2020-and-2021.

Williams, C. (1983). A Brief Introduction To Artificial Intelligence. Proceedings OCEANS '83.

Williams, L. C. (2022). The Army Wants Smarter Sensors To Ease Soldiers' 'Cognitive Burden' - Defence One. [Online] Defence One. https://www.defenseone.com/technology/2022/2009/army-wants-smarter-sensors-ease-soldiers-cognitive-burden/376632/.

Xu, Y., K. Lin, S. Wang, L. Wang, C. Cai, C. Song et al. (2019). Deep learning for molecular generation. Future Med. Chem. 11(6): 567–597.

Yamashita, R., M. Nishio, R. K. G. Do and K. Togashi. (2018). Convolutional neural networks: An overview and application in radiology. Insights into Imaging 9(4): 611–629.

Yang, Y., S. D. Walls, S. M. Gross, G. P. Schroth, R. G. Jarman and J. Hang. (2018). Targeted sequencing of respiratory viruses in clinical specimens for pathogen identification and genome-wide analysis. Methods Mol. Biol. 1838: 125–140.

Yang, Z. R. and Z. Yang (2014). Chapter 6—Artificial Neural Networks. Comprehensive Biomedical Physics. Brahme, A., Elsevier, 1–17. (Available at https://www.sciencedirect.com/science/article/pii/B9780444536327011011).

YCSung. (2017). [Online] Using R and Tensorflow to build CNN. (Available at https://www.kaggle.com/code/cd12631/using-r-and-tensorflow-to-build-cnn/report/; last accessed on 09/07/2023).

Ye, W. and Q. Li. (2020). Chatbot Security and Privacy in the Age of Personal Assistants. 2020 IEEE/ACM Symposium on Edge Computing (SEC).

Yom-Tov, E. (2021). Active syndromic surveillance of COVID-19 in Israel. Sci. Rep. 11(1): 24449.

Young, A. N. and B. Kairdolf. (2014). Nanotechnology in molecular diagnostics. Molecular Genetic Pathology: Second Edition, 383–398.

Zemčík, T. (2021). Failure of chatbot Tay was evil, ugliness and uselessness in its nature or do we judge it through cognitive shortcuts and biases? AI & SOCIETY 36(1): 361–367.

Zeng, W., M. Wu and R. Jiang. (2018). Prediction of enhancer-promoter interactions via natural language processing. BMC Genomics 19(Suppl 2): 84.

Zhang, W. E., Q. Z. Sheng, A. Alhazmi and C. Li. (2020). Adversarial attacks on deep-learning models in natural language processing: A survey. ACM Trans. Intell. Syst. Technol. 11(3): Article 24.

Zhang, X. -Y., C. -L. Liu and C. Y. Suen. (2020). Towards robust pattern recognition: A review. Proceedings of the IEEE 108(6): 894–922.

Zhu, S. and F. Chollet (2023). [Online] Working with RNNs. TensorFlow, https://www.tensorflow.org/guide/keras/rnn.

Chapter 2

Detection of Gastrointestinal Protists

Monica Santin,* Josephine S.Y. Ng-Hublin
and *Jenny G. Maloney*

Introduction

Infections of the gastrointestinal tract caused by parasitic protists are a major cause of morbidity and mortality worldwide (Troeger et al. 2018). Clinical symptoms and duration of parasitosis depend on the parasite and host factors such as immune status or age. For instance, cryptosporidiosis causes acute self-limiting gastroenteritis in immune-competent patients; while in immune-compromised patients severe, chronic disease may occur, and infection can be fatal (Chalmers and Davies 2010). Immunocompromised patients infected with *Cystoisospora belli* also experience a more severe disease than immunocompetent individuals (Dubey and Almeria 2019), while the higher occurrence of clinical giardiasis is observed in children younger than 5 years with those infections being associated with wasting and cognitive impairment (Cacciò and Lalle 2015). Diarrhea is the main symptom observed in most gastrointestinal parasitic infections, and differential diagnosis is important to properly identify the parasite responsible for the infection. Additionally, differential diagnoses with bacterial and viral infections, such as norovirus, rotavirus, *Campylobacter*, or *Salmonella*, that also share diarrhea as a main clinical symptom are necessary. However, gastrointestinal infections with protist parasites are not always associated with diarrhea; *Giardia duodenalis* has been found more often in non-diarrheal than diarrheal stools in children (Kotloff et al. 2018) while infections with *Blastocystis* sp. have similar occurrence in individuals with and without gastrointestinal disorders (Rojas-Velázquez et al. 2019). Similarly, infections with *Entamoeba histolytica* in most individuals remain asymptomatic; but in some instances, it causes amoebic colitis and disseminated disease (Kantor et al. 2018).

Environmental Microbial and Food Safety Laboratory, Agricultural Research Service, U.S. Department of Agriculture, 10300 Baltimore Ave, Beltsville, MD 20705, USA.
* Corresponding author: monica.santin-duran@usda.gov

The life cycles of gastrointestinal protists all have in common a stage where the organism is passed in the feces of infected persons (Table 1). Traditionally, the detection of protists from the gastrointestinal tract has relied on light microscopy for morphological determination of intestinal stages in the stool. However, an important limitation of conventional microscopic diagnostic methods is their inability to differentiate strains of the same parasite. Application of molecular techniques has not only allowed for the detection of lower numbers of parasites in a given sample, improving sensitivity and specificity, but also to genetically characterize isolates to determine species, genotypes, or subtypes that are morphologically indistinguishable (e.g., Fotedar et al. 2007, Xiao 2010, Li et al. 2019, Maloney et al. 2019, Dixon 2020).

Before testing any sample, it is important to obtain a complete anamnesis that could aid in discovering epidemiological risk factors which can be used to decide which diagnostic tests are appropriate (Garcia et al. 2018). Examples of risk factors to include in clinical history are travel or immunological status. History of travel to cyclosporiasis-endemic areas is associated with a risk of infection with *Cyclospora cayetanensis*; swimming or contact with calves is associated with a higher risk of *Cryptosporidium parvum* infections; drinking from streams is associated with *G. duodenalis* infections (Benedict et al. 2019, Almeria et al. 2019). Individuals with compromised immune systems are at higher risk for opportunistic protist pathogen infection, as such these organisms should be considered in differential diagnosis and additional tests may be needed for their identification (Wołyniec et al. 2018, Laksemi et al. 2019, Valenčáková and Sučik 2020). It is important to note that most diagnostic parasitological tests require personnel expertise and can be time-consuming.

With all techniques that require the manipulation of fresh feces, it is crucial that all necessary safety precautions are taken. Appropriate personal protective equipment (PPE) needs to be used as well as engineering controls, such as biological safety cabinets, to reduce or eliminate exposure to biohazards when working with stool samples.

Stool Specimen Collection

Proper specimen collection and preservation are crucial to securing a valid diagnosis of intestinal protist parasites. Diagnostic stages of intestinal protist parasites present in stool specimens include trophozoites, cysts, oocysts, and spores (Table 1). The stability of these stages must be considered when collecting and handling stool specimens to ensure that they are identifiable if present. Factors that are well recognized to influence the success of parasite detection include contamination of specimens with urine or water (e.g., damage trophozoites); the presence of drugs or compounds (e.g., antibiotics, antidiarrheal) in patient's stool specimens, number of specimens collected, and method of preservation used (Garcia 2007).

As many intestinal protozoan parasites, such as *Cryptosporidium* spp. and *G. duodenalis*, are known for shedding intermittently, the number and intervals of stool specimens collected for laboratory testing need to account for potential daily variation in shedding. Studies have shown that the probability of detecting

Table 1. Overview of diagnostic features of intestinal protist parasites.

Organism	Forms Identified in Stool	Size	Description	Microscopy Diagnostic Method
Balantidium coli	Trophozoite	50–70 μm	• Large, oval with tapering anterior end and covered with short cilia • Cytoplasm contains many vacuoles with ingested bacteria and debris • Contains two nuclei—a large bean-shaped macronucleus and a smaller round micronucleus • Motility is rotary and boring	• Motile trophozoites and cysts are easily seen on direct wet mounts on low magnification
	Cysts	45–65 μm	• Spherical or oval • Thick wall • Contains two nuclei—a large bean-shaped macronucleus and a smaller round micronucleus, which is difficult to see in unstained preparations • Older cysts appear granular, whereas macronucleus and contractile vacuole are visible in young cysts	
Blastocystis sp.	Cysts	6–40 μm	• Spherical to somewhat oval • Formed central body • Contains 1–4 nuclei that may be present around the central body	• Direct/iodine wet mount • Better sensitivity with permanent stains (trichrome, acid-fast stains)
	Vacuolar	5–30 μm	• Spherical or oval • Contains 1–4 nuclei (usually 1) • Contains a large central vacuole	
	Granular	6.5–8 μm	• Visually similar to vacuolar form but with granules in the central vacuole	

Table 1 contd. ...

...Table 1 contd.

Organism	Forms Identified in Stool	Size	Description	Microscopy Diagnostic Method
Cyclospora cayetanensis	Oocyst	8–10 µm	• Round, non-refractile spheres on a wet mount	• Fecal specimens should be concentrated to increase sensitivity
			• Morphologically similar to *Cryptosporidium* oocysts but can be differentiated based on size measurements	• Autofluorescence intense blue under UV light excitation 330–385 nm or strong green with 450–490 nm • Permanent stain (safranin, modified acid-fast, fluorescent stains) • Acid-fast variable
Cryptosporidium spp.	Oocyst	4–6 µm	• Round • Oocyst contains 4 "naked" sporozoites (no sporocysts)	• Fecal specimens should be concentrated before staining • Permanent stain (modified acid-fast stains or Giemsa) • Immunofluorescence antibody stain • Acid-fast
Cytoisospora belli	Oocyst	25–30 µm	• Ellipsoidal oocyst • The fecal diagnostic stage is usually an immature oocyst (unsporulated) that contains a zygote • Mature oocyst contains 2 sporocysts with 4 sporozoites each	• Concentration sedimentation • Modified acid-fast stains • Autofluoresces violet under UV light excitation 330–385 nm or green with 450–490 nm • Acid-fast
Entamoeba spp. (*E. histolytica/E. dispar/E. moshkovskii*)	Trophozoite	15–20 µm	• Finger shaped pseudopodia • Cytoplasm is fine, granular • The presence of RBC is diagnostic for *E. histolytica* (although rarely, RBC can also be present in some *E. dispar* strains)	• Direct wet mount to identify motile trophozoite • Permanent stains (trichrome or iron hematoxylin)
	Cyst	10–15 µm	• Spherical • Immature cysts contain 1–2 nucleus • A mature cyst contains 4 nuclei • Diagnosis based on morphology with or without RBC presence	

Table 1 contd. ...

Table 1 contd. ...

Organism	Forms Identified in Stool	Size	Description	Microscopy Diagnostic Method
Giardia duodenalis	Trophozoite	10–20 μm	• Teardrop shaped with large ventral disc • 4 pairs of flagella (2 lateral, 1 ventral, and 1 caudal)	• Direct wet mount to identify motile trophozoite
			• Contains 2 nuclei (visible only in stained preparations) • Motility is described as a "falling leaf" • Median bodies below the ventral disc	• Permanent stains (trichrome or iron hematoxylin, Giemsa) • Immunofluorescence antibody stain
	Cyst	8–15 μm	• Oval, ellipsoidal, may appear round • Contains 4 nuclei (visible only in stained preparations)	
Microsporidia	Spore	1–4 μm long	• Pyriform or oval with a polar tubule that usually appears as diagonal or horizontal "stripes" when stained	• Permanent stain (modified trichrome-stain, optical brightening agents) • Concentration of spores recommended especially for light infections

RBC: red blood cell.

protozoan parasite infection from a single stool specimen may be as low as 50%, while the examination of multiple stool samples, collected at separate intervals, can increase the detection probability to > 95% (Marti and Koella 1993, Hiatt et al. 1995, Garcia et al. 2018). For optimal diagnostic yield in the parasite examination, it is recommended that three stool specimens be collected, ideally on alternate days within a 10-day period, and submitted for examination prior to ruling out a parasitic infection (Guerrent et al. 2001, Garcia 2007, Garcia et al. 2018).

There are, however, several hurdles to the examination of multiple stool samples for parasite diagnosis. Multiple stool examinations are labor intensive, require a high level of technical expertise, and can be costly (Branda et al. 2006, Khan et al. 2020). To mitigate these hurdles without compromising diagnostic yield, alternative approaches and recommendations have been developed to limit the number of necessary tests. Alternative approaches include applying inferences to ascertain the number of specimens required based on clinical features (e.g., results of the first test and symptoms, length and persistence of diarrhea > 7 d, patient history and pre-existing conditions, and patients' immunological status), considering epidemiological features (e.g., travel history, exposure to unsafe drinking water), and/or taking into account the parasite prevalence in the population where in low-prevalence settings, examination of a single stool specimen is adequate (Morris et al. 1992, Branda et al. 2006, Furuno et al. 2006, Libman et al. 2008, Garcia 2007, Khan et al. 2020). Alternatively, pooling of multiple specimens and performing a single concentration prior to parasite examination are equally sensitive in detecting intestinal protists compared to examining multiple stool specimens individually (Peters et al. 1988, Wahlquist et al. 1991, Aldeen et al. 1993, McLaughlin et al. 1993, Libman et al. 2008, Garcia 2007, Gaafar 2011). The number of specimens needed for parasite detection may also be influenced by the testing method used as most of the above recommendations are based on ova and parasite microscopy examinations. In contrast, given the superior sensitivity of molecular detection methods, only one specimen may be required to achieve sensitivities equal to or greater than that of microscopy (Morgan et al. 1998, ten Hove et al. 2007, Bruijnesteijn van Coppenraet et al. 2009, Laude et al. 2016).

Stool Preservation

Unpreserved Specimens

Although parasite examinations can be carried out on either fresh or preserved stool specimens to ensure a reliable diagnosis, examinations of fresh specimens must be performed within a requisite time frame from the time of passage. Generally, diarrheic (loose or watery) stools should be examined within 30 minutes of passage, within 60 minutes of passage if stools are soft or semi-formed stools, and within 24 hours of passage for formed stools (Garcia 2007).

Fresh stool specimens are recommended, particularly for the detection of motile trophozoite stage of flagellates (*G. duodenalis*), amoebas (*E. histolytica, Dientamoeba fragilis*), and ciliates (*Balantidium coli*). Trophozoites are especially fragile and deteriorate rapidly as they do not multiply or encyst outside the body. Hence, microscopic examination of unpreserved stools within 30 minutes of passage is required for optimal recovery and detection of motile parasite forms (Garcia 2007, Garcia et al. 2018). The trophozoite stage is commonly found in diarrheic specimens and semi-formed stools are more likely to contain a mixture of trophozoites and cysts. For more robust parasitic stages that can survive for an extended time after passage, such as cysts of *Entamoeba* spp., *G. duodenalis* and *B. coli*, oocysts of *C. cayetanensis, Cryptosporidium* spp. and *C. belli*, and Microsporidia spores, examinations can be performed at any time within 24 hours after passage as structures of these stages should still be intact and detectable (Garcia 2007). To maintain parasites that are able to grow and develop in stools and to prevent further degeneration of cysts, unpreserved specimens should be refrigerated as soon as possible and not left at room temperature for more than 3 hours (Smith et al. 1997, Despommier et al. 2011).

Preserved Specimens

The use of preservatives for stool specimens is recommended if a delay is anticipated between the time stool is passed until it is received at the laboratory and examined.

Preservation of stool specimens retains the morphology of the stages of the parasite present in the specimen, preventing tissue degradation and further development of other intestinal protozoa. As fixation itself involves chemical modifications to proteins and nucleic acid structures (Srinivasan et al. 2002, Howat and Wilson 2014), the selection of the appropriate fixative is determined by the method used for the examination and downstream applications of other tests (e.g., antigen or nucleic acid test). A variety of fixatives are available for preserving stool specimens. Those that are commonly used include formalin, sodium acetate-acetic acid-formalin (SAF), Schaudin's solution (mercuric chloride-PVA), and modified PVA-based fixatives (zinc, copper, mercury). A summary of these fixatives can be found in Table 2. In the United States, the "gold standard" for stool specimen collection uses a two-vial system where each stool is preserved in two different preservatives of complementary advantages, with one vial containing 5% or 10% buffered formalin and the second vial containing mercuric chloride-PVA-based fixative (McHardy et al. 2014, Garcia et al. 2018). Both preservatives are excellent fixatives that allow for long-term preservation of parasitic stages in the stools. Formalin preserves the morphology of parasitic ova including protozoan cysts and oocysts and is suitable for concentration procedures and fecal immunoassays, whereas mercuric chloride-PVA provides optimal preservation of trophozoites and cysts and is used for permanent stain smear (Garcia 2007, Garcia et al. 2018).

Despite being the two most widely used preservatives, both formalin and mercuric chloride-PVA contain highly toxic chemicals that are both hazardous to the health of laboratory workers and the environment. Formalin contains formaldehyde which is a known carcinogen. PVA serves as an adhesive of stool material onto the slide, but the fixative component, Schaudinn's solution, contains mercuric chloride, which can form highly toxic vapors when exposed to heat and result in chronic mercury poisoning. Disposal of these chemicals is also tightly regulated and needs to follow strict local, state, and federal biosafety regulations. As many laboratories cannot dispose of materials contaminated with mercury or formalin, a licensed disposal agency must be contracted, thus incurring additional expenses. Because of these factors, the higher cost of two-vial systems compared to single-collection vials and the need to select specific fixatives for specific stains and downstream assays, laboratories are increasingly adopting alternative fixatives and single-vial collection systems (Garcia et al. 1992, 2018, Pietrzak-Johnston et al. 2009, McHardy et al. 2014).

Alternative Stool Preservatives

Sodium Acetate-Acetic Acid-Formalin (SAF)

SAF is a good substitute for mercury-based PVA fixative as it confers a long-shelf life and is suitable for concentration procedures and fecal immunoassays (Yang and Scholten 1977, Mank et al. 1995, Gaafar 2011). For optimal visualization of parasite morphology, SAF-fixed specimens are best stained with iron-hematoxylin stain (Garcia et al. 1993, Garcia 2007) or chlorazol black dye stain (Mank et al. 1995, Van Gool et al. 2003, Gaafar 2011). This, however, may not be an ideal option

Table 2. Summary of common fixatives used for the preservation of ova and parasites in stool specimens.

Preservative	Application	Advantages	Disadvantages
Formalin (5–10%)	• Concentration techniques (formalin-ethyl acetate sedimentation; flotations and centrifugations) • UV fluorescence microscopy • Can be used with acid-fast, safranin, and chromotrope stains • Compatible for use with IFA and other immunoassays	• Easy to prepare • Long shelf life • Good preservation of parasitic ova, larvae, protozoan cyst, oocyst, and spore morphology	• Can interfere with nucleic acid amplification assays after an extended fixation time • Poor preservation of trophozoite morphology • Not suitable for use with most permanent stains
SAF (Sodium Acetate Acetic Acid Formalin	• Permanent stains (works best with iron hematoxylin) • Concentrated wet mount • Suitable for acid-fast, safranin, and chromotrope stains • Compatible for use with IFA and other immunoassays	• Considered a gentler fixative compared to mercuric chloride (Schaudinn's fluid) • Contains no mercury compound • Easy to prepare • Long shelf life	• Requires additives for stool adhesion (e.g., albumin-glycerin) • Not suitable for nucleic acid amplification assays • Suboptimal trophozoite morphology • Permanent staining is suboptimal compared to PVA or Schaudinn's fixative; optimal morphology is achieved if stained with iron hematoxylin
Schaudinn's solution (mercuric chloride + PVA)	• Permanent stained smear and concentrated wet mount (rare) • Compatible for use with nucleic acid assays	• Excellent preservation of trophozoites and cysts • Long shelf life	• Fixative is highly toxic; contains a mercuric compound • *Giardia* cysts are not easily concentrated compared to formalin fixatives • Suboptimal preservation of Microsporidia and coccidia oocysts • Difficult and expensive to dispose of • Not suitable for concentration procedures and fecal immunoassays • Not compatible with acid-fast, safranin, and chromotrope stains

Table 2 contd. ...

...Table 2 contd.

Preservative	Application	Advantages	Disadvantages
Modified PVA (copper, zinc)	• Permanent stains • Suitable for concentration procedures	• Compatible for use in nucleic acid amplification assays • Zinc produces better results compared to copper	• Not suitable for immunoassays • Suboptimal quality of parasite morphology especially with copper • Zinc is better than copper but still not as good as mercuric chloride-PVA
Single-vial proprietary fixative formulations (e.g. EcoFix™, Parasafe, AlcorFix™, ProtoFix®, STF)	• Permanent stains • Concentrated wet mount • Compatible with some immunoassays and most nucleic acid assays	• A safer alternative to the two-vial system; no formalin or mercury	• Suboptimal quality of parasite morphology • Not all are suitable for immunoassays

PVA: Polyvinyl alcohol
IFA: Immunofluorescent antibody assay
Adapted from Garcia (2007), McHardy et al. (2014), and Garcia et al. (2018).

for laboratories that want to maintain the use of trichrome stain, which when used with SAF, has yielded poor quality results (Garcia et al. 1993, Pietrzak-Johnston et al. 2000). SAF also contains formalin and poses the same health and environmental concerns as 5% or 10% formalin fixatives, albeit minus the hazards of PVA as in a two-vial system.

Modified PVA Fixatives

To replace mercury-based PVA fixatives, alternative formulations using zinc and copper-based PVA have been developed and are commercially available (Garcia et al. 1983, 1993). Although these modified PVA fixatives do not convey the same quality of preservation and morphological clarity compared to the "gold standard" mercuric chloride-PVA, studies have shown that the detection sensitivity was only negligibly compromised. In a study where 106 paired specimens were analyzed, Garcia et al. (1993) showed that zinc sulfate was a suitable substitute with an overall agreement of 92.5% (87% if the rare organisms were included) on morphology and number of organisms detected. A comparative study on the performance of zinc sulfate-PVA with mercuric chloride-PVA for the detection and identification of five different parasites (*Blastocystis* sp., *E. histolytica* or *Entamoeba coli*, *Iodamoeba bütschlii*, and *Chilomastix mesnili*), also showed no significant difference in parasite recoveries between the two fixatives and that even though there were inconsistencies in the quality of parasite internal structures, in most cases, the parasites were still detectable (Jensen et al. 2000). For copper sulfate-PVA, however, Garcia et al. (1983) noted that the compound did not provide consistent fixation for adequate protozoan morphology and therefore only recommends the use of copper sulfate-PVA if mercuric chloride-PVA cannot be used and other fixatives are not available.

Commercially Available Stool Preservatives

There are many commercially produced single-vial preservative options to substitute for formalin and mercuric chloride-PVA as stool specimen preservatives for parasite examinations. Examples of some of these single-vial stool preservatives that have been developed and modified from mercuric chloride-PVA include fixatives that contain minimal formalin such as Proto-Fix® (AlphaTec, Vancouver, WA), those that contain PVA but are free of formalin and mercury, such as EcoFix™ (Meridian Bioscience, Inc, Cincinnati, Ohio), Parasafe (Cruinn Diagnostics, Dublin, Ireland) and AlcorFix™ (Apacor, Berkshire, England, UK), and fixatives that are free of PVA, mercury, and formalin such as Total-Fix® (Medical Chemical Corporation, Torrance, CA) and Streck Tissue Fixative™ (STF) (Streck Laboratories, Omaha, NE). Most of these preservatives, like EcoFix™ and STF, are compatible with some immunoassays and most nucleic acid tests (Nace et al. 1999, Fedorko et al. 2000, McHardy et al. 2014).

Although parasite recovery and quality of morphology are superior for specimens fixed in formalin and mercuric chloride-PVA, single-vial preservatives have shown adequate preservation qualities to replace the "gold standard" (Garcia and Shimizu 1998, Fedorko et al. 2000, Pietrzak-Johnston et al. 2000, Couturier et al. 2015). The performance of commercially available preservatives EcoFix™, SAF, Proto-Fix®, STF, and Parasafe was evaluated with 10% formalin and mercuric chloride-PVA at the Centers for Disease Control and Prevention (CDC, Atlanta, GA.) for diagnostic quality with concentrated wet mounts and permanently stained smear preparations. This study found that for concentration procedures and wet mounts, all fixatives, except for Parasafe, produced overall satisfactory preservation of morphologic quality, while for permanent stained smears, only EcoFix™ showed the best overall comparable results to mercuric chloride and formalin, producing quality morphological structures (Pietrzak-Johnston et al. 2000). Fedorko et al. (2000) also reported comparable performance between EcoFix™ preserved specimens and formalin and mercuric chloride-PVA; however, compared to concentrates prepared from formalin-fixed materials, recovery of *Blastocystis* sp. and *Endolimax nana* cyst was significantly lower from EcoFix™ concentrates. The manufacturer of EcoFix™ has also recommended the use of their proprietary stain, EcoStain® (Meridian Diagnostics, Inc.), although it has been shown that the use of conventional trichrome stain on EcoFix™ preserved specimens produces a comparable quality of morphology and stain retention (Garcia and Shimizu 1993).

The more recently available preservatives, Total-Fix® and AlcorFix™, are similar to EcoFix™ and can be used for concentration procedures and permanent stain smears, including special stains for *Cryptosporidium/Cytoisospora/Cyclospora* and Microsporidia as well as downstream immunoassays and nucleic acid tests for protists detection (Couturier et al. 2015, Garcia et al. 2018). AlcorFix™ has been reported to adequately preserve trophozoite, cyst, oocyst, and spore morphology when compared to conventional formalin and PVA preservative, with results from the wet mount and permanent stain preparations showing quality morphology and retention of trichrome and modified acid-fast stains (Couturier et al. 2015). Similarly, limits of detection for stool specimens preserved in Total-Fix® were found to be comparable to 10% formalin in a study that utilized a real-time PCR kit that amplifies *G. duodenalis*, *C. parvum* or *C. hominis*, and *E. histolytica* (DeBurger et al. 2018).

Fecal Examination

Macroscopic Examination

Macroscopic examination starts by observing the characteristics of a stool sample. It is important to record the odor, color, and consistency of the stool (formed, hard, soft, or watery) and whether there is the presence of mucus or blood. Stools should also be examined for the potential presence of adult nematodes or tapeworm proglottids.

Microscopy Examination

The microscopic examination for parasites in stool specimens, commonly referred to as ova and parasite examination (O&P), remains the cornerstone of routine diagnostic testing for intestinal protist parasites (Garcia et al. 2018). O&P examination techniques performed in a diagnostic laboratory include direct wet mount preparations, the concentration of stool specimens, and permanently stained smears. These techniques rely on visualization using bright-field or fluorescent microscopes to detect parasite life-cycle stages in the stool. An overview of parasite features and microscopy techniques used in diagnosis can be found in Table 1.

Life-cycle stages that are usually detected in stool specimens for parasite diagnosis vary by organism. For *E. histolytica/E. dispar*, *G. duodenalis*, and *B. coli*, the presence of either trophozoites and/or cysts are detected for a diagnosis (Fotedar et al. 2007, Garcia 2007, Schuster and Ramirez-Avila 2008). For *Cryptosporidium*, *C. cayetanensis*, and *C. belli*, the oocyst form is the only form detected in stool specimens for diagnosis, whereas for Microsporidia, diagnosis is based on observation of its spores. *Blastocystis* sp., however, is a polymorphic parasite and various morphologies including vacuolar, avacuolar, granular, amoeboid, and cyst forms, can be present in a stool specimen, but only vacuolar and cyst forms are observed in feces as other forms are usually lost during fecal sample processing (Navarro et al. 2008, Tan 2008). Due to the small sizes of oocysts and spores, concentration procedures and the use of specialized permanent stains are recommended to increase detection sensitivity. In contrast, for *B. coli*, which has a large cyst, staining (temporary or permanent) of this parasite is not recommended as its cyst is too large and thick, and examination for this parasite is best carried out using low magnification on the direct wet mount (Schuster and Ramirez-Avila 2008).

Despite being a routine diagnostic tool, microscopic methods are labor intensive and require skilled laboratory personnel to be able to evaluate morphological variations and differentiate parasite forms from common artifacts that may be present in the stool material examined (Ricciardi and Ndao 2015, Momčilović et al. 2019). Common artifacts present in stool material that may be mistaken for protist parasite life-cycle stages include epithelial cells, white blood cells such as eosinophils and macrophages, which are morphologically similar to trophozoites, plant cells, pollen, grains, or fungal spores that have similar appearances to cysts, oocysts, or spores (Garcia 2007, Ricciardi and Ndao 2015). Of note, *B. coli* with its large cyst (40 to 200 μm), can sometimes be mistaken for helminth ova and lead to misdiagnosis (Schuster and Ramirez-Avila 2008). A major limitation of O&P examinations is that the method is not able to distinguish between different species in a genus (e.g., *Cryptosporidium, Cyclospora, Entamoeba*), genotypes, assemblages, or subtypes within a species (e.g., *Blastocystis, Enterocytozoon bieneusi, G. duodenalis*) nor between pathogenic and commensal morphologically similar species (e.g., *E. histolytica* from *E. dispar*) (Pedraza-Díaz et al. 2000, Garcia 2002, Thompson and Monis 2004, Fotedar et al. 2007, Tan 2008, Giangaspero and Gasser 2019).

Direct Wet Mount Preparation

Direct wet mount (or direct microscopy) is a fast and simple approach to obtain a quick diagnosis and approximation of parasite burden. It can be prepared from unconcentrated or concentrated fresh stool specimens by mixing a small amount of stool material with a few drops of 0.85% saline solution. Direct wet mounts are used primarily to detect live motile trophozoites of *E. histolytica, G. duodenalis*, or *B. coli*, which are usually pale and transparent, appearing as a refractile object, and detected by their motility; this method is also used to detect protists cysts and oocysts (Fotedar et al. 2007, Garcia 2007, Schuster and Ramirez-Avila 2008, Singh et al. 2009). With a large cyst size, *B. coli* can readily be recognized on direct wet mounts, even at low magnification (x100). For preserved specimens, the formalin fixative replaces saline and can be used for a direct smear. To aid in the identification of protists cysts and oocysts, iodine solution, such as Lugol's or D'Antoni's iodine, can also be added to the wet mount. The addition of iodine to fresh stool specimens will cause trophozoites to lose their motility although, visualization of protists cysts will be enhanced as it stains glycogen, increases cyst nuclei visibility, and helps distinguish *Cryptosporidium* oocysts (which do not take up iodine stains) from yeast cells which they resemble on the saline wet mount (Garcia 2007).

One of the major limitations of direct wet mounts is that the method lacks sensitivity and does not convey optimal parasite recovery. In a study that examined 2,206 specimens, parasites were only detected in three specimens by direct wet mount compared to 14 positive specimens by the wet mount of concentrated specimens, 19 positives with Wheatley's trichrome staining, and 92 positives with concentration procedures and Wheatley's trichrome staining (Estevez and Levine 1985). Detection of protozoa, particularly *Cyclospora, Cryptosporidium*, and *Cytoisospora*, which have small oocyst sizes, is difficult, easily confused with artifacts, and may be visualized only in heavy infections (Zierdt 1984, Baron et al. 1989, Fotedar et al. 2007, Garcia 2007). Spores of Microsporidia are also not readily visible in a direct smear as they are too small (size range of 0.7 to 1 μm wide and 1.4 to 3 μm long) and morphologically can be mistaken for stool debris (Garcia 2007). Hence, although some protozoa can be definitively identified (cysts of *Giardia, Entamoeba*, and

Balantidium as well as *Cytoisospora* oocysts), results from direct wet mounts are often considered presumptive and subject to confirmation with concentration and permanently stained smear procedures (Garcia 2007). As there is often the need for downstream confirmation procedures, the value of performing direct wet mounts have been questioned (Estevez and Levine 1985, Watson et al. 1988, Neimeister et al. 1990). Therefore, to increase laboratory efficiency, it has been recommended that if stool specimens are in preservatives, concentration procedures and permanent staining of specimens be directly performed, instead of examining by direct wet mount (Garcia 2007, Garcia et al. 2018).

Autofluorescence – UV Fluorescence Microscopy

UV fluorescence microscopy (*syn.* epifluorescence microscopy) is an alternate method of detecting *Cyclospora*, *Cytoisospora,* and *Cryptosporidium* oocysts on wet mounts. This method takes advantage of the autofluorescence properties of *Cyclospora*, *Cytoisospora*, and *Cryptosporidium* oocysts, which fluoresces when exposed to light in the ultraviolet (UV) range (Varea et al. 1998, Bialek et al. 2002a, Harrington 2008, Garcia et al. 2018). At 365 nm (UV light), *Cyclospora* appears blue while under 405 nm (violet light) or 436 nm (blue light), oocysts appear green (Varea et al. 1998). Detection of *Cyclospora* oocysts by UV fluorescence microscopy is a highly sensitive and reliable method; the fluorescence, though limited to the outer cell wall, emits with strong intensity and has been reported to be superior to wet smears and staining procedures for *Cyclospora* oocyst detection (Berlin et al. 1998). This method, with its high sensitivity and simple preparation, is recommended by the CDC for the screening of *Cyclospora* in outbreak situations (Garcia et al. 2018). Epifluorescence detection of *Cytoisospora* oocysts has also been reported to be highly sensitive in comparison to iodine wet mount and permanent stained smear (Berlin et al. 1998, Bialek et al. 2002a, Dubey and Almeria 2019). *Cytoisospora* oocysts, however, have been reported to fluoresce a blue color under UV light (Bialek et al. 2002a, Dubey and Almeria 2019), instead of the green oocyst appearance previously reported at 365 nm by Varea et al. (1998). Despite reports of autofluorescence of *Cryptosporidium* oocysts (Varea et al. 1998, Harrington 2008), autofluorescence was not observed in reported attempts to detect *Cryptosporidium* oocysts using UV fluorescence microscopy (Garcia et al. 2018). This may be due to differences in the composition of *Cryptosporidium* oocyst wall proteins which may produce varying autofluorescence sensitivity (Mai et al. 2009).

Concentration Procedures

Fecal concentration methods have become a part of routine parasitological examinations as they remove fecal debris and increase parasite yield, particularly when the number of parasites in a specimen is too low for visualization by direct microscopy. Concentration procedures are only applicable to cysts, oocysts, and spores but not trophozoites, which can get distorted or destroyed during the process. There are two types of concentration techniques, flotation, and sedimentation.

Flotation concentration procedures use solutions that have higher specific gravity than the parasite stages in the specimen, allowing the cysts, oocysts, and spores to float to the top while fecal debris sinks to the bottom. This results in a cleaner preparation than the sedimentation procedure. Flotation procedures can be performed using fresh or formalinized stool specimens; although PVA-based preserved specimens can also be used, it is not recommended (Garcia 2007). Zinc sulfate or Sheather's sucrose flotation (SSF) procedures are the two most commonly used flotation methods (Garcia et al. 2018). The SSF method is particularly suited for the recovery of oocysts, which are concentrated at the top meniscus after centrifugation (Garcia et al. 1983, Kimura et al. 2004). McNabb et al. (1985) observed that SSF and formalin-ethyl acetate concentration had comparable recovery of *Cryptosporidium*, however, other parasites that were present and recovered by formalin-ethyl acetate concentration (*Giardia*, *Blastocystis*, *Entamoeba*, *Dientamoeba*, and *Endolimax*) were not recovered by SSF method. These flotation methods have also been reported to alter the morphology of the parasite, where collapsed cyst walls or lysis of oocysts have been observed, resulting in inhibition of staining procedures, thus hindering identification (Truant et al. 1981, Garcia 2007, Ahmed and Karanis 2018, Garcia et al. 2018).

Concentration by sedimentation is based on the use of solutions that have a lower specific density than the parasite, allowing the parasite to concentrate in the sediment while fecal debris floats to the top. The most common sedimentation technique used is the formalin-ethyl acetate concentration (FEC) technique, which is an easy method that recovers a broad range of parasites present by centrifugation into a fecal pellet (Ritchie 1948, Young et al. 1979). The addition of ethyl acetate to the fecal suspension of 0.85% saline and 10% formalin prior to concentration enables fat and fecal debris to be separated from the parasites which settle in the sediment at the bottom of the tube. The sediment is then pelleted by centrifugation and the supernatant is discarded. The removal of fat and debris from the stool specimen results in a cleaner preparation that is favorable for use in direct fluorescence antibody (DFA) microscopy (Pacheco et al. 2013, Garcia et al. 2018). However, significant loss of *Cryptosporidium* and *Cytoisospora* oocysts in the fat layer has been observed and hence, to avoid false-negative test results, slide preparations from both fecal pellet and fatty layer are required (Pacheco et al. 2013). To ensure consistency and standardization of concentration procedures, various commercially manufactured concentration kits are available, with studies reporting comparable parasite recovery for diagnostic use (Perry et al. 1990, Becker et al. 2011, Koltas et al. 2014, Cociancic et al. 2018, Khanna et al. 2018, Leméteil et al. 2019, Mewara et al. 2019).

Water-ether sedimentation (WES) method for stool specimens has also been described and recommended for the detection of Microsporidia spores using optical brighteners to counter formalin inhibition and increase detection sensitivity (van Gool et al. 1994, Harrington 2008). With WES, stool specimens are first homogenized in distilled water and filtered through a 300 μm mesh sieve. Ether is then added to the filtrate, mixed, and then centrifuged at 700 g for 2 minutes, after which the supernatant is decanted and the pellet resuspended in distilled water (van Gool et al. 1994).

The loss of parasite cysts and oocysts during stool concentration, with either flotation or sedimentation, is inevitable (Casemore 1991, Weber et al. 1992, Soares et al. 2020). Hence, to increase parasite recovery and diagnostic yield, concentration methods are best performed coupled with permanent staining to improve detection.

Permanent Stain Smear

The use of permanent stains on stool preparations is important for the accurate detection and identification of intestinal parasites and is often used to confirm parasites detected on wet mount preparations (Garcia 2007). Permanent stains provide contrasting colors for the background artifacts and parasites present, staining nuclear and cytoplasmic characteristics, which allow for recognition of detailed organism morphology and better visualization of smaller parasites that are easily missed on wet mount preparations (Garcia et al. 1983, Garcia et al. 2018). Although direct wet mounts are recommended for visualization of trophozoite motility, recovery, and detection of trophozoites were reported to be better when permanent stains are used (Garcia et al. 1979, Gardner et al. 1980). Examination of permanent stained smears is carried out with an oil immersion lens (100x objective; 1,000x magnification), and the prepared slides can be archived for downstream analysis. Permanent stain smears can be performed on stool specimens that are unpreserved or preserved in PVA (mercury or non-mercury based), SAF, or single-vial system fixatives. However, specimens preserved in formalin are not suitable for use for permanent staining procedures, unless concentrated (which dilutes the formalin), as it may result in poor adhesion of stool material onto the slide and poor chromatin staining (Garcia 2007).

There are several staining techniques available; however, Wheatley's trichrome stain (Wheatley 1951) and iron-hematoxylin stain (Tompkins and Miller 1947) are most widely used for routine diagnostic examinations for intestinal protist parasites, as these techniques are simple, less prone to error, and produce uniformly well-stained smears of intestinal protists, human cells, yeast cells, and artifact material in less than 1 hour (Garcia 2007). Both trichrome and iron-hematoxylin stains provide comparable recovery and identification for the detection of cysts and trophozoites of *Giardia* and *Entamoeba* (Shetty and Prabhu 1988). These stains have been shown to provide good recovery and detection of *Giardia*, *B. coli*, *Entamoeba*, *Cytoisospora*, and *Blastocystis* (Garcia et al. 1979, Thornton et al. 1983, Fotedar et al. 2007, Harrington 2008, Schuster and Ramirez-Avila 2008, Tan 2008). For *Cryptosporidium*, *Cyclospora*, and Microsporidia, however, the use of modified trichrome/iron-hematoxylin stains or other specialized stains is required for oocyst and spore detection due to their small sizes; visualization is generally more challenging (Harrington 2008, Dubey and Almeria 2019, Giangaspero and Gasser 2019).

Wheatley's trichrome and modified trichrome stains. The routine Wheatley's trichrome stain is a rapid staining procedure that is simple and does not require overstaining and differentiation, although this may be performed for enhanced morphological visualization. Compared to iron hematoxylin, the color contrast of trichrome stain is more diverse and allows for easier differentiation between organisms and artifacts. The varied color contrast of red, blue, purple, and green is usually seen; cytoplasm of well-stained cysts and trophozoites will appear blue-green with a purple tinge sometimes; nuclear chromatid, red blood cells, Charcot-Leyden crystals, and bacteria stain red while the background, yeast, and other artifacts generally stain green. Routine trichrome stain does not stain Microsporidia spores nor the oocysts of *Cryptosporidium* and *Cyclospora* which appear as unstained holes or "ghosts" in the background (Harrington 2008). Although trichrome stains can be performed on unpreserved and preserved stool specimens, staining with the specimens preserved in newer non-formalin, non-PVA fixatives yield the best results, while other stains are recommended for specimens fixed in SAF for better overall results (Garcia 2007, Garcia et al. 2018). A rapid trichrome staining method, which reduces processing time to less than 10 minutes per slide has also been developed (Flournoy et al. 1982) and may be used as an alternative, although comparative studies with this technique have not been conducted.

Modified trichrome stain (chromotrope 2R). The modified trichrome stain was developed for the detection of Microsporidia as spores do not stain with the routine trichrome stain. Two modifications were made to Wheatley's trichrome method where the chromotrope 2R was increased 10-fold and the staining time within the trichrome solution was extended to 90 min (Weber et al. 1992, Ryan et al. 1993). This provided good staining of microsporidial spores, which stain bright pink with clear zones or a belt-like stripe girding the spores diagonally or equatorially, against a faint green background. However, with the increased concentration of the chromotrope 2R, *Cryptosporidium* oocysts have also been observed to take up the dye and stain pink (Harrington 2008), and hence downstream confirmation of the pink structures using more *Cryptosporidium*-sensitive detection methods (e.g., acid-fast staining, immunoassays) is recommended.

To increase the efficiency of the technique, further modifications to the method of Weber et al. (1992) and Ryan et al. (1993) were made. By increasing the staining temperature to 50°C, Kokoskin et al. (1994) reduced the staining time to 10 minutes and found that not only was parasite recovery compared with the original technique, but the color of the spores appeared more vibrant against a sharper clearer background and morphological structures was less distorted. Didier et al. (1995) found that comparable results can also be achieved by modifying the staining temperature to a convenient temperature of 37°C for 30 minutes.

Iron-hematoxylin stain. The iron-hematoxylin stain is a regressive stain that requires the slides first be overstained and then differentiated. It was the stain used for most of the original morphological descriptions of intestinal protozoa found in humans (Faust et al. 1938, Garcia 2007). Iron-hematoxylin stains are also recommended for use with specimens that have been preserved in SAF as staining with Wheatley's trichrome stain has yielded poor quality results (Garcia et al. 1993, Pietrzak-Johnston et al. 2000). The iron-hematoxylin stain colors the background blue-gray with the organism staining bluish or grayish and nuclear structures as well as chromatoid bodies of cysts and inclusions, such as bacteria and red blood cells, in the cytoplasm of trophozoites stain black. An effective stain for the detection of intestinal protist parasites, the iron-hematoxylin stain, can be used with either fresh, SAF-preserved, PVA-preserved, or specimens preserved in a single-vial system. The method, however, can be time consuming and requires expertise for successful slide overstaining (Tompkins and Miller 1947). This has led to various modifications to the technique (Garcia et al. 2018). These modified methods allow for rapid staining to be performed. The iron-hematoxylin modification of Tompkins and Miller (1947) uses phosphotungstic acid to destain the parasites giving great results even for unskilled hands. This procedure, however, is best prepared with fresh fecal smears than with PVA-fixed stool specimens. The iron-hematoxylin technique has been reported to provide excellent staining, particularly for the detection of cyst and trophozoites stages of smaller intestinal protozoan parasites like *Giardia* and *Entamoeba* (Shetty and Prabhu 1988, Garcia 2007). *Cryptosporidium* and *Cyclospora* oocysts, however, are typically not identifiable on an iron-hematoxylin stain.

Giemsa stain. Routinely used for the detection of blood pathogens (Woods and Walker 1996), the Giemsa stain can also be used for the detection of *Cryptosporidium* (Ahmed and Karanis 2018) and Microsporidia spores (van Gool et al. 1990). *Cryptosporidium* oocyst appears faintly blue with reddish to purple eosinophilic granules appearing as dots, while Microsporidia spores are visible as broad oval structures with pale grayish-blue cytoplasm and deep purple nuclei (van Gool et al. 1990, Ahmed and Karanis 2018). The level of stain uptake can vary even though weak color contrast must be considered positive. In an evaluation of 15 different methods for *Cryptosporidium* detection in stool specimens, Garcia et al. (1983) found that Giemsa stain was the most effective method for the detection of specimens with few organisms present and that this method worked well with specimens preserved in formalin. This technique, however, has been reported as being time-consuming, although oocysts can be well differentiated and can be identified well with low magnification in heavy infections (Horen 1983, Baxby et al. 1984, Mata et al. 1984, Casemore et al. 1985, MacPherson and McQueen 1993). Giemsa staining techniques can also be used to detect *G. duodenalis*, staining flagella and nuclei reddish pink and the cytoplasm blue (Ament 1972, Wolfe 1975, Koehler et al. 2014).

Safranin stain. First developed for the detection of *Cryptosporidium*, safranin stain has since been shown to be compatible with the detection of *Cyclospora* and *Cytoisospora* in stool specimens. Briefly, the method developed by Baxby et al. (1984) for identifying *Cryptosporidium* using safranin stain involved heating of the slide in an acid-alcohol solution followed by staining with heated safranin and counterstaining with methylene blue. Results from the staining method showed better oocysts stain uptake with comparable recovery to smears stained with modified acid-fast stains (Baxby et al. 1984). When stained, the oocysts of *Cryptosporidium* appear as vivid orange-pink bodies whereas the sporozoites within the oocyst stain slightly darker and are sometimes arranged around the borders. Larger intestinal protozoa parasites, like *Giardia* and *Entamoeba*, were observed to take up the methylene blue counterstain, as do yeast, bacteria, and other fecal debris present (Baxby et al. 1984).

Experimenting for the detection of *Cyclospora*, Visvesvara et al. (1997) found that by replacing the heating step with microwave heating of fecal smear immersed in safranin, the safranin staining was superior to modified acid-fast staining and noted that staining was more uniform and that a higher number of oocysts were detected. A study comparing six different stains for the identification of *Cyclospora* oocysts also found that safranin stain was superior as all oocysts were stained uniformly (Negm 1998).

Modified acid-fast stains. Acid-fast staining, also known as Ziehl and Neelsen staining, is a type of differential staining method, used to distinguish between acid-fast and non-acid-fast bacteria. It uses the combination of three reagents: carbol fuschin (primary stain), acid alcohol (decolorizing agent), and methylene blue (counterstain). For parasite detection, modified acid-fast stains are used and have been found to be useful for the identification of *Cryptosporidium*, *Cystoisospora*, and *Cyclospora*, and Microsporidia spores, which may be difficult to detect with routine stains. The primary stain used is carbol fuchsin, which is lipid soluble and hence can penetrate oocyst wall lipids. The modified Ziehl-Neelsen acid-fast and modified Kinyoun's acid-fast methods are the two most commonly used. Unlike the modified Ziehl-Neelsen, the modified Kinyoun's method does not require heating and instead uses higher concentrations of carbol fuchsin and phenol. For these methods, a diluted sulfuric acid (1% to 3%) and no alcohol is used as a decolorizer and counterstained with either methylene blue (which will stain the background blue) or malachite green (which will stain the background green) (Garcia 2007). Bronsdon (1984) made a minor alteration to the technique by adding dimethyl sulfoxide (DMSO) to the phenol basic fuchsin and incorporating acetic acid with malachite green to create a combined decolorizer and counterstain. This method variation was reported to result in more detailed staining of oocyst internal structures compared to conventional modified Ziehl-Neelsen techniques.

With modified acid-fast staining, oocysts of *Cryptosporidium*, *Cystoisospora* and *Cyclospora* stain pink to red to deep purple while intestinal protist parasites that are not acid-fast (e.g., *Giardia*, *Entamoeba*, *Blastocystis*, or *B. coli*), parasites (trophozoites and cysts) stain with the counterstain used and can be recognized in stained smears. Although Microsporidia spores are also acid-fast and may take up the stain, identification is difficult due to their small size, thus the use of specialized stains is recommended (Garcia 2007). Pacheco et al. (2013) have found modified Ziehl-Neelsen stain is suitable for the diagnostic detection of *Cryptosporidium* and *C. belli* in clinical laboratories compared to safranin and auramine fluorescence staining. "Ghost" oocysts, which are oocysts that are poorly stained have been reported and have been associated with empty oocyst walls, continue to be shed during resolving infections or are attributed to variable levels of stain uptake (Bronsdon 1984, Visvesvara et al. 1997, Negm 1998, Harrington 2008, Pacheco et al. 2013). This variability in the staining pattern may result in the misidentification of the parasite and misdiagnosis.

Acid-fast modifications of routine trichrome and iron-hematoxylin stains. Modifications to the routine trichrome and iron-hematoxylin techniques, including an acid-fast stain step have also been developed to enable the simultaneous detection of Microsporidia and *Cryptosporidium*. Ignatius et al. (1997b) developed a combined acid-fast trichrome staining process that utilized Kinyoun's stain (10 minutes) and decolorization with hydrochloric acid (0.5%) and counterstaining with Didier's modified trichrome blue stain. This method yielded the comparable recovery of both parasites to those obtained by modified Kinyoun's and modified trichrome methods and in addition allowed for the detection of *C. cayetanensis* and *C. belli* (Ignatius et al. 1997b). Making minor modifications to this method, Reisner and Spring (2000) evaluated the combined acid-fast trichrome stain using only commercially prepared reagents and reported that Microsporidia could be identified and that results for *Cryptosporidium* were comparable with direct fluorescence assay.

Laboratories that use iron-hematoxylin stains with SAF-fixed materials can employ a combination staining technique that incorporates a carbol fuchsin acid-fast step with iron-hematoxylin staining procedures (Garcia 2007). This combination stain approach, however, is not recommended for specimens preserved in Schaudinn's fixative or any mercury-based PVA.

Fluorescent modified acid-fast stain. Although not as commonly used as the modified Kinyoun's or modified Ziehl-Neelsen stains, the auramine O fluorescent stain can be incorporated with the modified acid-fast staining techniques for the detection of *Cryptosporidium*, *Cytoisospora*, and *Cyclospora* (Garcia 2007). The stain fluoresces using blue light (490 nm) and provides a good contrast with stained oocysts fluorescing bright golden-orange-yellow against a dark background (Harrington 2008). Staining occurs intracellularly in *Cryptosporidium* oocysts and localizes in the sporozoites; whereas for *Cytoisospora*, the oocyst interior or sporocyst is stained (Hanscheid et al. 2008). An advantage of *Cryptosporidium* detection is that the fluorescing oocyst enables ease of reading and increased sensitivity compared to common staining. A study that compared six different microscopy techniques for *Cryptosporidium* detection reported that staining with auramine O fluorescent stain was quick to prepare and produced the highest diagnostic yield (MacPherson and McQueen 1993). Bronsdon (1984) also found that auramine O fluorescent stain conveyed greater sensitivity when compared to carbol fuchsin with the fluorescing oocysts enabling the detection of low numbers of oocysts in the fecal smear. The fluorescence of auramine O staining has been reported to be strong and lasting with *Cytoisospora* and *Cryptosporidium* oocysts but for oocysts of *Cyclospora*, variability in the intensity and lifespan of the fluorescent stain has been observed (Long et al. 1990, Cann et al. 2000, Hanscheid et al. 2008, Harrington 2008).

Optical brighteners. Optical brighteners are fluorescent compounds that bind to chitin in cell walls and fluoresce an intense bluish-white color when excited with ultraviolet or violet light, or fluoresce green with 510 nm, 520 nm, and 530 nm barrier filters in the fluorescent microscope light path, against a dark background (Harrington 2008, van Gool et al. 1993). With chitin present in Microsporidia spore walls, this staining method has been described as rapid and sensitive, enabling quick screening for diagnostic confirmation. The two fluorescent brighteners that have gained the most use in clinical parasitology laboratories are calcofluor white (CFW) and Uvitex 2B (Vávra et al. 1993, van Gool et al. 1994, Didier 2005, Harrington 2008). Both fluorescent brighteners are reported to be equally effective in staining

Microsporidia spores and are simpler and more sensitive than modified trichrome (Didier et al. 1995, Luna et al. 1995, Ignatius et al. 1997a, Harrington 2008, Garcia et al. 2018). For the detection of low numbers of Microsporidia spores, Ignatius et al. (1997a) reported a good correlation between Uvitex 2B and modified trichrome and suggested that both methods be used concurrently when very low numbers of spores are suspected.

Despite their sensitivity, these optical brighteners are not specific and will bind to other artifacts present in a stool specimen and fluoresce. Yeast and bacteria have been reported to fluoresce along with Microsporidia spores, although subtle differences in shape and color can be observed to distinguish them (Didier et al. 1995, Chioralia et al. 1998). Because of this low specificity, fluorescent brighteners are better suited as a quick screening method for Microsporidia to rule out negative samples while positives should be later confirmed using other stains or molecular methods (Valenčáková and Sučik 2020).

Detection of other intestinal protozoa may also be possible as two separate studies using Uvitex 2B for fluorescence of *Cryptosporidium* oocysts have reported fluorescence (van Gool et al. 1994, Ignatius et al. 1997a). Franzen et al. (1996) explored the use of Uvitex 2B for the diagnosis of *C. belli* and reported bright white-blue fluorescence of oocysts from two patients. The sensitivity of Uvitex 2B can be improved if carried out on specimens concentrated using the water-ether sedimentation technique (see "Concentration Procedures") (van Gool et al. 1994).

Immunofluorescence antibody stain. Immunofluorescence assay (IFA) is an immunological method that uses specific fluorescein-labeled monoclonal antibodies directed against parasite cell wall antigens to allow parasite visualization using a fluorescence microscope. The IFA assay includes direct immunofluorescence (DFA), where the fluorescent-labeled antibodies bind directly to the target antigen, and indirect immunofluorescence, which is a two-step assay where the primary unlabeled antibody is first allowed to bind to the target antigen followed by binding of a fluorescently labeled secondary antibody to the primary antibody used. IFA detects intact organisms and provides a definitive diagnosis of infection. A clear advantage of IFA is that fluorescent labeling of the parasite allows for rapid scanning of stained slides reducing the time required to analyze a sample. On the other hand, a curtail to the use of the IFA is the requirement for a microscope with epifluorescence capabilities, which may not be always available in diagnostic laboratories.

Detection of *Cryptosporidium* and *Giardia* using DFA assays is commonly used. Of the DFA assay detection kits that are commercially available, the Merifluor® *Cryptosporidium/Giardia* kit (Meridien Bioscience, Inc., Cincinnati, Ohio) has the highest sensitivity and is often used as a reference method when evaluating immunoassays for *Cryptosporidium* and *Giardia* (Weber et al. 1991, Garcia and Shimizu 1997, Fedorko et al. 2000, Johnston et al. 2003, Branda et al. 2006, Roellig et al. 2017). The assay includes a counterstain; parasites stain a bright green color while the background material in the specimen is counterstained dull orange to red which eases *Cryptosporidium* and *Giardia* detection. Compared to conventional staining methods, DFA assays for both *Cryptosporidium* and *Giardia* are highly sensitive and specific. For *Cryptosporidium*, the sensitivity ranges between

96–100% with a specificity of 98.5–100%, while for *Giardia*, the sensitivity ranges between 93–100% with a specificity of 99.8–100% (Weber et al. 1991, Garcia et al. 1992, Alles et al. 1995, Zimmerman and Needham 1995, Garcia and Shimizu 1997, Fedorko et al. 2000). Although the concentration of stool specimens will prepare a cleaner product and less background fluorescence, a study which used fresh fecal smears and compared DFA with routine stains for detection, found that *Giardia* and *Cryptosporidium* were still easily identifiable but noted that fluorescence of organisms recovered from formalin-ethyl acetate concentrated stool specimens was weaker and less intense (Weber et al. 1991, Alles et al. 1995).

There are also commercially manufactured monoclonal antibodies for indirect IFA detection of *Encephalitozoon intestinalis* and *E. bieneusi* in stool specimens (Bordier Affinity Products SA, Switzerland). These assays were found to be highly sensitive and specific for detecting and identifying these two species of Microsporidia (Ghoshal et al. 2016, Halánová et al. 2019). The ability to distinguish these two species will assist in the use of appropriate therapy for infected patients since *E. intestinalis* albendazole is a first-line therapy while *E. bieneusi* responds better to fumagillin or its analogues (Conteas et al. 2000).

Digital Diagnostic Test

There is a pressing concern about the shortage of skilled microscopists capable of reliably evaluating O&P. This is especially relevant in non-endemic areas in which laboratories come across low numbers of specimens harboring intestinal parasites, making it hard to preserve proficient technologists or train new technologists (McHardy et al. 2014). A novel approach to diagnosing parasites using digital technology was recently developed and could be helpful in addressing these skill-related challenges (Mathison et al. 2020). Techcyte Inc. (Linden, UT) offers the use of artificial intelligence (AI) to power digital diagnostic tests and assist laboratories with a more efficient diagnostic process. Their system uses a microscope scanner to scan and digitize samples on glass slides where the digitalized slides are stored automatically and pre-classified using AI to be reviewed later by laboratory experts. So far, Techcyte offers an O&P Fecal Test that uses deep machine learning analyses on slides prepared using trichrome stain to classify the following parasites: *G. duodenalis* (cysts and trophozoites), *Blastocystis, D. fragilis, E. coli, E. nana, E. histolytica/E. dispar, E. hartmanni, C. mesnili,* and *Iodamoeba butschlii*. This system, however, is currently only available for research purposes as it is not yet approved by the FDA for clinical use.

Fecal Immunoassays

Fecal immunoassays are used to detect parasite-specific antigens, and formats of these assays include direct fluorescent antibody (DFA), enzyme immunoassay (EIA), and immunochromatographic assay (ICA), also known as lateral flow assay (LFA) (dipstick like test). DFA is covered as an immunofluorescence stain in the microscopy section. In this section, EIA and ICA assays are covered. EIA provides a result by the obtained optical densities and can easily be used to screen a large number of samples (Church et al. 2005). ICAs are simple devices intended to detect the presence or absence of parasite antigens, and they have gained popularity as they are quick and easy to utilize.

Antigen detection methods have the advantage in comparison to microscopy of being able to be performed quickly as they do not require concentration prior to testing (in fact antigens will be lost during the concentration procedure), and they do not require experienced and skilled microscopists for an accurate diagnosis. In addition, the intermittent shedding of parasites in feces will have less impact on detecting parasite proteins in feces, thus making antigen detection assays more sensitive than microscopy-based methods (Sadaka et al. 2015, Van den Bossche et al. 2015, Silva et al. 2016). Although immunoassays are more sensitive and specific than microscopy, they are limited to a specific parasite or up to three parasites (*Cryptosporidium* and *Giardia*; *E. histolytica/E. dispar* group; *Cryptosporidium*, *Giardia*, and *Entamoeba*; and *Cryptosporidium*, *Giardia*, and *Entamoeba*).

There are many commercially available EIA kits for the detection of *Giardia*, *Cryptosporidium*, *Entamoeba*, and *Blastocystis* (Table 3). Similarly, there are many commercially available ICAs for the detection of *Giardia*, *Cryptosporidium*, *E. histolytica/E. dispar* group, and *E. hystolytica* (Table 4). Both EIA and ICA kits can detect individual parasites while others offer the possibility of detecting more than one parasite simultaneously including *Giardia* and *Cryptosporidium* or *Cryptosporidium*, *Giardia*, and *Entamoeba*.

Fresh, frozen, or preserved stool samples can be used for antigen detection testing. Some tests such as CoproELISA™ *Entamoeba* (Savyon Diagnostics) require fresh unpreserved fecal specimens (refrigerated up to 48 hours or frozen), while others such as CoproELISA™ *Giardia* (Savyon Diagnostics) accept formalin/SAF-preserved specimens. Thus, it is advised to always check if preserved specimens are accepted and which preservatives are accepted for each specific kit before use.

All kits have high specificities (90–100%) and sensitivities (63 to 100%) (Gonil and Trudel 2003, Garcia et al. 2018). However, commercially available antigen detection tests have differences in the performance described by manufacturers or in the literature. These differences can be attributed to using a different types of samples (fresh or preserved), methodology to process samples (direct or concentration of parasites), or gold standards used for the comparison. Thus, it is hard to compare assays not only among each other but also against other detection methods. A comparison of four ICAs (ImmunoCardSTAT!®CGE, Meridian Bioscience Inc.; *Crypto/Giardia* Duo-Strip, Coris Bioconcepts; RIDA®QUICK *Cryptosporidium/Giardia/Entamoeba* Combi, R-BioPharm; and *Giardia/Cryptosporidium* Quik Chek, Techlab Inc.), ELISAs (*G. lamblia* ProSpecT ELISA Microplate assay; *Cryptosporidium* ProSpecT ELISA Microplate; and *E. histolytica* ProSpecT ELISA Microplate that detects *E. histolytica* and *E. dispar*, Remel), microscopy (direct smears, wet mounts and carbon-fuchsin staining after formalin concentration, and iron-hematoxylin Kinyoun staining of SAF-fixed specimens), and PCR for the detection of *Giardia*, *Cryptosporidium*, and *E. histolytica* in feces found that sensitivities of the evaluated ICAs were excellent for *Cryptosporidium* and *E. histolytica* but variable for *Giardia*

Table 3. Commercially available enzyme immunological assay (EIA) kits to detect enteric protists in human stools.

Parasite Detected	EIA Kit	Manufacturer	Selected References
Blastocystis sp.	*Blastocystis* sp. ELISA Kit	Creative Diagnostics	NA
	CoproELISA™ *Blastocystis* test	Savyon® Diagnostics Ltd.	Dogruman-Al et al. (2015)
Cryptosporidium spp.	CoproELISA™ *Cryptosporidium*	Savyon® Diagnostics Ltd.	Salman et al. (2015), Tejashree et al. (2017)
	CRYPTOSPORIDIUM II™[a]	TechLab Inc.	Fleece et al. (2016)
	Cryptosporidium 2nd generation	Diagnostic Automation	Sadaka et al. (2015)
	Cryptosporidium (Fecal) ELISA Kit	Creative Diagnostics	NA
	Cryptosporidium parvum Antigen ELISA Assay Kit	EagleBio	NA
	IVD Cryptosporidium Stool Antigen Detection Microwell ELISA test	IVD Research, Inc.	NA
	ProSpecT™ *Cryptosporidium* ELISA Microplate[a]	ThermoFisher Scientific	Garcia and Shimizu 1997, Van den Bossche et al. (2015)
	RIDASCREEN® *Cryptosporidium*	R-Biopharm Diagnostic	Weitzel et al. (2006)
Giardia duodenalis	apDia *Giardia lamblia* ELISA	apDia	Sadaka et al. (2015)
	CoproELISA™ *Giardia*	Savyon® Diagnostics Ltd.	NA
	GIARDIA II™[a]	TechLab Inc.	Boone et al. (1999), Silva et al. (2016)
	Giardia lamblia Antigen ELISA Assay Kit	EagleBio	NA
	Giardia lamblia ELISA Kit	Creative Diagnostics	NA
	IVD *Giardia* Stool Antigen Detection Microwell ELISA test[a]	IVD Research, Inc.	NA
	Optimun®T *Cryptosporidium parvum* antigen EIA	Merlin	Bialek et al. (2002)
	ProSpecT™ *Giardia* Microplate assay[a]	ThermoFisher Scientific	Zimmerman and Needham 1995, Garcia and Shimizu 1997, Van den Bossche et al. (2015)
	RIDASCREEN® *Giardia*[a]	R-Biopharm Diagnostic	Weitzel et al. (2006), Goñi et al. (2012), Jahan et al. (2014), Singhal et al. (2015)

Table 3 contd. ...

... Table 3 contd.

Parasite Detected	EIA Kit	Manufacturer	Selected References
Entamoeba spp	CoproELISA™ *Entamoeba*	Savyon® Diagnostics Ltd.	NA
	E. HISTOLYTICA II™ᵃ	TechLab Inc.	Haque et al. (1995), Leo et al. (2006), Buss et al. (2008), Gaafar (2011)
	Entamoeba CELISA PATH	Cellabs	Stark et al. (2008)
	ProSpecT™ *Entamoeba histolytica* Microplate Assayᵃ	ThermoFisher Scientific	Van den Bossche et al. (2015), Verkeke et al. (2015)
	RIDASCREEN® *Entamoeba*	R-Biopharm Diagnostic	Buss et al. (2008)
G. duodenalis/ Cryptosporidium spp.	CoproELISA *Giardia/ Cryptosporidium*	Savyon® Diagnostics Ltd.	NA
	Giardia lamblia/ Cryptosporidium spp. ELISA Kit	Creative Diagnostics	NA
	GIARDIA/ CRYPTOSPORIDIUM CHEK®ᵃ	TechLab Inc.	Youn et al. (2009), Chalmers et al. (2011), Hawash (2014)
	IVD *Giardia/Cryptosporidium* Combo Stool Antigen Detection Microwell ELISA	IVD Research, Inc.	Chalmers et al. (2011)
	ProSpecT™ *Giardia/ Cryptosporidium* Microplate Assayᵃ	ThermoFisher Scientific	Srijan et al. (2005), Chalmers et al. (2011)
G. duodenalis/ Cryptosporidium spp./*Entamoeba* spp.	TRI-COMBO PARASITE SCREENᵃ	TechLab Inc.	Christy et al. (2012), Den Hartog et al. (2013)

NA: To our knowledge, no published reference for this kit is available.
ᵃ FDA-approved.

(Van den Bossche et al. 2015). However, the same study also found that specificity for the tested ICAs was excellent for *Giardia* and *Cryptosporidium* but not able to discriminate *E. histolytica* and *E. dispar*. Another comparison study aimed to compare the detection of *Cryptosporidium* and *Giardia* using ICA ImmunoCard STAT *Cryptosporidium/Giardia* (Meridian Bioscience Inc.) and two EIAs, one for *Giardia* (apDia Giardia lamblia EISA, apDia nv.) and one for *Cryptosporidium* (*Cryptosporidium* second generation EISA, Diagnotic Automation, Inc), and found that ICA detected the highest number of positive samples for both *Giardia* and *Cryptosporidium* while also being easier to use and to interpret and more rapid than EIAs (Sadaka et al. 2015). A study comparing EIA *CRYPTOSPORIDIUM* II™ (TechLab Inc.) and ICA QUIK CHEK™ (TechLab Inc.) to detect *Cryptosporidium*

Table 4. Commercially available immunochromatographic assays (ICA) to detect enteric protists in human stools.

Parasite	ICA Kit	Manufacturer	Selected Reference(s)
Cryptosporidium spp.	CerTest Crypto one step card test	CerTest Biotec	Manouana et al. (2020)
	CoproStrip™ *Cryptosporidium*	Savyon® Diagnostics Ltd.	NA
	Cryptosporidium Antigen Rapid Test Cassette	Screen Italia	NA
	Cryptosporidium Antigen Rapid Test Cassette	RealyTech	NA
	Cryptosporidium Ag Rapid Test	Creative Diagnostics	NA
	Cryptosporidium Rapid Test	Creative Diagnostics	NA
	Cryptosporidium-Strip®	Coris BioConcept	Weitzel et al. (2006), Agnamey et al. (2011)
	IVD *Cryptosporidium* Stool Antigen Detection Lateral Flow Test[a]	IVD Research, Inc.	NA
	RIDA QUICK *Cryptosporidium*	R-Biopharm Diagnostic	Weitzel et al. (2006), Agnamey et al. (2011), Chalmers et al. (2011), Goñi et al. 2012, Hawash et al. (2014b)
	Uni-Gold™ *Cryptosporidium*[a]	Trinity Biotech	NA
	Xpect™ *Cryptosporidium* Test[a]	ThermoFisher Scientific	Agnamey et al. (2011)
Entamoeba spp.	*E. histolytica* QUIK CHEK™[a]	TechLab Inc.	Verkerke et al. (2015)
	Entamoeba one-step card test	CerTest Biotec	NA
	Entamoeba Ag Rapid Test	Creative Diagnostics	NA
	Entamoeba Rapid Test Cassette	RealyTech	NA
	RIDA®QUICK *Entamoeba*	R-Biopharm Diagnostic	Goñi et al. (2012)
Giardia duodenalis	CerTest *Giardia*+ One Step Card Test	CerTest Biotec	NA
	CoproStrip™ Giardia	Savyon® Diagnostics Ltd.	NA
	Giardia lamblia Rapid Test Cassette	Screen Italia	NA
	Giardia lamblia Rapid Test Cassette	RealyTech	NA

Table 4 contd. ...

...Table 4 contd.

Parasite	ICA Kit	Manufacturer	Selected Reference(s)
	Giardia intestinalis One Step Assay	Novamen	NA
	Giardia-Strip®	Coris BioConcept	Oster et al. (2006), Weitzel et al. (2006), Nguyen et al. (2012)
	IVD *Giardia* Stool Antigen Detection Lateral Flow test[a]	IVD Research, Inc.	NA
	RIDA® QUICK *Giardia*	R-Biopharm Diagnostic	Weitzel et al. (2006), Goñi et al. (2012), Hawash et al. (2014b)
	Uni-Gold™ *Giardia*[a]	Trinity Biotech	NA
	Xpect™ *Giardia* Test[a]	ThermoFisher Scientific	NA
G. duodenalis/ Cryptosporidium spp.	CerTest Crypto + *Giardia* One Step Combo Card Test	CerTest Biotec	Gutiérrez-Cisneros et al. (2011)
	CoproStrip™ *Giardia/ Cryptosporidium*	Savyon® Diagnostics Ltd.	NA
	Crypto-*Giardia intestinalis* One Step Assay	Novamed	NA
	Crypto + *Giardia* dipstick	CLONIT	NA
	Crypto/Giardia Duo-Strip	Coris BioConcept	Van den Bossche et al. (2015), Bitilinyu-Bangoh et al. (2019)
	ImmunoCard STAT!® *Crypto/ Giardia* test	Meridian Bioscience, Inc.	Garcia et al. (2003), Agnamey et al. (2011), Minak et al. (2012), Sadaka et al. (2015)
	GIARDIA/ CRYPTOSPORIDIUM QUIK CHEK®[a]	TechLab Inc.	Minak et al. (2012), Alexander et al. (2013), Van den Bossche et al. (2015), Bitilinyu-Bangoh et al. (2019)
	RIDA® QUICK *Cryptosporidium/Giardia* Combi	R-Biopharm Diagnostic	Weitzel et al. (2006), Goñi et al. (2012), Bitilinyu-Bangoh et al. (2019)
	Sure-Vue Signature Crypto/ GI Test Kit	Fisher Healthcare	NA
	Stick Crypto-Giardia	Operon	Gutierrez-Cisero et al. (2011), Abd El Kader et al. (2012)
	Xpect™ *Giardia/ Cryptosporidium* Test[a]	ThermoFisher Scientific	Minak et al. (2012)

Table 4 contd. ...

...Table 4 contd.

Parasite	ICA Kit	Manufacturer	Selected Reference(s)
G. duodenalis/ Cryptosporidium spp./*Entamoeba* spp.	CerTest Crypto + *Giardia* + *Entamoeba* One Step Combo Card Test	CerTest Biotec	NA
	Crypto/Giardia/Entamoeba Ag Rapid Test (strip)	DRG International, Inc	NA
	ImmunoCard STAT!® CGE	Meridian Bioscience, Inc.	Formenti et al. (2015), Van den Bossche et al. (2015)
	RIDA® QUICK *Cryptosporidium/Giardia/ Entamoeba* Combi Test	R-Biopharm Diagnostic	Goñi et al. (2012), Van den Bossche et al. (2015)
	Triage Micro Parasite Panel[a]	Biosite	Pillai and Kain (1999), Garcia et al. (2000), Gaafar (2011), Swierczewski et al. (2012)

NA: To our knowledge, no published reference for this kit is available.

[a] FDA-approved.

in diarrheal stool samples collected from a cohort of children in Bangladesh found comparable sensitivity and specificity with the advantage of lateral flow being rapid, reliable, and very easy to use in the field (Fleece et al. 2016).

Overall, immunoassay tests are a useful tool for rapid screening and great alternatives for laboratories with little expertise in microscopy or not being able to implement molecular diagnostic methods. The capability of testing simultaneously for multiple parasites can reduce turnaround time decreasing the time patients wait to receive results, allowing for quick use of a more specific treatment, if available. From a public health perspective, immunoassays may assist with potential outbreak situations by providing prompt reporting of a notifiable disease. However, as with microscopy, antigen detection of protists does not allow for the identification of species, genotypes, or subtypes responsible for the infection.

Stool Culture

In a clinical diagnostic laboratory setting, cultivation plays a minor role in parasite detection as this method is limited in sensitivity and specificity (Clark and Diamond 2002). Many organisms still cannot be cultured while others require special sample handling after sample collection to maintain viability. These requirements include the use of specific media or laboratory procedures that cannot always be performed in all collection settings such as small or resource-limited laboratories. In addition, culture can be time consuming as most organisms require several days to grow to a level that will allow detection (Roberts et al. 2011, Saidin et al. 2019). Therefore, cultures are mostly used as research tools rather than as diagnostic tools.

Parasites can be cultured in xenic and axenic cultures. In an axenic culture, the parasite grows as a pure culture without any other organisms present, while in xenic culture, parasites grow in conjunction with unknown microbiota. When the parasite grows in a xenic culture in the presence of a single additional species, it is called a monoxenic culture. A major problem that arises during cultivation is the overgrowth of other organisms, thus to successfully culture intestinal parasitic protists controlling/eliminating bacterial and fungal growth is crucial.

To establish a protist in culture, an inoculum is placed in the appropriate medium for the growth of the organism that is suspected to be the source of the infection. After 48 hours, the sediment of the culture is microscopically examined. If no parasite is observed, sediment will be transferred to a new vial and a fresh medium will be added. After incubating for another 48 hours, if the sample is negative, the same replenishment procedure will be performed a final time. If after an additional 48 hours of incubation, the culture is still negative, that sample will be considered negative (Clark and Diamond 2002). However, a negative culture cannot definitively determine the absence of a parasite in the sample due to sensitivity and specificity issues of culture methods (Garcia et al. 2018).

To isolate *Entamoeba*, the most frequently used media are modified Boeckand Drbohlav's egg slant medium, Robinson's medium, and Diamond's TYSGM-9 (Diamond 1982; Robinson 1968). Further axenization of *Entamoeba* is possible using TYI-S-33, but it is a tedious process (Clark and Diamond 2002). For primary isolation from feces, higher success was reported using diphasic media than with Diamond's TYSGM-9 (Clark and Diamond 2002). The culture of *Entamoeba* serves only as a complementary method of diagnosis and should not replace diagnosis by microscopy, PCR, or fecal antigen immunoassay. Axenic culture of *Entamoeba* using TYI-S-33 is commonly used. *Entamoeba* stool culture coupled with isoenzyme analysis used to be the gold standard approach to distinguish *E. histolytica* and *E. dispar* (Clark and Diamond 2002). This method has several difficulties, which have led to it not being commonly used as a diagnostic tool; it is laborious and expensive, culturing is not always successful (success rate 50–70%), and growing trophozoites can be tedious, taking 4–10 days to produce the necessary numbers to perform the analysis (Clark and Diamond 2002, Haque and Petri 2006, Carrero et al. 2020). Hence, this technique is mostly used for research (Saidin et al. 2019).

For *G. duodenalis*, modified TYI-S-33 is currently the medium used almost exclusively for its axenic cultivation (Clark and Diamond 2002). Xenic media is used for *D. fragilis*, *B. coli*, and *Blastocystis* culture (Clark and Diamond 2002). *Blastocystis* can be easily established in culture by inoculation of fecal samples in xenic media such as Jones or Robinson's media. In fact, short-term xenic *in vitro* culture was considered the gold standard method for its detection. However, molecular tools are currently used instead as a culture still requires 2–3 days for diagnosis and could allow preferential growth of one subtype over another if more than one subtype is present in the stool.

For Microsporidia, *E. intestinalis* has been established in culture using different cell lines. However, only short-term culture is possible for *E. bieneusi*, which is the most frequently identified microsporidian in AIDS patients with diarrhea, as all efforts for continuous *in vitro* culture have not been successful (Visvesvara 2002, Garcia et al. 2018).

Although culture is not practical for diagnosis, it is an important tool for research. It allows the production of large numbers of parasites, that in the case of axenic cultures, are free of other organisms. Cultures are used to achieve cell numbers suitable for producing whole genomes as well as for *in vitro* or *in vivo* studies of biochemistry, immune response, vaccination, or therapeutic drug efficacy screens.

Molecular Detection Methods

Molecular techniques are progressively replacing conventional microscopy to diagnose intestinal protists as the first-line diagnostic method in laboratories particularly in industrialized countries (Van Lieshout and Roestenberg 2015). The development of molecular methods, predominantly those based on the polymerase chain reaction (PCR), has provided new tools for improved detection of low levels of parasites while also allowing molecular typing. Correct identification of parasites at the species level is essential especially when morphologically identical species have different clinical importance. This is the case, for example, for intestinal amebiasis caused by *E. histolytica* for which a correct diagnosis at the species level is critical to avoid unnecessary treatment to patients harboring commensal *Entamoeba* species and to control the spread of the parasite (Carrero et al. 2020). Microscopic examination is unable to distinguish cysts of pathogenic *E. histolytica* from morphologically identical but nonpathogenic *Entamoeba* species, while PCR amplification and analysis of genetic variants can be used to discriminate *Entamoeba* species (e.g., Nuñez et al. 2001, Roy et al. 2005, Hamzah et al. 2006). Overall, molecular methods offer several advantages over microscopy such as increased sensitivity and specificity, the option for molecular typing, and optimized turnaround time when PCR is coupled to automated DNA extraction (Verweij and Stensvold 2014).

DNA Extraction and Purification

Molecular assays are greatly impacted by the quality and quantity of DNA, therefore an efficient DNA extraction method needs to be carefully selected. It is essential to utilize DNA extraction procedures that maximize the rupture of parasite forms, which possess robust cell walls, to release DNA. Extraction methods should also eliminate potential inhibitors present in fecal samples (e.g., urea, bilirubin, or bile salts) that when co-extracted with parasite DNA, can interfere with obtaining the high-quality DNA that is required for consistent and reproducible results in molecular assays (Paulos et a. 2016). To increase parasite DNA yield and limit contaminant DNA from other material present in feces, pre-extraction procedures to concentrate parasite forms (e.g., salt flotation or formol-ether concentration techniques) are used, but concentration processes could also result in some loss of parasite forms. Additionally, procedures such as heating, boiling, or freeze-thawing are also frequently incorporated in pre-DNA extraction to break the strong parasite walls (Adamska et al. 2010).

In-house methods (e.g., phenol-chloroform or guanidinium thiocyanate-silica) and commercial kits for DNA extraction are available based on chemical, enzymatic, and/or mechanical lysis (e.g., Subrungruang et al. 2004, Adamska et al. 2010, Elwin et al. 2014, Paulos et al. 2016). Although most commercial kits were originally developed for DNA extraction from pathogens other than enteric protists, many have been found suitable for protist DNA extraction (e.g., Hawash 2014a, Paulos et al. 2016). A comparative study of five commonly used commercially available kits, QIAamp DNA stool mini (QIAGEN), SpeedTools DNA extraction (Biotools), DNAExtract-VK (Vacunek), PowerFecal DNA isolation (MoBio), and Wizard magnetic DNA purification system (Promega Corporation) to assess their efficacy in obtaining DNA of relevant enteric protists (*Cryptosporidium*, *Giardia*, *E. histolytica*, and *E. dispar*) found that all yielded amplifiable amounts of DNA of the pathogens tested (Paulos et al. 2016). Another study compared 12 protocols for DNA extraction of *Giardia* cysts that included additional steps taken before extraction in order to destroy the cysts' walls (Adamska et al. 2010). The best protocol was found to include pre-treating, freezing in liquid nitrogen, and incubation in the water bath at 100°C three times, and then performing the extraction using QIAamp DNA Tissue Mini Kit (QIAGEN) with overnight incubation with proteinase K at 56°C. Thus, some experimentation may be required to determine the ideal conditions for the extraction of a particular parasite with a particular DNA extraction kit.

DNA extraction may be carried out manually or automatically using DNA extraction systems such as QIAsimphony (QIAGEN), EasyMag (BioMerieux), Liaison IXT/Arrow (DiaSorin) MagNA Pure 96 (Roche), or Bullet Pro (DiaSorin). Manual processing of large batches of specimens is labor intensive and automatic extraction systems offer the advantage of processing up to 96 specimens at a time, reducing hands-on time and costs. Additionally, automatic extraction systems can facilitate the increased throughput, reproducibility, standardization, and quality control needed in clinical diagnostic laboratories.

PCR-Based Detection

PCR is a fast and inexpensive technique used to amplify fragments of DNA leading to millions of exact copies of the original DNA fragment. In the PCR process, DNA is first heated to separate it into two single strands (denaturation), followed by a decrease in temperature to enable primers to attach to the template DNA (annealing), and finally a rise in temperature in which the enzyme *Taq polymerase* synthesizes two new strands of DNA using the original strands as templates (extension). The process is repeated as many as 30 to 40 times with a doubling of the number of target DNA copies in each round of the reaction. Identification of the target is based on the expected size of the PCR product. In conventional PCR, the amplification product is then subjected to agarose gel electrophoresis and visualized using ethidium bromide (which incorporates into the DNA and fluoresces with UV light) or other safer alternative dyes (SYBR Green or Gel Red). Detection of PCR products can also be achieved using capillary electrophoresis systems such as the QIAxcel (QIAGEN), a fully automated system designed to overcome the bottlenecks of gel electrophoresis that can process up to 96 samples per run.

PCR can be impacted by the presence of inhibitors co-extracted with DNA that can reduce or prevent PCR amplification, impact the sensitivity of the assay, or even produce false-negative results. Different strategies are used to overcome inhibition. One effective option is the dilution of the template, but this strategy has the drawback of lowering the sensitivity of the PCR as the concentration of target DNA is decreased. Another option is the addition of bovine serum albumin to the PCR reaction, which is an effective and inexpensive method used to address potential PCR inhibition (Kreader 1996, Abu Al-Soud and Rådström 2000).

There are multiple PCR-based molecular methods including PCR, nested PCR, multiplex PCR, or real-time PCR with many primers sets available targeting numerous genes for the detection of gastrointestinal protists (e.g., Buckholt et al. 2002, Xiao 2010, Santín et al. 2011, Feng and Xiao 2011, Cacciò 2018). The most commonly used genes for detection are the small subunit (*SSU*) and the internal transcriber spacer (ITS) of the rRNA (Dacal et al. 2020). These genes are also used as genotyping tools, for example, the *SSU* rRNA gene and ITS are the most commonly used DNA sequences for the differentiation of *Cryptosporidium* species/ genotypes and *E. bieneusi* genotypes, respectively (Xiao et al. 1999, Santín and Fayer 2009, Xiao 2010).

Nested PCR was designed to improve the sensitivity and specificity of conventional PCR and involves two reactions as the product of the first reaction is used as a template for the second reaction. In the semi-nested (or hemi-nested), a variation of nested PCR, one of the primers from the first PCR amplification reaction is used also in a second PCR amplification reaction. Nested PCR protocols are often used to detect intestinal protists as they provide increased sensitivity for parasite DNA, which often represents only a small percentage of the total DNA present in a fecal sample (e.g., Xiao et al. 1999, Buckholt et al. 2002, Sulaiman et al. 2003, Read et al. 2004, Lalle et al. 2005). However, nested PCR procedures suffer from longer turnaround times, as they require two rounds of amplification; they are difficult to automate; more importantly, they are susceptible to amplicon contamination due to first PCR reaction product contamination of the second reaction PCR reagents, so great care must be exercised when performing it. For these reasons, they are not considered suitable for routine diagnostics in clinical laboratories and are mainly used for research purposes (Verweij and Stensvold 2014).

Multiplex PCR allows for the identification of multiple parasites in a single reaction by including multiple sets of primers that target different DNA fragments for each parasite in the assay. Primers are designed to produce amplicons with different sizes allowing for the identification of more than one parasite in a single analysis (Santín and Zarlenga 2009). However, optimization is difficult and preferential amplification of smaller products is a common issue. As such, multiplex PCRs are not commonly used for routine diagnosis in clinical laboratories.

Both direct PCR and nested PCR followed by direct sequencing using first-generation sequencing based on the Sanger chain termination method is currently the main technique used for genotyping of gastrointestinal protists. In fact, it is the most widely used method in epidemiological studies for molecular characterization of specimens to determine species, genotypes, or subtypes (Xiao 2010, Feng and Xiao 2011, Stensvold 2013, Stensvold et al. 2018, Li et al. 2019). Additionally, PCR or nested PCR can be combined with restriction fragment length polymorphism (RFLP) analysis to discriminate species or genotypes by comparing polymorphisms in targeted nucleotide sequences to distinguish genetic variants (Xiao et al. 1999, Johnson and Clark 2000, Cacciò et al. 2002, Khairnar et al. 2007).

Real-time PCR

Real-time PCR assays have become very popular in clinical settings as they allow for rapid and sensitive detection of protists in a sample. In real-time PCR, the amplification of a targeted DNA molecule is monitored in real time during the PCR and not at the end as in conventional PCR. The monitoring of DNA amplification in real time has the clear advantage of expediting results. Real-time PCR can also be used to quantify pathogens in a sample. In a real-time quantitative PCR (qPCR) assay, DNA amplification is detected by the accumulation of fluorescent signal, where the cycle threshold (Ct) is the number of cycles required for the fluorescent signal to cross the threshold (background level). Thus, the Ct value is inversely proportional to the amount of starting DNA templates in a sample; the higher the Ct value the smaller the number of DNA templates in the sample. By creating a standard curve using pre-quantified amounts of control DNA, the number of DNA templates in a sample can be estimated. It is the norm in qPCR assays to use the averaged Ct values from replicates of a sample to accurately calculate the amount of template DNA present. Numerous real-time PCR methods have been described for the detection of gastrointestinal protists including non-specific staining of double-stranded DNA using intercalating dyes and highly specific fluorescence-labeled DNA probes (Verweij et al. 2003, Stensvold et al. 2012, Hijjawi et al. 2018).

Multiplex real-time PCR assays have been developed for the simultaneous detection of various parasites representing a cost-effective option for clinical laboratories (Bruijnesteijn van Coppenraet et al. 2009, Stark et al. 2011, Friesen et al. 2018, Parčina et al. 2018). In addition, this format can be used to perform comprehensive gastrointestinal disease-causing pathogen panels, which can detect not only parasites but also bacteria and viruses in one assay, making them extremely cost-effective (Verweij and Stensvold 2014). There are many commercially available multiplex molecular assays that detect gastrointestinal protists (Table 5). Some of the assays can also be used for quantification such as the recently launched syndromic testing system QIAstat-Dx that by providing Ct values, instead of just endpoint detection of PCR products, can provide quantitation of the detected pathogens (Hannet et al. 2019, Boers et al. 2020).

There are four FDA-cleared multiplexed assays available for use in clinical laboratories including BioFire® FilmArray Gastrointestinal Panel, xTAG® Gastrointestinal Pathogen Panel, BD MAX™ Enteric Parasite Panels, and BioCode®

Table 5. Commercially available multiplex molecular assays for the detection of gastrointestinal protists.

Multiplex Assay Kit	Manufacturer	Parasites Detected	Incorporates Automatic DNA Extraction	Includes Detection of Bacteria and Viruses	Selected References
Allplex™ GI-Parasite Assay	Seegene	*Blastocystis* sp. *Cryptosporidium* spp. *C. cayetanensis* *D. fragilis* *E. histolytica* *G. duodenalis*	Yes	No	Paulos et al. (2019), Yoo et al. (2019), Autier et al. (2020)
BD MAX™ Enteric Parasite Panel[a]	BD	*C. parvum/C. hominis* *E. histolytica* *G. duodenalis*	Yes	No	Batra et al. (2016), Madison-Antenucci et al. (2016), Mölling et al. (2016), Perry et al. (2017), Autier et al. (2018), Formenti et al. (2018), Parčina et al. (2018), Yoo et al. (2019), Akgun and Celik (2020)
BioCode® Gastrointestinal Pathogen Panel[a]	Applied BioCode	*C. parvum/C. hominis* *E. histolytica* *G. duodenalis*	Yes	No	NA
Biofire® FilmArray Gastrointestinal[a]	BioFire	*Cryptosporidium* spp. *C. cayetanensis* *E. histolytica* *G. duodenalis*	Yes	Yes	Khare et al. (2014), Spina et al. (2015), Beal et al. (2017), Connor et al. (2018), Cybulski et al. (2018), Buss et al. (2019), Hannet et al. (2019), Zhang et al. (2015), Bateman et al. (2020), Gingras and Maggiore (2020), Machiels et al. (2020), Zhan et al. (2020)
EasyScreen™ Enteric Protozoan	Genetic Signatures	*Blastocystis* sp. *Cryptosporidium* spp. *D. fragilis* *E. histolytica* *G. duodenalis*	Optional	No	Stark et al. (2014), Cao et al. (2019), Dirani et al. (2019), Gough et al. (2019)

Enteric Bacteria and Parasites Panel T-Plex	Aus Diagnostics	Blastocystis sp. Cyclospora spp. Cryptosporidium spp. D. fragilis E. histolytica G. duodenalis	Yes	Yes	NA
EntericBio Gastro® Panel 2	Serosep	C. parvum/C. hominis G. duodenalis	Yes	Yes	McAuliffe et al. (2017)
FTD® Stool Parasites	Fast-Track Diagnostics	Cryptosporidium spp. E. histolytica G. duodenalis	No	No	Paulos et al. (2019)
G-DiaPara™	Diagenode	C. parvum/C. hominis E. histolytica G. duodenalis	No	No	Autier et al. (2018), Paulos et al. (2019)
Gastro Finder™ Smart17 Fast	PathoFinder	Cryptosporidium spp. D. fragilis E. histolytica G. duodenalis	No	Yes	NA
GI-MAP®	Diagnostic Solutions Laboratory	Blastocystis sp. Chilomastix mesnelli Cryptosporidium spp. C. cayetanensis D. fragilis Endolimax nana E. coli E. histolytica G. duodenalis Pentatrichomonas hominis G. duodenalis Pentatrichomonas hominis	Yes	Yes	Gingras and Maggiore (2020)

Table 5 contd. ...

...Table 5 contd.

Multiplex Assay Kit	Manufacturer	Parasites Detected	Incorporates Automatic DNA Extraction	Includes Detection of Bacteria and Viruses	Selected References
LIGHTMIX® Gastro Parasites	Roche	*Blastocystis* sp. *Cryptosporidium* spp. *D. fragilis E. histolytica G. duodenalis*	Yes	No	Friesen et al. (2018)
NanoCHIP® GIP Combi I and II	Savyon Diagnostics	*Blastocystis* sp.[b] *Cryptosporidium* spp. *D. fragilis*[b] *E. histolytica G. duodenalis*	No	Yes	Perry et al. (2014)
QIAstat-Dx® Gastrointestinal Panel	QIAGEN	*Cryptosporidium* spp. *C. cayetanensis E. histolytica G. duodenalis*	Yes	Yes	Hamnet et al. (2019), Boers et al. (2020)
RIDA® GENE Parasitic Stool Panel I and II	R-Biopharm	*Cryptosporidium* spp. *D. fragilis*[c] *E. histolytica G. duodenalis*	No	No	Autier et al. (2018), Paulos et al. (2019)
xTAG® Gastrointestinal Pathogen Panel[a]	Luminex	*C. parvum/C. hominis E. histolytica G. duodenalis*	Yes	Yes	Navidad et al. (2013), Claas et al. (2013), Khare et al. (2014), Wessels et al. (2014), Perry et al. (2014), Zhang et al. (2015), Albert et al. (2016), Hawash et al. (2017), Yoo et al. (2019), Wang et al. (2020), Zhan et al. (2020)

NA: To our knowledge, no published reference for this kit is available.

[a] FDA-approved.

[b] not included in Panel I.

[c] not included in Panel II.

Gastrointestinal Pathogen Panel. Multiplex commercial assays differ in the number of pathogens the assay detects, the throughput of the assay, the overall time to results, regulatory status, and the complexity of the assay (Table 5; Ryan et al. 2017, Dacal et al. 2020). Of the commercial multiplex assays some are considered comprehensive syndromic (virus, bacteria, and parasite) while others only detect members of a specific class of pathogens (Table 5). One of the most popular syndromic assays is the first FDA-approved multiplex assay, xTAG® Gastrointestinal Pathogen Panel, which simultaneously detects multiple viruses (adenovirus 40/41, norovirus GI/GII, and rotavirus A), parasites (*C. parvum, C. hominis, E. histolytica*, and *G. duodenalis*), and bacteria (*Campylobacter jejuni, Campylobacter coli, Campilobacter lari, Clostridium difficile, Escherichia coli* O157, enterotoxigenic *E. coli, Salmonella,* Shiga-like toxin-producing *E. coli, Shigella boydii, Shigella sonnei, Shigella flexneri, Shigella dysenteriae*, and *Vibrio cholerae*) in human stool specimens (fresh and frozen or in transport media) from individuals with signs and symptoms of infectious colitis or gastroenteritis (Navidad et al. 2013, Khare et al. 2014, Perry et al. 2014, Zhang et al. 2015, Albert et al. 2016, Hawash et al. 2017, Yoo et al. 2019, Wang et al. 2020).

The xTAG® Gastrointestinal Pathogen Panel was evaluated and compared to conventional and molecular methods available at the Milwaukee Health Department Laboratory for routine clinical diagnostics. The evaluation concluded that this pathogen panel was a great tool for public health laboratories as the assay offers high sensitivity and specificity for screening and identification of the major pathogens responsible for the acute diarrheal disease (Navidad et al. 2013). Using the xTAG® Gastrointestinal Pathogen Panel, laboratories can obtain results for 15 pathogens in a quick, streamlined workflow that eliminates the complexity of managing multiple samples and testing methods. Another commonly used syndromic FDA-approved panel, BioFire® FilmArray® Gastrointestinal Panel, can test for 22 of the most common pathogens associated with gastroenteritis including four parasites (*Cryptosporidium, C. cayetanensis, E. histolytica, G. duodenalis*) (Khare et al. 2014, Cybulski et al. 2018, Hannet et al. 2019, Bateman et al. 2020, Gingras and Maggiore 2020). Using BioFire® FilmArray® Gastrointestinal Panel, increased detection of *E. histolytica* and *G. duodenalis* compared to the microscopic examination of the same specimen and detection of viral or parasitic pathogens in specimens for which specific diagnostic tests for them were not ordered was observed, reducing the need for further testing to achieve diagnoses (Cybulski et al. 2018). Rapid identification of a broad range of pathogens, which may not have otherwise been detected, improves patient care by providing appropriate treatment leading to a reduction in hospital length and by reducing unnecessary use of antibiotics for viral and parasitic infections (Beal et al. 2017).

Evaluation of the non-syndromic FDA-approved BD MAX™ Enteric Parasite Panel demonstrated that it is significantly faster than microscopy and allows laboratory workflows to be streamlined with high sensitivity and specificity for the diagnosis of the three predominant protozoan parasites causing enteritis, *C. parvum/ C. hominis, E. histolytica*, and *G. duodenalis* (Batra et al. 2016, Madison-Antenucci et al. 2016, Perry et al. 2017, Parčina et al. 2018). However, careful interpretation when comparing performance characteristics (sensitivity and specificity) of panels conducted at different laboratories is needed as often methods used for comparison have different performance characteristics. For example, comparing panels with microscopy to establish performance will likely produce different results than the use of culture or conventional PCR (Zhang et al. 2015, Yoo et al. 2019). Overall, these evaluations have shown that molecular techniques, especially those in multiplex formats, have significantly improved workflow and diagnostic output for diagnosing gastrointestinal infections (Laude et al. 2016). It is important to note that comprehensive gastrointestinal pathogen panels have the potential to lead to increased recognition of the role of protist parasites in causing infections and disease in humans. An example of this recognition comes from a recent *Cyclospora* outbreak where results from the BioFire® FilmArray® Gastrointestinal Panel, which includes *C. cayetanensis* detection, substantially contributed to the recognition of a *Cyclospora* outbreak in Wisconsin in 2018 as most positive specimens early in the outbreak were FilmArray-positive specimens (Bateman et al. 2020). This early recognition of an outbreak is vital to assist public health authorities with a prompt intervention that could slow down the spread of the pathogen reducing the number of people impacted by the outbreak.

Loop-Mediated Isothermal Amplification (LAMP)

Although the use of LAMP in the detection of intestinal parasites is mainly used in research laboratories, this robust and highly sensitive technique has the potential for use in routine clinical diagnostics. It is a cost-effective alternative for parasite detection that is rapid and only requires simple equipment (e.g., water bath and heating block) (Mori et al. 2001, Njiru 2012, Becherer et al. 2020). LAMP methods developed for the detection of *Cryptosporidium*, *G. duodenalis*, and *E. histolytica* have demonstrated superior sensitivity compared to PCR assays and are able to detect the equivalent concentration of one *Cryptosporidium* and *Entamoeba* parasites and four to six *G. duodenalis* parasites (Karanis et al. 2007, Plutzer and Karanis 2009, Adeyemo et al. 2018, Foo et al. 2020, Liang et al. 2009). The technique is based on auto-cycling strand displacement DNA synthesis facilitated by a DNA polymerase with high strand displacement activity (e.g., *Bst* DNA polymerase) and up to six specially designed primers that recognize six distinct regions within the target DNA (Notomi et al. 2000, Nagamine et al. 2002). The reaction is performed under isothermal conditions ranging from 60°C to 65°C and is able to amplify as few as six copies of DNA to 10^9 copies in less than an hour (Notomi et al. 2000). Rapid end point detection of LAMP products is enabled by a large amount of double-stranded DNA formed and the precipitation of magnesium pyrophosphate, a by-product of the reaction, from which turbidity can be measured in real-time or visualized by the naked eye (Notomi et al. 2000, Mori et al. 2001). Other detection methods also include visual fluorescence under UV light in the presence of intercalating dyes or by gel electrophoresis (Njiru et al. 2012, Becherer et al. 2020). The high tolerance of LAMP to PCR-inhibitors also makes this method suitable for the analysis of stool specimens, which contain inhibitory compounds such as bile salts, heme, and complex carbohydrates and may result in false negatives (Holland et al. 2000, Kaneko et al. 2007, Karanis et al. 2007, Liang et al. 2009).

Next Generation Sequencing

PCR amplification and Sanger sequencing of different gene regions have been widely used as a method for exploring the prevalence and genetic diversity of enteric parasites from humans, animals, and environmental samples from around the world. Comparisons between these sequences have been used to describe species/genotypes/ subtypes within parasite genera which have allowed for important distinctions in host specificity and public health importance within these parasite groups (Koehler et al. 2014, Feng et al. 2018, Li et al. 2019, Saidin et al. 2019). Just as the advent of PCR and Sanger sequencing ushered in a sea change in how we quantify and distinguish parasite infections, the development of second and third-generation sequencing technologies represents a new era in parasite detection.

Second-generation sequencing technologies, often referred to as next-generation sequencing (NGS), offer fast, sensitive, and high-throughput sequencing of both whole genomes and individual gene targets providing a cost-effective way to study genetic variations. NGS is currently used for two types of parasite detection, shot-gun metagenomics, which provides an untargeted profile of the entire diversity of parasites present within a given sample and amplicon-based sequencing which provides targeted detection of a specific gene or gene segment (Ryan et al. 2017). These two techniques have both advantages and challenges for use in the detection of enteric protist parasites and are currently only available at research facilities.

Shot-gun metagenomics allows for the characterization of the complex communities of microbes that reside in the intestinal track of humans and other animals (Simner et al. 2018). This technique, in theory, offers the advantage of a less biased pathogen detection methodology and can define the full diversity of organisms present in a given sample through direct sequencing of the specimen's extracted DNA; this includes rare or unculturable organisms which can be overlooked using traditional detection methods (Schneeberger et al. 2016, Wylezich et al. 2019). However, shot-gun metagenomics is currently not widely used in parasite detection, in part, due to the lack of parasite reference genomes that are needed to identify parasite sequences from the expansive data sets generated by NGS (Ryan et al. 2017). As more enteric parasite reference genomes become available it is likely that shot-gun metagenomics will be used to study the full diversity of parasites present in individual hosts. Furthermore, as intestinal protist parasites can represent a relatively small percentage of the total organisms present in a sample, it is possible that their presence could be missed using an untargeted approach like shot-gun metagenomics (Schneeberger et al. 2016). Thus, a targeted approach using NGS of amplicon may provide a more sensitive method for parasite detection.

Next-generation amplicon sequencing leverages the massively parallel sequencing capability of NGS to provide the sequencing depth needed to uncover complex mixtures of parasite DNA in complex matrixes such as fecal samples. In fact, NGS has been successfully used to explore intra-host parasite diversity for several enteric protists including *Blastocystis*, *Cryptosporidium*, *Entamoeba*, and *Giardia* (Grinberg et al. 2013, Maloney et al. 2019, 2020a, Paparini et al. 2015, Vlčková et al. 2018). These studies all demonstrate the suitability of individual parasite-specific amplicons for both detections of these parasites and for exploring intra-host parasite diversity. While within host-parasite diversity reported in these studies vary, they all find that NGS detects more diversity than PCR and Sanger sequencing, demonstrating the improved sensitivity NGS provides. A broader but still targeted parasite detection approach using amplicon-based metagenomics utilizing the 18S rRNA gene has been used to demonstrate that NGS can successfully detect enteric protists from water samples (Moreno et al. 2018). However, the use of this broader approach will likely result in some parasites not being detected, thus discounting the diversity of parasites present. A study using a eukaryotic 18S NGS method demonstrated inadequate sensitivity for detecting intestinal parasites in wastewater that is expected in low abundance (Zahedi et al. 2019). It was reported that *Cryptosporidium* was easily detected in water samples using a parasite-specific NGS approach but was not detected in the same samples using non-specific amplicon NGS (Zahedi et al. 2019). Thus, a parasite-specific gene target may be the more accurate and sensitive NGS detection method for enteric protist parasites.

The newest generation of sequencing technology, sometimes called third-generation sequencing, also provides fast, sensitive, and high-throughput sequencing and can be used to sequence both whole genomes and individual gene targets. The main advantage this new generation of sequencers offers over previous technologies is the ability to produce extremely long individual DNA sequences from 10s to 100s kilobases in length (Calarco et al. 2020, Jain et al. 2018). While early iterations of some third-generation sequencing platforms suffered from high error rates, recent software improvements now yield individual read accuracies of 85–95% and consensus accuracies > 99% (Kono and Arakawa 2019). To our knowledge, there are no published detection methods for enteric protist parasites using third-generation sequencers. However, this sequencing technology has been recently used to aide in the production of novel full-length reference sequences of *Blastocystis* (Maloney et al. 2020b). Furthermore, detection methods using third-generation sequencing for parasites, including protozoa and nematodes, have been reported (Imai et al. 2017, Knot et al. 2020). Therefore, it is likely only a matter of time before third-generation sequencing is employed for enteric parasite detection.

NGS (including both second and third-generation sequencing technologies) has produced several exciting emerging tools for exploring enteric protist parasite prevalence and diversity. However, barriers still exist to its widespread use. NGS requires access to specialized equipment, is expensive, and requires bioinformatic capabilities, which may not be easily available to many diagnostic laboratories (Ryan et al. 2017, Sekse et al. 2017, Simner et al. 2018). NGS however, is increasingly becoming affordable; in fact, it may be cheaper than traditional PCR and sequencing when large numbers of samples containing multiple variants of the same parasite are being sequenced (Maloney et al. 2019, Paparini et al. 2015). As the use of these new technologies expands bringing with them more sensitive parasite detection and improved detection of complex parasite mixtures within individual hosts, they are helping to usher in a new era of sequencing and analysis which is sure to expand our understanding of enteric protist parasite epidemiology.

Other Specimens from the Intestinal Tract

In the event of persisting gastrointestinal symptoms despite a negative O&P examination of stool for parasites, other specimens from the intestinal tract such as duodenal aspirations or biopsies and sigmoidoscopy specimens can be evaluated. For example, oocysts of *C. belli* are not always found in O&P examination of stool, and examination of duodenal specimens collected by biopsy or string test may be necessary (McHardy et al. 2014). Examinations of these materials are a sensitive diagnostic method; however, these specimens are collected using invasive procedures, are time sensitive, and need to be examined immediately. Biopsy and aspirate specimens can be examined for *Giardia, Cryptosporidium, Cyclospora, Cytoisospora*, and Microsporidia (DeGirolami et al. 1996, Bown et al. 1996, Garcia 2002, Garcia et al. 2018, Dubey et al. 2019) by microscopy, immunoassays, and nucleic acid tests. Examination by microscopy, however, is advantageous, as it may reveal the presence of other pathogens and should be considered especially in the diagnosis of travelers with diarrhea and patients with compromised or suppressed immune systems.

Biopsy specimens are collected during an endoscopy procedure, preferably from multiple duodenal-jejunal sites. The specimen needs to be examined immediately and must be transported to the laboratory in isotonic saline solution at room temperature. Duodenal fluid may also be aspirated during the endoscopy; the aspirated fluid needs to remain at room temperature without any preservatives and be sent to the laboratory for immediate examination. When evaluating for *Giardia, Cryptosporidium, Cyclospora*, or Microsporidia, duodenal aspirates may require concentration by centrifugation (10 minutes at 500 x g) prior to microscopic examinations on wet mounts for motile organisms and permanent stains (Garcia 2007; Garcia et al. 2018). Alternatively, the collection of duodenal fluids can also be performed without endoscopy using the string test. Marketed commercially as the Entero-Test®, the string test consists of a gelatin capsule attached to a weighted nylon string of the appropriate length (length differs for children and adults) that is swallowed by the patient. The gelatin dissolves once in the stomach and the weight carries the string into the duodenum. The string is left in position for a minimum of 4 hours and upon retrieval, the bile-stained mucus can be scraped off or "milked" between the thumb and index finger for examination on a direct wet mount and permanent stain.

If routine stool examinations are negative and amebiasis is suspected in patients with persistent gastrointestinal symptoms, biopsy or scrapings of the sigmoid can collect and evaluated for the diagnosis of *E. histolytica* during sigmoidoscopy or colonoscopy (Tanyuksel and Petri 2003, Fleming et al. 2015, Garcia et al. 2018). The procedure allows for visualization of the rectum and sigmoid flexure of the colon with a lighted tube and may reveal characteristic ulcers in more severe cases of intestinal amebiasis. Scrapings or aspirations of the mucosa should be collected from at least six representative areas of the mucosa and lesions on the mucosa should be targeted for specimen collection (Garcia 2007, Garcia et al. 2018). Biopsy specimens should be processed immediately for examination by the direct wet mount. For histological examination, specimens can be stored in 10% buffered formalin, whereas for permanent staining procedures, preservation of specimens in PVA-based fixatives or single-vial fixatives is recommended (Garcia 2007).

Serology

Although active gastrointestinal parasite infections are currently diagnosed by analysis of stool specimens, tests have also been developed for the detection of anti-parasite antibodies in serum. However, the difficulty of differentiating an active infection from a past infection has considerably limited its use to identify parasites in a clinical environment (Pacheco et al. 2020). In fact, serology has been mainly used for seroepidemiological studies of gastrointestinal parasites (Ungar et al. 1988, Cox et al. 2005, Cedillo-Rivera et al. 2009, Sak et al. 2010, Alvarado-Esquivel et al. 2015, Mosites et al. 2018, Arnold et al. 2019, Pacheco et al. 2020).

Important information can be obtained from seroprevalence studies such as measuring the overall exposure of a population or understanding the dynamics of infections that can be useful for the planning of preventive measures. A seroepidemiological study using ELISA to detect antibodies to *Cryptosporidium* in 389 children and adults in Peru and 84 children in Venezuela found that 64% of subjects had detectable levels of anti-*Cryptosporidium* IgG indicating infection sometimes in life; furthermore, there was an increased percentage in children of 2–3 years of age suggesting that this is a common age for infection with *Cryptosporidium* in these populations (Ungar et a. 1988). Similarly, IgG seropositivity from 512 samples including 39 pairs of maternal-cord sera obtained from a suburban population in Brazil was low in infants but quickly increased to 60% by 5 years and then remained constant at 80% after the age of 10 years (Cox et al. 2005). A cross-sectional study using an ELISA to determine *E. histolytica* IgG antibodies in 282 adults living in a rural population in Mexico that included association with the socio-demographic, housing conditions, and behavioral characteristics of the subjects studied showed that *E. histolytica* exposure was positively associated with a source of drinking water and education status of the head of the family (Alvarado-Esquivel et al. 2015).

Commercially available kits to test for antibodies against protist parasites are shown in Table 6. They are available for *Giardia*, *Cryptosporidium*, and *Entamoeba* as ELISA and latex agglutination assays. Non-commercial assays have also been used for research purposes but not for clinical diagnosis. These include approaches such as a multiplex bead assay that simultaneously detects specific human IgG antibodies to *Cryptosporidium* and *Giardia* surface antigens (Priest et al. 2010, Mosites et al. 2018) or assays that use a lysate of *Cryptosporidium* oocysts or *Giardia* trophozoite

Table 6. Commercially available serology kits to detect enteric protists in human serum or plasma.

Parasite Detected	Enzyme Immunological Assay (EIA) kits	Manufacturer	Selected Reference
Cryptosporidium spp.	*Cryptosporidium* Antibody ELISA Kit	MyBioSource	NA
Entamoeba spp.	Amoebiasis Serology Microwell ELISA	LMD Laboratories	Hira et al. (2001), Gatti et al. (2002)
	Bichro-Latex Amibe Fumouze Test	Laboratoires Fumouze Diagnostics	Van Doorn et al. (2005)
	Entamoeba histolytica IgG ELISA Kit	Bordier Affinity Products	Beyls et al. (2018)
	Entamoeba histolytica IgG (Amebiasis) ELISA Kit	Creative Diagnostics	NA
	Entamoeba histolytica IgG ELISA[a]	DRG International Inc.	NA
	Entamoeba histolytica IgG ELISA	MyBioSource	NA
	Entamoeba histolytica Serum Detection Microwell ELISA	IVD Research, Inc.	NA
	RIDASCREEN® *Entamoeba histolytica* IgG	R-Biopharm	Knappik et al. (2005), Dhanalakshmi and Parija (2016)
Giardia duodenalis	Anti-Giardia *lamblia* IgM ELISA Assay Kit	EagleBio	NA
	Anti-Giardia *lamblia* IgG ELISA Assay Kit	EagleBio	NA
	Anti-Giardia *lamblia* IgA ELISA Assay Kit	EagleBio	NA

NA: To our knowledge, no published reference for this kit is available.
[a] FDA-approved.

antigens or specific parasite antigens (e.g., *Cryptosporidium* gp15 or p23 antigens) to coat microplates to detect IgG and/or IgM antibodies (Winiecka et al. 1984, Ungar et al. 1986, Zu et al. 1994, Robin et al. 2001, Teixeira et al. 2007, Borad et al. 2012, Lazarus et al. 2015).

References

Abd El Kader, N. M., M. -A. Blanco, M. Ali-Tammam, A. E. R. B. Abd El Ghaffar, A. Osman, N. El Sheikh et al. (2012). Detection of *Cryptosporidium parvum* and *Cryptosporidium hominis* in human patients in Cairo, Egypt. Parasitol. Res. 110: 161–166.

Abu Al-Soud, W. and P. Rådström. (2000). Effects of amplification facilitators on diagnostic PCR in the presence of blood, feces, and meat. J. Clin. Microbiol. 38: 4463–4470.

Adamska, M., A. Leońska-Duniec, A. Maciejewska, M. Sawczuk and B. Skotarczak. (2010). Comparison of efficiency of various DNA extraction methods from cysts of *Giardia intestinalis* measured by PCR and TaqMan real time PCR. Parasite 17: 299–305.

Adeyemo, F. E., G. Singh, P. Reddy and T. A. Stenström. (2018). Methods for the detection of *Cryptosporidium* and *Giardia*: From microscopy to nucleic acid based tools in clinical and environmental regimes. Acta Trop. 184: 15–28.

Agnamey, P., C. Sarfati, C. Pinel, M. Rabodoniriina, N. Kapel, E. Dutoit et al. (2011). Evaluation of four commercial rapid immunochromatographic assays for detection of *Cryptosporidium* antigens in stool samples: A blind multicenter trial. J. Clin. Microbiol. 49: 1605–1607.

Ahmed, S. A. and P. Karanis. (2018). Comparison of current methods used to detect *Cryptosporidium* oocysts in stools. Int. J. Hyg. Environ. Health. 221: 743–763.

Akgun, S. and T. Celik. (2020). Evaluation of *Giardia intestinalis, Entamoeba histolytica* and *Cryptosporidium hominis/Cryptosporidium parvum* in human stool samples by the BD MAXTM Enteric Parasite Panel. Folia Parasitol. (Praha). 67: 2020.020.

Albert, M. J., V. O. Rotimi, J. Iqbal and W. Chehadeh. (2016). Evaluation of the xTAG gastrointestinal pathogen panel assay for the detection of enteric pathogens in Kuwait. Med. Princ. Pract. 25: 472–476.

Aldeen, W. E., J. Shisenant, D. Hale, J. Matsen and K. Carroll. (1993). Comparison of pooled formalin-preserved fecal specimens with three individual samples for detection of intestinal parasites. J. Clin. Microbiol. 31: 144–145.

Alexander, C. L., M. Niebel and B. Jones. (2013). The rapid detection of *Cryptosporidium* and *Giardia* species in clinical stools using the Quik Chek immunoassay. Parasitol. Int. 62: 552–553.

Alles, A. J., M. A. Waldron, L. S. Sierra and A. R. Mattia. (1995). Prospective comparison of direct immunofluorescence and conventional staining methods for detection of *Giardia* and *Cryptosporidium* spp. in human fecal specimens. J. Clin. Microbiol. 33: 1632–1634.

Almeria, S., H. N. Cinar and J. P. Dubey. (2019). *Cyclospora cayetanensis* and cyclosporiasis: An update. Microorganisms 7: 317.

Alvarado-Esquivel, C., J. Hernandez-Tinoco and L. F. Sanchez-Anguiano. (2015). Seroepidemiology of *Entamoeba histolytica* infection in general population in rural Durango, Mexico. J. Clin. Med. Res. 7: 435–439.

Ament, M. E. (1972). Diagnosis and treatment of giardiasis. J. Pediatr. 80: 633–637.

Arnold, B. F., D. L. Martin, J. Juma, H. Mkocha, J. B. Ochieng, G. M. Cooley et al. (2019). Enteropathogen antibody dynamics and force of infection among children in low-resource settings. Elife 8: e45594.

Autier, B., J. P. Gangneux and F. Robert-Gangneux. (2020). Evaluation of the Allplex™ Gastrointestinal panel-parasite assay for protozoa detection in stool samples: A retrospective and prospective study. Microorganisms 8: 569.

Autier, B., S. Belaz, R. Razakandrainibe, J. P. Gangneux and F. Robert-Gangneux. (2018). Comparison of three commercial multiplex PCR assays for the diagnosis of intestinal protozoa. Parasite 25: 48.

Baron, E. J., C. Schenone and B. Tanenbaum. (1989). Comparison of three methods for detection of *Cryptosporidium* oocysts in a low-prevalence population. J. Clin. Microbiol. 27: 223–224.

Bateman, A. C., Y. J. Kim, A. I. Guaracao, J. L. Mason, R. F. Klos and D. M. Warshauer. (2020). Performance and impact of the BioFire FilmArray Gastrointestinal Panel on a large *Cyclospora* outbreak in Wisconsin. 2018. J. Clin. Microbiol. 58: e01415–19.

Batra, R., E. Judd, J. Eling, W. Newsholme and S. D. Goldenberg. (2016). Molecular detection of common intestinal parasites: A performance evaluation of the BD Max™ Enteric Parasite Panel. Eur. J. Clin. Microbiol. Infect. Dis. 35: 1753–1757.

Baxby, D., N. Blundell and C. A. Hart. (1984). The development and performance of a simple, sensitive method for the detection of *Cryptosporidium* oocysts in faeces. J. Hyg. (Lond). 93: 317–323.

Beal, S. G., E. E. Tremblay, S. Toffel, L. Velez and K. H. Rand. (2017). A gastrointestinal PCR panel improves clinical management and lowers health care costs. J. Clin. Microbiol. 56: e01457–17.

Becherer, L., N. Borst, M. Bakheit, S. Frischmann, R. Zengerle and F. Von Stetten. (2020). Loop-mediated isothermal amplification (LAMP)-review and classification of methods for sequence-specific detection. Anal. Methods 12: 717–746.

Becker, S. L., L. K. Lohourignon, B. Speich, L. Rinaldi, S. Knopp, E. K. N'goran et al. (2011). Comparison of the FLOTAC-400 dual technique and the formalin-ether concentration technique for diagnosis of human intestinal protozoon infection. J. Clin. Microbiol. 49: 2183–2190.

Benedict, K. M., S. A. Collier, E. P. Marder, M. C. Hlavsa, K. E. Fullerton and J. S. Yoder. (2019). Case-case analyses of cryptosporidiosis and giardiasis using routine national surveillance data in the United States - 2005–2015. Epidemiol. Infect. 147: e178.

Berlin, O. G., J. B. Peter, C. Gagne, C. N. Conteas and L. R. Ash. (1998). Autofluorescence and the detection of *Cyclospora* oocysts. Emerg. Infect. Dis. 4: 127–128.

Beyls, N., O. Cognet, J. -P. Stahl, O. Rogeaux and H. Pelloux. (2018). Serodiagnosis of extraintestinal amebiasis: Retrospective evaluation of the diagnostic performance of the Bordier® ELISA Kit. Korean J. Parasitol. 56: 71–74.

Bialek, R., N. Binder, K. Dietz, J. Knobloch and U. E. Zelck. (2002a). Comparison of autofluorescence and iodine staining for detection of *Isospora belli* in feces. Am. J. Trop. Med. Hyg. 67: 304–305.

Bialek, R., N. Binder, K. Dietz, A. Joachim, J. Knobloch and U. E. Zelck. (2002b). Comparison of fluorescence, antigen and PCR assays to detect *Cryptosporidium parvum* in fecal specimens. Diagn. Microbiol. Infect. Dis. 43: 283–288.

Bitilinyu-Bangoh, J., W. Voskuijl, J. Thitiri, S. Menting, N. Verhaar, L. Mwalekwa et al. (2019). Performance of three rapid diagnostic tests for the detection of *Cryptosporidium* spp. and *Giardia duodenalis* in children with severe acute malnutrition and diarrhoea. Infect. Dis. Poverty 8: 96.

Boers, S. A., C. J. A. Peters, E. Wessels, W. J. G. Melchers and E. C. J. Claas. (2020). Performance of the QIAstat-Dx Gastrointestinal Panel for diagnosing infectious gastroenteritis. J. Clin. Microbiol. 58: e01737–19.

Boone, J. H., T. D. Wilkins, T. E. Nash, J. E. Brandon, E. A. Macias, R. C. Jerris et al. (1999). TechLab and Alexon *Giardia* enzyme-linked immunosorbent assay kits detect cyst wall protein 1. J. Clin. Microbiol. 37: 611–614.

Borad, A. J., G. M. Allison, D. Wang, S. Ahmed, M. M. Karim and A. V. Kane. (2012). Systemic antibody responses to the immunodominant p23 antigen and p23 polymorphisms in children with cryptosporidiosis in Bangladesh. Am. J. Trop. Med. Hyg. 86: 214–222.

Bown, J. W., T. J. Savides, C. Mathews, J. Isenberg, C. Behling and K. D. Lyche. (1996). Diagnostic yield of duodenal biopsy and aspirate in AIDS-associated diarrhea. Am. J. Gastroenterol. 91: 2289–2292.

Branda, J. A., T. Y. D. Lin, E. S. Rosenberg, E. F. Halpern and M. J. Ferrero. (2006). A rational approach to the stool ova and parasite examination. Clin. Infect. Dis. 42: 972–978.

Bronsdon, M. A. (1984). Rapid dimethyl sulfoxide-modified acid-fast stain of *Cryptosporidium* oocysts in stool specimens. J. Clin. Microbiol. 19: 952–953.

Bruijnesteijn van Coppenraet, L. E. S., J. A. Wallinga, G. J. H. M. Ruijs, M. J. Bruins and J. J. Verweij. (2009). Parasitological diagnosis combining an internally controlled real-time PCR assay for the detection of four protozoa in stool samples with a testing algorithm for microscopy. Clin. Microbiol. Infect. 15: 869–874.

Buckholt, M. A., J. H. Lee and S. Tzipori. (2002). Prevalence of *Enterocytozoon bieneusi* in swine: An 18-month survey at a slaughterhouse in Massachusetts. Appl. Environ. Microbiol. 68: 2595–2599.

Buss, S., M. Kabir, W. A. Petri and R. Haque. (2008). Comparison of two immunoassays for detection of *Entamoeba histolytica*. J. Clin. Microbiol. 46: 2778–2779.

Buss, S. N., A. Leber, K. Chapin, P. D. Fey, M. J. Bankowski, M. K. Jones et al. (2015). Multicenter evaluation of the BioFire FilmArray gastrointestinal panel for etiologic diagnosis of infectious gastroenteritis. J. Clin. Microbiol. 53: 915–25.

Cacciò, S. M. (2018). Molecular epidemiology of *Dientamoeba fragilis*. Acta Trop. 184: 73–77.

Cacciò, S. M. and S. M. Lalle. (2015). Giardiasis. pp. 175–193. *In*: Xiao, L., U. Ryan and Y. Feng (eds.). Biology of Foodborne Parasites. Boca Raton: CRC Press.

Cacciò, S. M., M. De Giacomo and E. Pozio. (2002). Sequence analysis of the beta-giardin gene and development of a polymerase chain reaction-restriction fragment length polymorphism assay to genotype *Giardia duodenalis* cysts from human faecal samples. Int. J. Parasitol. 32: 1023–1030.

Calarco, L., J. Barratt and J. Ellis. (2020). Detecting sequence variants in clinically important protozoan parasites. Int. J. Parasitol. 50: 1–18.

Cann, K. J., R. M. Chalmers, G. Nichols and S. J. O'Brien. (2000). *Cyclospora* infections in England and Wales: 1993 to 1998. Commun. Dis. public Heal. 3: 46–49.

Cao, M., J. T. Ellis, D. Marriott, J. Harkness and D. Stark. (2019). Evaluation of the easyscreen protozoan detection kit for the diagnosis of *Entamoeba histolytica*. Pathology 51: 426–428.

Carrero, J. C., M. Reyes-López, J. Serrano-Luna, M. Shibayama, J. Unzueta, N. León-Sicairos et al. (2020). Intestinal amoebiasis: 160 years of its first detection and still remains as a health problem in developing countries. Int. J. Med. Microbiol. 310: 151358.

Casemore, D. P. (1991). ACP Broadsheet 128: June 1991. Laboratory methods for diagnosing cryptosporidiosis. J. Clin. Pathol. 44: 445–451.

Casemore, D. P., M. Armstrong and R.L. Sands. (1985). Laboratory diagnosis of cryptosporidiosis. J. Clin. Pathol. 38: 1337–1341.

Cedillo-Rivera, R., Y. A. Leal, L. Yépez-Mulia, A. Gómez-Delgado, G. Ortega-Pierres, R. Tapia-Conyer et al. (2009). Seroepidemiology of giardiasis in Mexico. Am. J. Trop. Med. Hyg. 80: 6–10.

Chalmers, R. M. and A. P. Davies (2010). Minireview: Clinical cryptosporidiosis. Exp. Parasitol. 124: 138–146.

Chalmers, R. M., B. M. Campbell, N. Crouch, A. Charlett and A. P. Davies. (2011). Comparison of diagnostic sensitivity and specificity of seven *Cryptosporidium* assays used in the UK. J. Med. Microbiol. 60: 1598–1604.

Chioralia, G., T. Trammer, H. Kampen and H. M. Seitz. (1998). Relevant criteria for detecting microsporidia in stool specimens. J. Clin. Microbiol. 36: 2279–2283.

Christy, N. C. V., J. D. Hencke, A. Escueta-De Cadiz, F. Nazib, H. von Thien, K. Yagita et al. (2012). Multisite performance evaluation of an enzyme-linked immunosorbent assay for detection of *Giardia, Cryptosporidium,* and *Entamoeba histolytica* antigens in human stool. J. Clin. Microbiol. 50: 1762–1763.

Church, D., K. Miller, A. Lichtenfeld, H. Semeniuk, B. Kirkham, K. Laupland et al. (2005). Screening for *Giardia/Cryptosporidium* infections using an enzyme immunoassay in a centralized regional microbiology laboratory. Arch. Pathol. Lab. Med. 129: 754–759.

Claas, E. C., C. A. Burnham, T. Mazzulli, K. Templeton and F. Topin. (2013). Performance of the xTAG® gastrointestinal pathogen panel, a multiplex molecular assay for simultaneous detection of bacterial, viral, and parasitic causes of infectious gastroenteritis. J. Microbiol. Biotechnol. 23: 1041–1045.

Clark, C. G. and L. S. Diamond. (2002). Methods for cultivation of luminal parasitic protists of clinical importance. Clin. Microbiol. Rev. 15: 329–341.

Cociancic, P., L. Rinaldi, M. L. Zonta and G. T. Navone. (2018). Formalin-ethyl acetate concentration, FLOTAC Pellet and anal swab techniques for the diagnosis of intestinal parasites. Parasitol. Res. 117: 3567–3573.

Connor, B. A., M. Rogova and O. Whyte. (2018). Use of a multiplex DNA extraction PCR in the identification of pathogens in travelers' diarrhea. J. Travel. Med. 25(1).

Conteas, C. N., O. G. Berlin, L. R. Ash and J. S. Pruthi. (2000). Therapy for human gastrointestinal microsporidiosis. Am. J. Trop. Med. Hyg. 63: 121–127.

Couturier, B. A., R. Jensen, N. Arias, M. Heffron, E. Gubler, K. Case et al. (2015). Clinical and analytical evaluation of a single-vial stool collection device with formalin-free fixative for improved processing and comprehensive detection of gastrointestinal parasites. J. Clin. Microbiol. 53: 2539–2548.

Cox, M. J., K. Elwin, E. Massad and R. S. Azevedo. (2005). Age-specific seroprevalence to an immunodominant *Cryptosporidium* sporozoite antigen in a Brazilian population. Epidemiol. Infect. 133: 951–956.

Cybulski, R. J. Jr., A. C. Bateman, L. Bourassa, A. Bryan, B. Beall, J. Matsumoto et al. (2018). Clinical impact of a multiplex gastrointestinal polymerase chain reaction panel in patients with acute gastroenteritis. Clin. Infect. Dis. 67: 1688–1696.

Dacal, E., P. C. Köster and D. Carmena. (2020). Diagnóstico molecular de parasitosis intestinales. Enferm. Infecc. Microbiol. Clin. 38 Suppl. 1: 24–31.

Despommier, D. D., D. O. Griffin, R. W. Gwadz, P. J. Hotez and C. A. Knirsch. (2011). Parasitic Diseases. 7th ed. A. (Harrie) Bickle, editor. Parasites Without Borders, Inc., New York. 72: 74 pp.

Diamond, L. S. (1982). A new liquid medium for xenic cultivation of *Entamoeba histolytica* and other lumen-dwelling protozoa. J. Parasitol. 68: 958–959.

Didier, E. S. (2005). Microsporidiosis: An emerging and opportunistic infection in humans and animals. Acta Trop. 94: 61–76.

Didier, E. S., J. M. Orenstein, A. Aldras, D. Bertucci, L. B. Rogers and F. A. Janney. (1995). Comparison of three staining methods for detecting microsporidia in fluids. J. Clin. Microbiol. 33: 3138–3145.

Den Hartog, J., L. Rosenbaum, Z. Wood, D. Burt and W. A. Petri. (2013). Diagnosis of multiple enteric protozoan infections by enzyme-linked immunosorbent assay in the Guatemalan highlands. Am. J. Trop. Med. Hyg. 88: 167–171.

DeGirolami, P. C., C. R. Ezratty, G. Desai, A. McCullough, D. Asmuth, C. Wanke et al. (1995). Diagnosis of intestinal microsporidiosis by examination of stool and duodenal aspirate with Weber's modified trichrome and Uvitex 2B strains. J. Clin. Microbiol. 33: 805–810.

Dhanalakshmi, S. and S. Parija. (2016). Seroprevalence of *Entamoeba histolytica* from a tertiary care hospital, South India. Trop. Parasitol. 6: 78–81.

Dirani, G., S. Zannoli, E. Paesini, P. Farabegoli, B. Dalmo, C. Vocale et al. (2019). Easyscreen™ Enteric Protozoa Assay for the detection of intestinal parasites: a retrospective bi-center study. J. Parasitol. 105: 58–63.

Dixon, B. R. 2020. *Giardia duodenalis* in humans and animals—Transmission and disease. Res. Vet. Sci. (Online ahead of print, https://doi.org/10.1016/j.rvsc.2020.09.034).

Dogruman-Al, F., S. Turk, G. Adiyaman-Korkmaz, A. Hananel, L. Levi, J. Kopelowitz et al. (2015). A novel ELISA test for laboratory diagnosis of *Blastocystis* spp. in human stool specimens. Parasitol. Res. 114: 495–500.

Dubey, J. P. and S. Almeria. (2019). *Cystoisospora belli* infections in humans: The past 100 years. Parasitology 146: 1490–1527.

Dubey, J. P., K. J. Evason and Z. Walther. (2019). Endogenous development of *Cystoisospora belli* in intestinal and biliary epithelium of humans. Parasitology 146: 865–872.

Elwin, K., H. V. Fairclough, S. J. Hadfield and R. M. Chalmers. (2014). *Giardia duodenalis* typing from stools: A comparison of three approaches to extracting DNA, and validation of a probe-based real-time PCR typing assay. J. Med. Microbiol. 63: 38–44.

Estevez, E. G. and J. A. Levine. (1985). Examination of preserved stool specimens for parasites: Lack of value of the direct wet mount. J. Clin. Microbiol. 22: 666–667.

Faust, E. C., J. S. D'Antoni, V. Odom, M. F. Miller, C. Peres, W. Sawitz et al. (1938). A critical study of clinical laboratory technics for the diagnosis of protozoan cysts and helminth eggs in feces. Am. J. Trop. Med. Hyg. 18: 169–183.

Fedorko, D. P., E. C. Williams, N. A. Nelson, L. B. Calhoun and S. S. Yan. (2000). Performance of three enzyme immunoassays and two direct fluorescence assays for detection of *Giardia lamblia* in stool specimens preserved in ECOFIX. J. Clin. Microbiol. 38: 2781–2783.

Feng, Y., U. M. Ryan and L. Xiao. (2018). Genetic diversity and population structure of *Cryptosporidium*. Trends Parasitol. 34: 997–1011.

Feng, Y. and L. Xiao. (2011). Zoonotic potential and molecular epidemiology of *Giardia* species and giardiasis. Clin. Microbiol. Rev. 24: 110–140.

Fleece, M. E., J. Heptinstall, S. S. Khan, M. Kabir, J. Herbein, R. Haque et al. (2016). Evaluation of a rapid lateral flow point-of-care test for detection of *Cryptosporidium*. Am. J. Trop. Med. Hyg. 95: 840–841.

Fleming, R., C. J. Cooper, R. Ramirez-Vega, A. Huerta-Alardin, D. Boman and M. J. Zuckerman. (2015). Clinical manifestations and endoscopic findings of amebic colitis in a United States-Mexico border city: A case series. BMC Res. Notes 8: 781.

Flournoy, D. J., S. J. McNabb, E. D. Dodd and M. H. Shaffer. (1982). Rapid trichrome stain. J. Clin. Microbiol. 16: 573–574.

Foo, P. C., A. B. Nurul Najian, N. A. Muhamad, M. Ahamad, M. Mohamed, C. Yean Yean et al. (2020). Loop-mediated isothermal amplification (LAMP) reaction as viable PCR substitute for diagnostic applications: a comparative analysis study of LAMP, conventional PCR, nested PCR (nPCR) and real-time PCR (qPCR) based on *Entamoeba histolytica* DNA derived from faecal sample. BMC Biotechnol. 20: 34.

Formenti, F., F. Perandin, S. Bonafini, M. Degani and Z. Bisoffi. (2015). Evaluation of the new ImmunoCard STAT!® CGE test for the diagnosis of Amebiasis. Bull. Soc. Pathol. Exot. 108: 171–174.

Formenti, F., C. Piubelli, R. Narra, D. Buonfrate, B. Pajola, G. Lunghi et al. (2018). Preliminary comparison of an in-house real-time PCR with the automated BD Max Enteric Parasite Panel for the detection of *Giardia intestinalis*. J. Parasitol. 104: 702–704.

Fotedar, R., D. Stark, N. Beebe, D. Marriott, J. Ellis and J. Harkness. (2007). Laboratory diagnostic techniques for *Entamoeba* species. Clin. Microbiol. Rev. 20: 511–532.

Franzen, C., A. Muller, B. Salzberger, P. Hartmann, V. Diehl and G. Fatkenheuer. (1996). Uvitex 2B stain for the diagnosis of *Isospora belli* infections in patients with the acquired immunodeficiency syndrome. Arch. Pathol. Lab. Med. 120: 1023–1025.

Friesen, J., J. Fuhrmann, H. Kietzmann, E. Tannich, M. Müller and R. Ignatius. (2018). Evaluation of the Roche LightMix Gastro parasites multiplex PCR assay detecting *Giardia duodenalis*, *Entamoeba histolytica*, cryptosporidia, *Dientamoeba fragilis*, and *Blastocystis hominis*. Clin. Microbiol. Infect. 24: 1333–1337.

Furuno, J. P., J. H. Maguire, H. P. Green, J. A. Johnson, R. Heimer, S. P. Johnston et al. (2006). Clinical utility of multiple stool ova and parasite examinations in low-prevalence patient populations. Clin. Infect. Dis. 43: 795–796.

Gaafar, M. R. (2011). Use of pooled sodium acetate acetic acid formalin-preserved fecal specimens for the detection of intestinal parasites. J. Clin. Lab. Anal. 25: 217–222.

Garcia, L. S. (2002). Laboratory identification of the microsporidia. J. Clin. Microbiol. 40: 1892–1901.

Garcia, L. S. (2007). Diagnostic Medical Parasitology. 5th ed. ASM Press, Washington D.C.

Garcia, L. S. and R. Y. Shimizu. (1997). Evaluation of nine immunoassay kits (enzyme immunoassay and direct fluorescence) for detection of *Giardia lamblia* and *Cryptosporidium parvum* in human fecal specimens. J. Clin. Microbiol. 35: 1526–1529.

Garcia, L. S. and R. Y. Shimizu. (1998). Evaluation of intestinal protozoan morphology in human fecal specimens preserved in EcoFix: Comparison of Wheatley's trichrome stain and EcoStain. J. Clin. Microbiol. 36: 1974–1976.

Garcia, L. S., A. C. Shum and D. A. Bruckner. (1992). Evaluation of a new monoclonal antibody combination reagent for direct fluorescence detection of *Giardia* cysts and *Cryptosporidium* oocysts in human fecal specimens. J. Clin. Microbiol. 30: 3255–3257.

Garcia, L. S., D. A. Bruckner, T. C. Brewer and R. Y. Shimizu. (1983). Techniques for the recovery and identification of *Cryptosporidium* oocysts from stool specimens. J. Clin. Microbiol. 18: 185–190.

Garcia, L. S., M. Arrowood, E. Kokoskin, G. P. Paltridge, D. R. Pillai, G. W. Procop et al. (2018). Laboratory diagnosis of parasites from the gastrointestinal tract. Clin. Microbiol. Rev. 31: e00025–17.

Garcia, L. S., R. Y. Shimizu and C. N. Bernard. (2000). Detection of *Giardia lamblia*, *Entamoeba histolytica/Entamoeba dispar*, and *Cryptosporidium parvum* antigens in human fecal specimens using the triage parasite panel enzyme immunoassay. J. Clin. Microbiol. 38: 3337–3340.

Garcia, L. S., R. Y. Shimizu, A. Shum and D. A. Bruckner. (1993). Evaluation of intestinal protozoan morphology in polyvinyl alcohol preservative: Comparison of zinc sulfate- and mercuric chloride-based compounds for use in Schaudinn's fixative. J. Clin. Microbiol. 31: 307–310.

Garcia, L. S., R. Y. Shimizu, S. Novak, M. Carroll and F. Chan. (2003). Commercial assay for detection of *Giardia lamblia* and *Cryptosporidium parvum* antigens in human fecal specimens by rapid solid-phase qualitative immunochromatography. J. Clin. Microbiol. 41: 209–212.

Garcia, L. S., T. C. Brewer and D. A. Bruckner. (1979). A comparison of the formalin-ether concentration and trichrome-stained smear methods for the recovery and identification of intestinal protozoa. Am. J. Med. Technol. 45: 932–935.

Gardner, B. B., D. J. Del Junco, J. Fenn and J. H. Hengesbaugh. (1980). Comparison of direct wet mount and trichrome staining techniques for detecting *Entamoeba* species trophozoites in stools. J. Clin. Microbiol. 12: 656–658.

Gatti, S., G. Swierczynski, F. Robinson, M. Anselmi, J. Corrales, J. Moreira et al. (2002). Amebic infections due to the *Entamoeba histolytica-Entamoeba dispar* complex: A study of the incidence in a remote rural area of Ecuador. Am. J. Trop. Med. Hyg. 67: 123–127.

Ghoshal, U., S. Khanduja, P. Pant and U. C. Ghoshal. (2016). Evaluation of Immunoflourescence antibody assay for the detection of *Enterocytozoon bieneusi* and *Encephalitozoon intestinalis*. Parasitol. Res. 115: 3709–3713.

Giangaspero, A. and R. B. Gasser. (2019). Human cyclosporiasis. Lancet Infect. Dis. 19: e226–e236.

Gingras, B. A. and J. A. Maggiore. (2020). Performance of a new molecular assay for the detection of gastrointestinal pathogens. Access Microbiol. 2: acmi000160.

Gonin, P. and L. Trudel. (2003). Detection and differentiation of *Entamoeba histolytica* and *Entamoeba dispar* isolates in clinical samples by PCR and enzyme-linked immunosorbent assay. J. Clin. Microbiol. 41: 237–41.

Goñi, P., B. Martín, M. Villacampa, A. García, C. Seral, F. J. Castillo et al. (2012). Evaluation of an immunochromatographic dip strip test for simultaneous detection of *Cryptosporidium* spp, *Giardia duodenalis*, and *Entamoeba histolytica* antigens in human faecal samples. Eur. J. Clin. Microbiol. 31: 2077–2082.

Gough, R., J. Ellis and D. Stark. (2019). Comparison and recommendations for use of *Dientamoeba fragilis* real-time PCR assays. J. Clin. Microbiol. 57: e01466–18.

Grinberg, A., P. J. Biggs, V. S. R. Dukkipati and T. T. George. (2013). Extensive intra-host genetic diversity uncovered in *Cryptosporidium parvum* using Next Generation Sequencing. Infect. Genet. Evol. 15: 18–24.

Guerrant, R. L., T. Van Gilder, L. Slutsker, R. V. Tauxe, T. Hennessy et al. (2001). Practice guidelines for the management of infectious diarrhea. Clin. Infect. Dis. 32: 331–351.

Gutiérrez-Cisneros, M. J., R. Martínez-Ruiz, M. Subirats, F. J. Merino, R. Millán and I. Fuentes. (2011). [Assessment of two commercially available immunochromatographic assays for a rapid diagnosis of *Giardia duodenalis* and *Cryptosporidium* spp. in human fecal specimens]. Enferm. Infecc. Microbiol. Clin. 29: 201–203.

Halánová, M., A. Valenčáková, P. Jarčuška, M. Halán, O. Danišová, I. Babinská et al. (2019). Screening of opportunistic *Encephalitozoon intestinalis* and *Enterocytozoon bieneusi* in immunocompromised patients in Slovakia. Cent. Eur. J. Public Health 27: 330–334.

Hamzah, Z., S. Petmitr, M. Mungthin, S. Leelayoova and P. Chavalitshewinkoon-Petmitr. (2006). Differential detection of *Entamoeba histolytica*, *Entamoeba dispar*, and *Entamoeba moshkovskii* by a single-round PCR assay. J. Clin. Microbiol. 44: 3196–200.

Hannet, I., A. L. Engsbro, J. Pareja, U. V. Schneider, J. G. Lisby, B. Pružinec-Popović et al. (2019). Multicenter evaluation of the new QIAstat Gastrointestinal Panel for the rapid syndromic testing of acute gastroenteritis. Eur. J. Clin. Microbiol. Infect. Dis. 38: 2103–2112.

Hanscheid, T., J. M. Cristino and M. J. Salgado. (2008). Screening of auramine-stained smears of all fecal samples is a rapid and inexpensive way to increase the detection of coccidial infections. Int. J. Infect. Dis. 12: 47–50.

Haque, R., L. M. Neville, P. Hahn and W. A. J. Petri. (1995). Rapid diagnosis of *Entamoeba* infection by using *Entamoeba* and *Entamoeba histolytica* stool antigen detection kits. J. Clin. Microbiol. 33: 2558–2561.

Haque, R. and W. A. Jr. Petri. (2006). Diagnosis of amebiasis in Bangladesh. Arch. Med. Res. 37: 273–276.

Harrington, B. J. (2008). Microscopy of 4 pathogenic enteric protozoan parasites: A review. Lab. Med. 39: 231–238.

Hawash, Y. (2014a). DNA extraction from protozoan oocysts/cysts in feces for diagnostic PCR. Korean J. Parasitol. 52: 263–271.

Hawash, Y. (2014b). Evaluation of an immunoassay-based algorithm for screening and identification of *Giardia* and *Cryptosporidium* antigens in human faecal specimens from Saudi Arabia. J. Parasitol. Res. 2014: 213745.

Hawash, Y. A., K. A. Ismail and M. Almehmadi. (2017). High frequency of enteric protozoan, viral, and bacterial potential pathogens in community-acquired acute diarrheal episodes: Evidence based on results of Luminex Gastrointestinal Pathogen Panel Assay. Korean J. Parasitol. 55: 513–521.

Hiatt, R. A., E. K. Markell and E. Ng. (1995). How many stool examinations are necessary to detect pathogenic intestinal protozoa? Am. J. Trop. Med. Hyg. 53: 36–39.

Hijjawi, N., R. Yang, R. Hatmal, Y. Yassin, T. Mharib, R. Mukbel et al. (2018). Comparison of ELISA, nested PCR and sequencing and a novel qPCR for detection of *Giardia* isolates from Jordan. Exp. Parasitol. 185: 23–28.

Hira, P. R., J. Iqbal, R. Al-Ali, R. Philip, S. Grover, E. D'Almeida et al. (2001). Invasive amebiasis: Challenges in diagnosis in a non-endemic country (Kuwait). Am. J. Trop. Med. Hyg. 65: 341–345.

Holland, J. L., L. Louie, A. E. Simor and M. Louie. (2000). PCR detection of *Escherichia coli* O157: H7 directly from stools: Evaluation of commercial extraction methods for purifying fecal DNA. J. Clin. Microbiol. 38: 4108–4113.

Horen, W. P. (1983). Detection of *Cryptosporidium* in human fecal specimens. J. Parasitol. 69: 622–624.

Howat, W. J. and B. A. Wilson. (2014). Tissue fixation and the effect of molecular fixatives on downstream staining procedures. Methods 70: 12–19.

Ignatius, R., S. Henschel, O. Liesenfeld, U. Mansmann, W. Schmidt, S. Köppe et al. (1997a). Comparative evaluation of modified trichrome and Uvitex 2B stains for detection of low numbers of microsporidial spores in stool specimens. J. Clin. Microbiol. 35: 2266–2269.

Ignatius, R., M. Lehmann, K. Miksits, T. Regnath, M. Arvand, E. Engelmann et al. (1997b). A new acid-fast trichrome stain for simultaneous detection of *Cryptosporidium parvum* and microsporidial species in stool specimens. J. Clin. Microbiol. 35: 446–449.

Imai, K., N. Tarumoto, K. Misawa, L. R. Runtuwene, J. Sakai, K. Hayashida et al. (2017). A novel diagnostic method for malaria using loop-mediated isothermal amplification (LAMP) and MinIONTM nanopore sequencer. BMC Infect. Dis. 17: 621.

Jahan, N., R. Khatoon and S. Ahmad. (2014). A comparison of microscopy and enzyme linked immunosorbent assay for diagnosis of *Giardia lamblia* in human faecal specimens. J. Clin. Diagn. Res. 8: DC04–DC6.

Jain, M., S. Koren, K. H. Miga, J. Quick, A. C. Rand, T. A. Sasani et al. (2018). Nanopore sequencing and assembly of a human genome with ultra-long reads. Nat. Biotechnol. 36: 338–345.

Jensen, B., W. Kepley, J. Guarner, K. Anderson, D. Anderson, J. Clairmont et al. (2000). Comparison of polyvinyl alcohol fixative with three less hazardous fixatives for detection and identification of intestinal parasites. J. Clin. Microbiol. 38: 1592–1598.

Johnson, J. A. and C. G. Clark. (2000). Cryptic genetic diversity in *Dientamoeba fragilis*. J. Clin. Microbiol. 38: 4653–4654.

Johnston, S. P., M. M. Ballard, M. J. Beach, L. Causer and P. P. Wilkins. (2003). Evaluation of three commercial assays for detection of *Giardia* and *Cryptosporidium* organisms in fecal specimens. J. Clin. Microbiol. 41: 623–626.

Kaneko, H., T. Kawana, E. Fukushima and T. Suzutani. (2007). Tolerance of loop-mediated isothermal amplification to a culture medium and biological substances. J. Biochem. Biophys. Methods 70: 499–501.

Kantor, M., A. Abrantes, A. Estevez, A. Schiller, J. Torrent, J. Gascon et al. (2018). *Entamoeba histolytica*: Updates in clinical manifestation, pathogenesis, and vaccine development. Can. J. Gastroenterol. Hepatol. 2018: 4601420.

Karanis, P., O. Thekisoe, K. Kiouptsi, J. Ongerth, I. Igarashi and N. Inoue. (2007). Development and preliminary evaluation of a loop-mediated isothermal amplification procedure for sensitive detection of *Cryptosporidium* oocysts in fecal and water samples. Appl. Environ. Microbiol. 73: 5660–5662.

Khairnar, K., S. C. Parija and R. Palaniappan. (2007). Diagnosis of intestinal amoebiasis by using nested polymerase chain reaction-restriction fragment length polymorphism assay. J. Gastroenterol. 42: 631–640.

Khan, M. Q., N. Gentile, Y. Zhou, B. A. Smith, R. B. Thomson and E. F. Yen. (2020). An audit of inpatient stool ova and parasite (O&P) testing in a multi-hospital health system. J. Community Hosp. Intern. Med. Perspect. 10: 204–209.

Khanna, V., S. Sagar, R. Khanna and K. Chawla. (2018). A comparative study of formalin-ethyl acetate sedimentation technique and Mini Parasep® solvent-free method in the rapid diagnosis of intestinal parasites. Trop. Parasitol. 8: 29–32.

Khare, R., M. J. Espy, E. Cebelinski, D. Boxrud, L. M. Sloan, S. A. Cunningham et al. (2014). Comparative evaluation of two commercial multiplex panels for detection of gastrointestinal pathogens by use of clinical stool specimens. J. Clin. Microbiol. 52: 3667–3673.

Kimura, K., S. Kumar Rai, K. Takemasa, Y. Ishibashi, M. Kawabata, M. Belosevic et al. (2004). Comparison of three microscopic techniques for diagnosis of *Cyclospora cayetanensis*. FEMS Microbiol. Lett. 238: 263–266.

Knappik, M., U. Börner and T. Jelinek. (2005). Sensitivity and specificity of a new commercial enzyme-linked immunoassay kit for detecting *Entamoeba histolytica* IgG antibodies in serum samples. Eur. J. Clin. Microbiol. Infect. Dis. 24: 701–703.

Knot, I. E., G. D. Zouganelis, G. D. Weedall, S. A. Wich and R. Rae. (2020). DNA barcoding of nematodes using the MinION. Front. Ecol. Evol. 8: 100.

Koehler, A. V., A. R. Jex, S. R. Haydon, M. A. Stevens, and R. B. Gasser. (2014). *Giardia*/giardiasis—A perspective on diagnostic and analytical tools. Biotechnol. Adv. 32: 280–289.

Kokoskin, E., T. W. Gyorkos, A. Camus, L. Cedilotte, T. Purtill and B. Ward. (1994). Modified technique for efficient detection of microsporidia. J. Clin. Microbiol. 32: 1074–1075.

Koltas, I. S., I. Akyar, G. Elgun and T. Kocagoz. (2014). Feconomics®; a new and more convenient method, the routine diagnosis of intestinal parasitic infections. Parasitol. Res. 113: 2503–2508.

Kono, N. and K. Arakawa. (2019). Nanopore sequencing: Review of potential applications in functional genomics. Dev. Growth Differ. 61: 316–326.

Kotloff, K. L., J. P. Nataro, W. C. Blackwelder, D. Nasrin, T. H. Farag, S. Panchalingam et al. (2013). Burden and aetiology of diarrhoeal disease in infants and young children in developing countries (the Global Enteric Multicenter Study, GEMS): A prospective, case-control study. Lancet 382: 209–222.

Kreader, C. A.(1996). Relief of amplification inhibition in PCR with bovine serum albumin or T4 gene 32 protein. Appl. Environ. Microbiol. 62: 1102–1106.

Laksemi, D. A., L. T. Suwanti, M. Mufasirin, K. Suastika and M. Sudarmaja. (2019). Opportunistic parasitic infections in patients with human immunodeficiency virus/acquired immunodeficiency syndrome: A review. Vet. World 13: 716–725.

Lalle, M., E. Pozio, G. Capelli, F. Bruschi, D. Crotti and S. M. Cacciò. (2005). Genetic heterogeneity at the beta-giardin locus among human and animal isolates of *Giardia duodenalis* and identification of potentially zoonotic subgenotypes. Int. J. Parasitol. 35: 207–213.

Laude, A., S. Valot, G. Desoubeaux, N. Argy, C. Nourrisson, C. Pomares et al. (2016). Is real-time PCR-based diagnosis similar in performance to routine parasitological examination for the identification of *Giardia intestinalis*, *Cryptosporidium parvum/Cryptosporidium hominis* and *Entamoeba histolytica* from stool samples? Evaluation of a new commercial multiplex PCR assay and literature review. Clin. Microbiol. Infect. 22: 190.e1–190.e8.

Lazarus, R. P., S. S. R. Ajjampur, R. Sarkar, J. C. Geetha, A. D. Prabakaran and V. Velusamy. (2015). Serum anti-cryptosporidial gp15 antibodies in mothers and children less than 2 years of age in India. Am. J. Trop. Med. Hyg. 93: 931–938.

Leméteil, D., G. Gargala, R. Razakandrainibe, J. J. Ballet, L. Favennec and D. Costa. (2019). Comparative evaluation of commercial concentration procedures for human intestinal parasite detection. Lab. Med. 50: 243–248.

Leo, M., R. Haque, M. Kabir, S. Roy, R. M. Lahlou, D. Mondal et al. (2006). Evaluation of *Entamoeba histolytica* antigen and antibody point-of-care tests for the rapid diagnosis of amebiasis. J. Clin. Microbiol. 44: 4569–4571.

Li, W., Y. Feng, M. Santin. (2019). Host specificity of *Enterocytozoon bieneusi* and public health implications. Trends Parasitol. 35: 436–451.

Liang, S. -Y., Y. -H. Chan, K. -T. Hsia, J. -L. Lee, M. -C. Kuo, K. -Y. Hwa et al. (2009). Development of loop-mediated isothermal amplification assay for detection of *Entamoeba histolytica*. J. Clin. Microbiol. 47: 1892–1895.

Libman, M. D., T. W. Gyorkos, E. Kokoskin and J. D. MacLean. (2008). Detection of pathogenic protozoa in the diagnostic laboratory: Result reproducibility, specimen pooling, and competency assessment. J. Clin. Microbiol. 46: 2200–2205.

Liu, J., F. Kabir, J. Manneh, P. Lertsethtakarn, S. Begum, J. Gratz et al. (2014). Development and assessment of molecular diagnostic tests for 15 enteropathogens causing childhood diarrhoea: A multicentre study. Lancet Infect. Dis. 14: 716–724.

Long, E. G., A. Ebrahimzadeh, E. H. White, B. Swisher and C. S. Callaway. (1990). Alga associated with diarrhea in patients with acquired immunodeficiency syndrome and in travelers. J. Clin. Microbiol. 28: 1101–1104.

Luna, V. A., B. K. Stewart, D. L. Bergeron, C. R. Clausen, J. J. Plorde and T. R. Fritsche. (1995). Use of the fluorochrome calcofluor white in the screening of stool specimens for spores of microsporidia. Am. J. Clin. Pathol. 103: 656–659.

Machiels, J. D., A. J. H. Cremers, M. C. G. T. van Bergen-Verkuyten, S. J. M. Paardekoper-Strijbosch, K. C. J. Frijns, H. F. L. Wertheim et al. (2020). Impact of the BioFire FilmArray gastrointestinal panel on patient care and infection control. PLoS One 15: e0228596.

MacPherson, D. W. and R. McQueen. (1993). Cryptosporidiosis: multiattribute evaluation of six diagnostic methods. J. Clin. Microbiol. 31: 198–202.

Madison-Antenucci, S., R. F. Relich, L. Doyle, N. Espina, D. Fuller, T. Karchmer et al. (2016). Multicenter evaluation of BD Max Enteric Parasite Real-Time PCR Assay for detection of *Giardia duodenalis*, *Cryptosporidium hominis*, *Cryptosporidium parvum*, and *Entamoeba histolytica*. J. Clin. Microbiol. 54: 2681–2688.

Mai, K., P. A. Sharman, R. A. Walker, M. Katrib, D. de Souza, M. J. McConville et al. (2009). Oocyst wall formation and composition in coccidian parasites. Mem. Inst. Oswaldo Cruz. 104: 281–289.

Maloney, J. G., A. Molokin and M. Santin. (2019). Next generation amplicon sequencing improves detection of *Blastocystis* mixed subtype infections. Infect. Genet. Evol. 73: 119–125.

Maloney, J. G., A. Molokin and M. Santin. (2020a). Assessment of next generation amplicon sequencing of the beta-giardin gene for the detection of *Giardia duodenalis* assemblages and mixed infections. Food Waterborne Parasitol. 21: e00098.

Maloney, J. G., A. Molokin and M. Santin. (2020b). Use of Oxford Nanopore MinION to generate full-length sequences of the *Blastocystis* small subunit (SSU) rRNA gene. Parasit. Vectors 13: 595.

Mank, T. G., J. O. Zaat, J. Blotkamp and A. M. Polderman. (1995). Comparison of fresh versus sodium acetate acetic acid formalin preserved stool specimens for diagnosis of intestinal protozoal infections. Eur. J. Clin. Microbiol. Infect. Dis. 14: 1076–1081.

Manouana, G. P., E. Lorenz, M. Mbong Ngwese, P. A. Nguema Moure, O. Maiga Ascofaré, C. W. Akenten et al. (2020). Performance of a rapid diagnostic test for the detection of *Cryptosporidium* spp. in African children admitted to hospital with diarrhea. PLoS Negl. Trop. Dis. 14: e0008448.

Marti, H. and J. C. Koella. (1993). Multiple stool examinations for ova and parasites and rate of false-negative results. J. Clin. Microbiol. 31: 3044–3045.

Mata, L., H. Bolaños, M. Vives and D. Pizarro. (1984). Cryptosporidiosis in children from some highland Costa Rican rural and urban areas. Am. J. Trop. Med. Hyg. 33: 24–29.

Mathison, B. A., J. L. Kohan, J. F. Walker, R. B. Smith, O. Ardon and M. R. Couturier. (2020). Detection of intestinal protozoa in trichrome-stained stool specimens by use of a deep convolutional neural network. J. Clin. Microbiol. 58: e02053–19.

McAuliffe, G., L. Bissessor, D. Williamson, S. Moore, J. Wilson, M. Dufour et al. (2017). Use of the EntericBio Gastro Panel II in a diagnostic microbiology laboratory: challenges and opportunities. Pathology 49: 419–422.

McHardy, I. H., M. Wu, R. Shimizu-Cohen, M. R. r Couturier and R. M. Humphries. (2014). Detection of intestinal protozoa in the clinical laboratory. J. Clin. Microbiol. 52: 712–720.

McLaughlin, J. C., S. K. Rasmussen, L. J. Nims, D. A. Madar and C. R. Yazzie. (1993). Evaluation of reliability of pooling stool specimens from different patients and detection of *Giardia lamblia* antigen by microtiter enzyme-linked immunosorbent assay. J. Clin. Microbiol. 31: 2807–2808.

McNabb, S. J., D. M. Hensel, D. F. Welch, H. Heijbel, G. L. McKee and G. R. Istre. (1985). Comparison of sedimentation and flotation techniques for identification of *Cryptosporidium* sp. oocysts in a large outbreak of human diarrhea. J. Clin. Microbiol. 22: 587–589.

Mewara, A., S. Khurana, S. Gupta, V. S. Munda, S. Singh and R. Sehgal. (2019). Diagnostic performance of mini parasep® solvent-free foecal parasite concentrator for the diagnosis of intestinal parasitic infections. Indian J. Med. Microbiol. 37: 381–386.

Minak, J., M. Kabir, I. Mahmud, Y. Liu, L. Liu, R. Haque et al. (2012). Evaluation of rapid antigen point-of-care tests for detection of *Giardia* and *Cryptosporidium* species in human fecal specimens. J. Clin. Microbiol. 50: 154–156.

Mölling, P, P. Nilsson, T. Ennefors, J. Ögren, K. Florén, S. Thulin Hedberg et al. (2016). Evaluation of the BD Max Enteric Parasite Panel for clinical diagnostics. J. Clin. Microbiol. 54: 443–444.

Momčilović, S., C. Cantacessi, V. Arsić-Arsenijević, D. Otranto and S. Tasić-Otašević. (2019). Rapid diagnosis of parasitic diseases: Current scenario and future needs. Clin. Microbiol. Infect. 25: 290–309.

Moreno, Y., L. Moreno-Mesonero, I. Amorós, R. Pérez, J. A. Morillo and J. L. Alonso. (2018). Multiple identification of most important waterborne protozoa in surface water used for irrigation purposes by 18S rRNA amplicon-based metagenomics. Int. J. Hyg. Environ. Health 221: 102–111.

Morgan, U. M., L. Pallant, B. W. Dwyer, D. A. Forbes, G. Rich and R. C. A. Thompson. (1998). Comparison of PCR and microscopy for detection of *Cryptosporidium parvum* in human fecal specimens: Clinical trial. J. Clin. Microbiol. 36: 995–998.

Mori, Y., K. Nagamine, N. Tomita and T. Notomi. (2001). Detection of loop-mediated isothermal amplification reaction by turbidity derived from magnesium pyrophosphate formation. Biochem. Biophys. Res. Commun. 289: 150–154.

Morris, A. J., M. L. Wilson and L. B. Reller. (1992). Application of rejection criteria for stool ovum and parasite examinations. J. Clin. Microbiol. 30: 3213–3216.

Mosites, E., K. Miernyk, J. W. Priest, D. Bruden, D. Hurlburt, A. Parkinson et al. (2018). *Giardia* and *Cryptosporidium* antibody prevalence and correlates of exposure among Alaska residents, 2007–2008. Epidemiol. Infect. 146: 888–894.

Nace, E. K., F. J. Steurer and M. L. Eberhard. (1999). Evaluation of Streck tissue fixative, a nonformalin fixative for preservation of stool samples and subsequent parasitologic examination. J. Clin. Microbiol. 37: 4113–4119.

Nagamine, K., T. Hase and T. Notomi. (2002). Accelerated reaction by loop-mediated isothermal amplification using loop primers. Mol. Cell. Probes 16: 223–229.

Navarro, C., M. V. Dominguez-Marquez, M. M. Garijo-Toledo, S. Vega-Garcia, S. Fernandez-Barredo, M. T. Perez-Gracia et al. (2008). High prevalence of *Blastocystis* sp. in pigs reared under intensive growing systems: frequency of ribotypes and associated risk factors. Vet. Parasitol. 153: 347–358.

Navidad, J. F., D. J. Griswold, M. S. Gradus and S. Bhattacharyya. (2013). Evaluation of Luminex xTAG gastrointestinal pathogen analyte-specific reagents for high-throughput, simultaneous detection of bacteria, viruses, and parasites of clinical and public health importance. J. Clin. Microbiol. 51: 3018–3024.

Negm, A. Y. (1998). Identification of *Cyclospora cayetanensis* in stool using different stains. J. Egypt. Soc. Parasitol. 28: 429–436.

Neimeister, R., A. L. Logan, J. H. Egleton and B. Kleger. (1990). Evaluation of direct wet mount parasitological examination of preserved fecal specimens. J. Clin. Microbiol. 28: 1082–1084.

Nguyen, T. K. T., H. Kherouf, V. Blanc-Pattin, E. Allais, Y. Chevalier, A. Richez et al. (2012). Evaluation of an immunochromatographic assay: *Giardia*-Strip® (Coris BioConcept) for detection of *Giardia intestinalis* in human fecal specimens. Eur. J. Clin. Microbiol. 31: 623–625.

Njiru, Z. K. (2012). Loop-mediated isothermal amplification technology: Towards point of care diagnostics. PLoS Negl. Trop. Dis. 6: e1572.

Notomi, T., H. Okayama, H. Masubuchi, T. Yonekawa, K. Watanabe, N. Amino et al. (2000). Loop-mediated isothermal amplification of DNA. Nucleic Acids Res. 28: E63.

Núñez, Y. O., M. A. Fernández, D. Torres-Núñez, J. A. Silva, I. Montano, J. J. Maestre et al. (2001). Multiplex polymerase chain reaction amplification and differentiation of *Entamoeba histolytica* and *Entamoeba dispar* DNA from stool samples. Am. J. Trop. Med. Hyg. 64: 293–297.

Oster, N., H. Gehrig-Feistel, H. Jung, J. Kammer, J. E. McLean and M. Lanzer. (2006). Evaluation of the immunochromatographic CORIS *Giardia*-Strip test for rapid diagnosis of *Giardia lamblia*. Eur. J. Clin. Microbiol. 25: 112–115.

Pacheco, F. T. F., R. K. N. R. Silva, A. S. Martins, R. R. Oliveira, N. M. Alcântara-Neves, M. P. Silva et al. (2013). Differences in the detection of *Cryptosporidium* and *Isospora* (*Cystoisospora*) oocysts according to the fecal concentration or staining method used in a clinical laboratory. J. Parasitol. 99: 1002–1008.

Pacheco, F. T. F., S. S. de Carvalho, S. A. Santos, G. M. T. das Chagas, M. C. Santos, J. G. C. Santos et al. (2020). Specific IgG and IgA antibody reactivities in sera of children by enzyme-linked immunoassay and comparison with *Giardia duodenalis* diagnosis in feces. Ann. Lab. Med. 40: 382–389.

Paparini, A., A. Gofton, R. Yang, N. White, M. Bunce and U. M. Ryan. (2015). Comparison of Sanger and next generation sequencing performance for genotyping *Cryptosporidium* isolates at the 18S rRNA and actin loci. Exp. Parasitol. 151-152: 21–27.

Parčina, M., I. Reiter-Owona, F. P. Mockenhaupt, V. Vojvoda, J. B. Gahutu, A. Hoerauf et al. (2018). Highly sensitive and specific detection of *Giardia duodenalis*, *Entamoeba histolytica*, and *Cryptosporidium* spp. in human stool samples by the BD MAX™ Enteric Parasite Panel. Parasitol. Res. 117: 447–451.

Paulos, S., M. Mateo, A. de Lucio, M. Hernández-de Mingo, B. Bailo, J. M. Saugar et al. (2016). Evaluation of five commercial methods for the extraction and purification of DNA from human faecal samples for downstream molecular detection of the enteric protozoan parasites *Cryptosporidium* spp., *Giardia duodenalis*, and *Entamoeba* spp. J. Microbiol. Methods 127: 68–73.

Paulos, S., J. M. Saugar, A. de Lucio, I. Fuentes, M. Mateo and D. Carmena. (2019). Comparative performance evaluation of four commercial multiplex real-time PCR assays for the detection of the diarrhoea-causing protozoa *Cryptosporidium hominis/parvum, Giardia duodenalis* and *Entamoeba histolytica*. PLoS One 14: e0215068.

Pedraza-Díaz, S., C. Amar and J. McLauchlin. (2000). The identification and characterisation of an unusual genotype of *Cryptosporidium* from human faeces as *Cryptosporidium meleagridis*. FEMS Microbiol. Lett. 189: 189–194.

Peters, C. S., L. Hernandez, N. Sheffield, A. L. Chittom-Swiatlo and F. E. Kocka. (1988). Cost containment of formalin-preserved stool specimens for ova and parasites from outpatients. J. Clin. Microbiol. 26: 1584–1585.

Perry, J. L., J. S. Matthews and G. R. Miller. (1990). Parasite detection efficiencies of five stool concentration systems. J. Clin. Microbiol. 28: 1094–1097.

Perry, M. D., S. A. Corden and R. A. Howe. (2014). Evaluation of the Luminex xTAG gastrointestinal pathogen panel and the savyon diagnostics gastrointestinal infection panel for the detection of enteric pathogens in clinical samples. J. Med. Microbiol. 63: 1419–1426.

Perry, M. D., S. A. Corden and P. Lewis White. (2017). Evaluation of the BD MAX enteric parasite panel for the detection of *Cryptosporidium parvum/hominis, Giardia duodenalis* and *Entamoeba histolytica*. J. Med. Microbiol. 66: 1118–1123.

Pietrzak-Johnston, S. M., H. Bishop, S. Wahlquist, H. Moura, N. de Oliveira da Silva, S. Pereira da Silva et al. (2000). Evaluation of commercially available preservatives for laboratory detection of helminths and protozoa in human fecal specimens. J. Clin. Microbiol. 38: 1959–1964.

Pillai, D. R. and K. C. Kain. (1999). Immunochromatographic strip-based detection of *Entamoeba histolytica-E. dispar* and *Giardia lamblia* coproantigen. J. Clin. Microbiol. 37: 3017–3019.

Plutzer, J. and P. Karanis. (2009). Rapid identification of *Giardia duodenalis* by loop-mediated isothermal amplification (LAMP) from faecal and environmental samples and comparative findings by PCR and real-time PCR methods. Parasitol. Res. 104: 1527–1533.

Priest, J. W., D. M. Moss, G. S. Visvesvara, C. C. Jones, A. Li and J. L. Isaac-Renton. (2010). Multiplex assay detection of immunoglobulin G antibodies that recognize *Giardia intestinalis* and *Cryptosporidium parvum* antigens. Clin. Vaccine Immunol. 17: 1695–1707.

Read, C. M., P. T. Monis and R. C. Thompson. (2004). Discrimination of all genotypes of *Giardia duodenalis* at the glutamate dehydrogenase locus using PCR-RFLP. Infect. Genet. Evol. 4: 125–130.

Reisner, B. S. and J. Spring. (2000). Evaluation of a combined acid-fast-trichrome stain for detection of microsporidia and *Cryptosporidium parvum*. Arch. Pathol. Lab. Med. 124: 777–779.

Ricciardi, A. and M. Ndao. (2015). Diagnosis of parasitic infections: what's going on? J. Biomol. Screen. 20: 6–21.

Ritchie, L. S. (1948). An ether sedimentation technique for routine stool examinations. Bull. U.S. Army Med. Dep. United States. Army. Med. Dep. 8: 326.

Roberts, T., J. Barratt, J. Harkness, J. Ellis and D. Stark. (2011). Comparison of microscopy, culture, and conventional polymerase chain reaction for detection of *Blastocystis* sp. in clinical stool samples. Am. J. Trop. Med. Hyg. 84: 308–312.

Robin, G., D. Fraser, N. Orr, T. Sela, R. Slepon, R. Ambar et al. (2001). *Cryptosporidium* infection in Bedouin infants assessed by prospective evaluation of anticryptosporidial antibodies and stool examination. Am. J. Epidemiol. 153: 194–201.

Robinson, G. L. (1968). The laboratory diagnosis of human parasitic amoebae. Trans. R. Soc. Trop. Med. Hyg. 62: 285–94.

Roellig, D. M., J. S. Yoder, S. Madison-Antenucci, T. J. Robinson, T. T. Van, S. A. Collier et al. (2017). Community laboratory testing for *Cryptosporidium*: Multicenter study retesting public health surveillance stool samples positive for *Cryptosporidium* by rapid cartridge assay with direct fluorescent antibody testing. PLoS One 12: e0169915.

Rojas-Velázquez, L., J. G. Maloney, A. Molokin, P. Morán, A. Serrano-Vázquez, E. González et al. (2019). Use of next-generation amplicon sequencing to study *Blastocystis* genetic diversity in a rural human population from Mexico. Parasit. Vectors 12: 566.

Roy, S., M. Kabir, D. Mondal, I. K. Ali, W. A. Jr. Petri and R. Haque. (2005). Real-time-PCR assay for diagnosis of *Entamoeba histolytica* infection. J. Clin. Microbiol. 43: 2168–2172.

Ryan, N. J., G. Sutherland, K. Coughlan, M. Globan, J. Doultree, J. Marshall et al. (1993). A new trichrome-blue stain for detection of microsporidial species in urine, stool, and nasopharyngeal specimens. J. Clin. Microbiol. 31: 3264–3269.

Ryan, U., A. Paparini and C. Oskam. (2017). New technologies for detection of enteric parasites. Trends Parasitol. 33: 532–546.

Sadaka, H. A., M. R. Gaafar, R. F. Mady and N. N. Hezema. (2015). Evaluation of ImmunoCard® STAT test and ELISA versus light microscopy in diagnosis of giardiasis and cryptosporidiosis. Parasitol. Res. 114: 2853–2863.

Saidin, S., N. Othman and R. Noordin. (2019). Update on laboratory diagnosis of amoebiasis. Eur. J. Clin. Microbiol. Infect. Dis. 38: 15–38.

Sak, B., Z. Kucerova, M. Kvac, D. Kvetonova, M. Rost and E. W. Secor. (2010). Seropositivity for *Enterocytozoon bieneusi*, Czech Republic. Emerg. Infect. Dis. 16: 335–337.

Salman, Y. J., W. S. Sadek and Z. K. Rasheed. (2015). Prevalence of *Cryptosporidium parvum* among Iraqi displaced people in Kirkuk city using direct microscopy, flotation technique and ELISA-copro antigen test. 4: 559–572.

Santín, M. and D. S. Zarlenga. (2009). A multiplex polymerase chain reaction assay to simultaneously distinguish *Cryptosporidium* species of veterinary and public health concern in cattle. Vet. Parasitol. 166: 32–37.

Santín, M. and R. Fayer. (2009). *Enterocytozoon bieneusi* genotype nomenclature based on the internal transcribed spacer sequence: A consensus. J. Eukaryot. Microbiol. 56: 34–8.

Santín, M., M. T. Gómez-Muñoz, G. Solano-Aguilar and R. Fayer. (2011). Development of a new PCR protocol to detect and subtype *Blastocystis* spp. from humans and animals. Parasitol. Res. 109: 205–212.

Schneeberger, P. H. H., S. L. Becker, J. F. Pothier, B. Duffy, E. K. N'Goran, C. Beuret et al. (2016). Metagenomic diagnostics for the simultaneous detection of multiple pathogens in human stool specimens from Côte d'Ivoire: A proof-of-concept study. Infect. Genet. Evol. 40: 389–397.

Schuster, F. L. and L. Ramirez-Avila. (2008). Current world status of *Balantidium coli*. Clin. Microbiol. Rev. 21: 626–638.

Sekse, C., A. Holst-Jensen, U. Dobrindt, G. S. Johannessen, W. Li, B. Spilsberg et al. (2017). High throughput sequencing for detection of foodborne pathogens. Front. Microbiol. 8: 2029.

Shetty, N. and T. Prabhu. (1988). Evaluation of faecal preservation and staining methods in the diagnosis of acute amoebiasis and giardiasis. J. Clin. Pathol. 41: 694–699.

Silva, R. K., F. T. Pacheco, A. S. Martins, J. F. Menezes, H. Jr. Costa-Ribeiro, T. C. Ribeiro et al. (2016). Performance of microscopy and ELISA for diagnosing *Giardia duodenalis* infection in different pediatric groups. Parasitol. Int. 65: 635–640.

Simner, P. J., S. Miller and K. C. Carroll. (2018). Understanding the promises and hurdles of metagenomic next-generation sequencing as a diagnostic tool for infectious diseases. Clin. Infect. Dis. 66: 778–788.

Singh, A., E. Houpt and W. A. Petri. (2009). Rapid diagnosis of intestinal parasitic protozoa, with a focus on *Entamoeba histolytica*. Interdiscip. Perspect. Infect. Dis. 2009: 1–8.

Smith, H. V., C. A. Paton, M. M. A. Mtambo and R. W. A. Girdwood. (1997). Sporulation of *Cyclospora* sp. oocysts. Appl. Environ. Microbiol. 63: 1631–1632.

Soares, F. A., A. D. N. Benitez, B. M. Dos Santos, S. H. N. Loiola, S. L. Rosa, W. B. Nagata et al. (2020). A historical review of the techniques of recovery of parasites for their detection in human stools. Rev. Soc. Bras. Med. Trop. 53: 1–9.

Spina, A., K. G. Kerr, M. Cormican, F. Barbut, A. Eigentler, L. Zerva et al. (2015). Spectrum of enteropathogens detected by the FilmArray GI Panel in a multicentre study of community-acquired gastroenteritis. Clin. Microbiol. Infect. 21: 719–728.

Singhal, S., V. Mittal, V. Khare and Y. Singh. (2015). Comparative analysis of enzyme-linked immunosorbent assay and direct microscopy for the diagnosis of *Giardia intestinalis* in fecal samples. Indian J. Pathol. Microbiol. 58: 69–71.

Srijan, A., B. Wongstitwilairoong, C. Pitarangsi, O. Serichantalergs, C. D. Fukuda, L. Bodhidatta et al. (2005). Re-evaluation of commercially available enzyme-linked immunosorbent assay for the detection of *Giardia lamblia* and *Cryptosporidium* spp. from stool specimens. Southeast Asian J. Trop. Med. Public Health. 36 Suppl 4: 26–29.

Srinivasan, M., D. Sedmak and S. Jewell. (2002). Effect of fixatives and tissue processing on the content and integrity of nucleic acids. Am. J. Pathol. 161: 1961–1971.

Stark, D., S. E. Al-Qassab, J. L. Barratt, K. Stanley, T. Roberts, D. Marriott et al. (2011). Evaluation of multiplex tandem real-time PCR for detection of *Cryptosporidium* spp., *Dientamoeba fragilis*, *Entamoeba histolytica*, and *Giardia intestinalis* in clinical stool samples. J. Clin. Microbiol. 49: 257–262.

Stark, D., S. van Hal, R. Fotedar, A. Butcher, D. Marriott, J. Ellis et al. (2008). Comparison of stool antigen detection kits to PCR for diagnosis of amebiasis. J. Clin. Microbiol. 46: 1678–1681.

Stark, D., T. Roberts, J. T. Ellis, D. Marriott and J. Harkness. (2014). Evaluation of the EasyScreen™ enteric parasite detection kit for the detection of *Blastocystis* spp., *Cryptosporidium* spp., *Dientamoeba fragilis*, *Entamoeba* complex, and *Giardia intestinalis* from clinical stool samples. Diagn. Microbiol. Infect. Dis. 78: 149–152.

Stensvold, C. R. (2013). *Blastocystis*: Genetic diversity and molecular methods for diagnosis and epidemiology. Trop. Parasitol. 3: 26–34.

Stensvold, C. R., U. N. Ahmed, L. O. Andersen and H. V. Nielsen. (2012). Development and evaluation of a genus-specific, probe-based, internal-process-controlled real-time PCR assay for sensitive and specific detection of *Blastocystis* spp. J. Clin. Microbiol. 50: 1847–1851.

Stensvold, C. R., J. Winiecka-Krusnell, T. Lier and M. Lebbad. (2018). Evaluation of a PCR method for detection of *Entamoeba polecki*, with an overview of its molecular epidemiology. J. Clin. Microbiol. 56: e00154–18.

Sulaiman, I. M., R. Fayer, C. Bern, R. H. Gilman, J. M. Trout, P. M. Schantz et al. (2003). Triosephosphate isomerase gene characterization and potential zoonotic transmission of *Giardia duodenalis*. Emerg. Infect. Dis. 9: 1444–1452.

Subrungruang, I., M. Mungthin, P. Chavalitshewinkoon-Petmitr, R. Rangsin, T. Naaglor and S. Leelayoova. (2004). Evaluation of DNA extraction and PCR methods for detection of *Enterocytozoon bienuesi* in stool specimens. J. Clin. Microbiol. 42: 3490–3494.

Swierczewski, B., E. Odundo, J. Ndonye, R. Kirera, C. Odhiambo and E. Oaks. (2012). Comparison of the Triage Micro Parasite Panel and microscopy for the detection of *Entamoeba histolytica/Entamoeba dispar*, *Giardia lamblia*, and *Cryptosporidium parvum* in stool samples collected in Kenya. J. Trop. Med. 2012: 564721.

Tan, K. S. W. (2008). New insights on classification, identification, and clinical relevance of *Blastocystis* spp. Clin. Microbiol. Rev. 21: 639–665.

Tanyuksel, M. and W. A. J. Petri. (2003). Laboratory diagnosis of amebiasis. Clin. Microbiol. Rev. 16: 713–729.

Teixeira, M. C., M. L. Barreto, C. Melo, L. R. Silva, L. R. Moraes and N. M. Alcântara-Neves. (2007). A serological study of *Cryptosporidium* transmission in a periurban area of a Brazilian Northeastern city. Trop. Med. Int. Health 12: 1096–1104.

Tejashree, A., P. B. Pooja and K. S. Babu. (2017). Comparative evaluation of microscopy and ELISA in diagnosis of cryptosporidiosis in HIV and non-HIV Patients. Int. J. Curr. Microbiol. Appl. Sci. 6: 232–239.

Ten Hove, R., T. Schuurman, M. Kooistra, L. Möller, L. van Lieshout and J. J. Verweij. (2007). Detection of diarrhoea-causing protozoa in general practice patients in The Netherlands by multiplex real-time PCR. Clin. Microbiol. Infect. 13: 1001–1007.

Thompson, R. C. A. and P. T. Monis. (2004). Variation in *Giardia*: Implications for taxonomy and epidemiology. Adv. Parasitol. 58: 69–137.

Thornton, S. A., A. H. West, H. L. Dupont and L. K. Pickering. (1983). Comparison of methods for identification of *Giardia lamblia*. Am. J. Clin. Pathol. 80: 858–860.

Tompkins, V. N. and J. K. Miller. (1947). Staining intestinal protozoa with iron-hematoxylin-phosphotungstic acid. Am. J. Clin. Pathol. 17: 755–758.

Troeger, C., B. F. Blacker, I. A. Khalil, P. C. Rao, S. Cao, S. R. Zimsen et al. (2018). Estimates of the global, regional, and national morbidity, mortality, and aetiologies of diarrhoea in 195 countries: A systematic analysis for the Global Burden of Disease Study 2016. Lancet. Infect. Dis. 18: 1211–1228.

Truant, A. L., S. H. Elliott, M. T. Kelly and J. H. Smith. (1981). Comparison of formalin-ethyl ether sedimentation, formalin-ethyl acetate sedimentation, and zinc sulfate flotation techniques for detection of intestinal parasites. J. Clin. Microbiol. 13: 882–884.

Ungar, B. L., R. Soave, R. Fayer and T. E. Nash. (1986). Enzyme immunoassay detection of immunoglobulin M and G antibodies to *Cryptosporidium* in immunocompetent and immunocompromised persons. J. Infect. Dis. 153: 570–578.

Ungar, B. L., R. H. Gilman, C. F. Lanata and I. Perez-Schael. (1988). Seroepidemiology of *Cryptosporidium* infection in two Latin American populations. J. Infect. Dis. 157: 551–556.

Valenčáková A. and M. Sučik. (2020). Alternatives in molecular diagnostics of *Encephalitozoon* and *Enterocytozoon* infections. J. Fungi. (Basel). 6: 114.

Van den Bossche, D., L. Cnops, J. Verschueren and M. Van Esbroeck. (2015). Comparison of four rapid diagnostic tests, ELISA, microscopy and PCR for the detection of *Giardia lamblia*, *Cryptosporidium* spp. and *Entamoeba histolytica* in feces. J. Microbiol. Methods 110: 78–84.

Van Doorn, H. R., H. Hofwegen, R. Koelewijn, H. Gilis, R. Peek, J. C. F. M. Wetsteyn et al. (2005). Use of rapid dipstick and latex agglutination tests and enzyme-linked immunosorbent assay for serodiagnosis of amebic liver abscess, amebic colitis, and *Entamoeba histolytica* cyst passage. J. Clin. Microbiol. 43: 4801–4806.

Van Gool, T., E. U. Canning and J. Dankert. (1994). An improved practical and sensitive technique for the detection of microsporidian spores in stool samples. Trans. R. Soc. Trop. Med. Hyg. 88: 189–190.

Van Gool, T., R. Weijts, E. Lommerse and T. G. Mank. (2003). Triple Faeces Test: an effective tool for detection of intestinal parasites in routine clinical practice. Eur. J. Clin. Microbiol. Infect. Dis. 22: 284–290.

Van Gool, T., W. S. Hollister, W. E. Schattenkerk, M. A. Van den Bergh Weerman, W. J. Terpstra, R. J. van Ketel et al. (1990). Diagnosis of *Enterocytozoon bieneusi* microsporidiosis in AIDS patients by recovery of spores from faeces. Lancet (London, England) 336: 697–698.

van Gool, T., F. Snijders, P. Reiss, J. K. Eeftinck Schattenkerk, M. A. Van Den Bergh Weermann, J. F. Bartelsman et al. (1993). Diagnosis of intestinal and disseminated microsporidial infections in patients with HIV by a new rapid fluorescence technique. J. Clin. Pathol. 46: 694–699.

Van Lieshout, L. and M. Roestenberg. (2015). Clinical consequences of new diagnostic tools for intestinal parasites. Clin. Microbiol. Infect. 21: 520–528.

Varea, M., A. Clavel, O. Doiz, F. J. Castillo, M. C. Rubio and R. Gómez-Lus. (1998). Fuchsin fluorescence and autofluorescence in *Cryptosporidium*, *Isospora* and *Cyclospora* oocysts. Int. J. Parasitol. 28: 1881–1883.

Vávra, J., R. Dahbiová, W. S. Hollister and E. U. Canning. (1993). Staining of microsporidian spores by optical brighteners with remarks on the use of brighteners for the diagnosis of AIDS associated human microsporidioses. Folia Parasitol. (Praha). 40: 267–272.

Verkerke, H. P., B. Hanbury, A. Siddique, A. Samie, R. Haque, J. Herbein et al. (2015). Multisite clinical evaluation of a rapid test for *Entamoeba histolytica* in stool. J. Clin. Microbiol. 53: 493–497.

Verweij, J. J., D. Laeijendecker, E. A. Brienen, L. van Lieshout and A. M. Polderman. (2003). Detection of *Cyclospora cayetanensis* in travellers returning from the tropics and subtropics using microscopy and real-time PCR. Int. J. Med. Microbiol. 293: 199–202.

Verweij, J. J. and C. R. Stensvold. (2014). Molecular testing for clinical diagnosis and epidemiological investigations of intestinal parasitic infections. Clin. Microbiol. Rev. 27: 371–418.

Visvesvara, G. S., H. Moura, E. Kovacs-Nace, S. Wallace and M. L. Eberhard. (1997). Uniform staining of *Cyclospora* oocysts in fecal smears by a modified safranin technique with microwave heating. J. Clin. Microbiol. 35: 730–733.

Visvesvara, G. S. (2002). *In vitro* cultivation of microsporidia of clinical importance. Clin. Microbiol. Rev. 15: 401–413.

Vlčková, K., J. Kreisinger, B. Pafčo, D. Čížková, N. Tagg, A. B. Hehl et al. (2018). Diversity of *Entamoeba* spp. in African great apes and humans: an insight from Illumina MiSeq high-throughput sequencing. Int. J. Parasitol. 48: 519–530.

Wahlquist, S. P., R. M. Williams, H. Bishop, D. G. Addiss, J. M. Stewart, R. J. Finton et al. (1991). Use of pooled formalin-preserved fecal specimens to detect *Giardia lamblia*. J. Clin. Microbiol. 29: 1725–1726.

Wang, C., X. Zhou, M. Zhu, H. Yin, J. Tang, Y. Huang et al. (2020). The application research of xTAG GPP multiplex PCR in the diagnosis of persistent and chronic diarrhea in children. BMC Pediatr. 20: 309.

Watson, B., M. Blitzer, H. Rubin and I. Nachamkin. (1988). Direct wet mounts versus concentration for routine parasitological examination: are both necessary? Am. J. Clin. Pathol. 89: 389–391.

Weber, R., R. T. Bryan, H. S. Bishop, S. P. Wahlquist, J. J. Sullivan and D. D. Juranek. (1991). Threshold of detection of *Cryptosporidium* oocysts in human stool specimens: evidence for low sensitivity of current diagnostic methods. J. Clin. Microbiol. 29: 1323–1327.

Weber, R., R. T. Bryan, R. L. Owen, C. M. Wilcox, L. Gorelkin and G. S. Visvesvara. (1992). Improved light-microscopical detection of microsporidia spores in stool and duodenal aspirates. The Enteric Opportunistic Infections Working Group. N. Engl. J. Med. 326: 161–166.

Weitzel, T., S. Dittrich, I. Möhl, E. Adusu and T. Jelinek. (2006). Evaluation of seven commercial antigen detection tests for *Giardia* and *Cryptosporidium* in stool samples. Clin. Microbiol. Infect. 12: 656–659.

Wessels, E., L. G. Rusman, M. J. van Bussel and E. C. Claas. (2014). Added value of multiplex Luminex Gastrointestinal Pathogen Panel (xTAG® GPP) testing in the diagnosis of infectious gastroenteritis. Clin. Microbiol. Infect. 20: O182–7.

Wheatley, W. B. (1951). A rapid staining procedure for intestinal amoebae and flagellates. Am. J. Clin. Pathol. 21: 990–991.

Winiecka, J., W. Kasprzak, W. Kociecka, J. Płotkowiak and P. Myjak. (1984). Serum antibodies to *Giardia intestinalis* detected by immunofluorescence using trophozoites as antigen. Tropenmed. Parasitol. 35: 20–22.

Wylezich, C., A. Belka, D. Hanke, M. Beer, S. Blome and D. Höper. (2019). Metagenomics for broad and improved parasite detection: a proof-of-concept study using swine faecal samples. Int. J. Parasitol. 49: 769–777.

Wolfe, M. S. (1975). Giardiasis. JAMA 233: 1362–1365.

Wołyniec, W., M. Sulima, M. Renke and A. Dębska-Ślizień. (2018). Parasitic infections associated with unfavourable outcomes in transplant recipients. Medicina (Kaunas) 54: 27.

Woods, G. L. and D. H. Walker. (1996). Detection of infection or infectious agents by use of cytologic and histologic stains. Clin. Microbiol. Rev. 9: 382–404.

Xiao, L. (2010). Molecular epidemiology of cryptosporidiosis: An update. Exp. Parasitol. 124: 80–89.

Xiao, L., L. Escalante, C. Yang, I. Sulaiman, A. A. Escalante, R. J. Montali et al. (1999). Phylogenetic analysis of *Cryptosporidium* parasites based on the small-subunit rRNA gene locus. Appl. Environ. Microbiol. 65: 1578–1583.

Yang, J. and T. Scholten. (1977). A fixative for intestinal parasites permitting the use of concentration and permanent staining procedures. Am. J. Clin. Pathol. 67: 300–304.

Yoo, J., J. Park, H. K. Lee, J. K. Yu, G. D. Lee, K. G. Park et al. (2019). Comparative evaluation of seegene allplex gastrointestinal, Luminex xTAG gastrointestinal pathogen panel, and BD MAX enteric assays for detection of gastrointestinal pathogens in clinical stool specimens. Arch. Pathol. Lab. Med. 143: 999–1005.

Youn, S., M. Kabir, R. Haque and W. A. Petri. (2009). Evaluation of a screening test for detection of *Giardia* and *Cryptosporidium*. Parasites. J. Clin. Microbiol. 47: 451–452.

Young, K. H., S. L. Bullock, D. M. Melvin and C. L. Spruill. (1979). Ethyl acetate as a substitute for diethyl ether in the formalin-ether sedimentation technique. J. Clin. Microbiol. 10: 852–853.

Zahedi, A., T. L. Greay, A. Paparini, K. L. Linge, C. A. Joll and U. M. Ryan. (2019). Identification of eukaryotic microorganisms with 18S rRNA next-generation sequencing in wastewater treatment plants, with a more targeted NGS approach required for *Cryptosporidium* detection. Water Res. 158: 301–312.

Zhan, Z., J. Guo, Y. Xiao, Z. He, X. Xia, Z. Huang et al. (2020). Comparison of BioFire FilmArray gastrointestinal panel versus Luminex xTAG Gastrointestinal Pathogen Panel (xTAG GPP) for diarrheal pathogen detection in China. Int. J. Infect. Dis. 99: 414–420.

Zhang, H., S. Morrison and Y. W. Tang. (2015). Multiplex polymerase chain reaction tests for detection of pathogens associated with gastroenteritis. Clin. Lab. Med. 35: 461–86.

Zierdt, W. S. (1984). Concentration and identification of *Cryptosporidium* sp. by use of a parasite concentrator. J. Clin. Microbiol. 20: 860–861

Zimmerman, S. K. and C. A. Needham. (1995). Comparison of conventional stool concentration and preserved-smear methods with Merifluor *Cryptosporidium/Giardia* Direct Immunofluorescence assay and ProSpecT Giardia EZ Microplate Assay for detection of *Giardia lamblia*. J. Clin. Microbiol. 33: 1942–1943.

Zu, S. X., J. F. Li, L. J. Barrett, R. Fayer, S. Y. Shu, J. F. McAuliffe et al. (1994). Seroepidemiologic study of *Cryptosporidium* infection in children from rural communities of Anhui, China and Fortaleza, Brazil. Am. J. Trop. Med. Hyg. 51: 1–10.

Chapter 3

Methods Used for Diagnosis of Malaria and their Strengths and Limitations

Samaly Souza Svigel,[1,*] *Venkatachalam Udhayakumar,*[1]
Michael Aidoo,[1] *Gireesh Subramaniam*[2] and
Naomi W. Lucchi[1]

Introduction

Malaria is a major vector-transmitted blood-borne disease with about 229 million reported cases globally in 2019 (WHO 2019b). The disease results from the infection of the host with protozoan parasites of the genus *Plasmodium*, intracellular parasites that reside mainly in the host's red blood cells (RBCs). Malaria in humans is caused by at least five *Plasmodium* species: *Plasmodium falciparum, Plasmodium vivax, Plasmodium malariae, Plasmodium ovale,* and *Plasmodium knowlesi*; currently considered a zoonotic malaria parasite restricted to Southeast Asia (WHO 2021b). At present, the control and prevention of malaria rely primarily on interventions for vector control as well as drugs for case management. Early diagnosis is important in disease management and critical for prompt treatment and preventing severe disease and mortality. The World Health Organization (WHO) recommends treatment of malaria based on confirmation of the presence of parasites, rather than by clinical symptoms only. Laboratory diagnosis is by morphologic identification of parasites in RBCs on stained blood smears and by detecting parasite antigens or DNA in the blood. This chapter discusses current malaria diagnostic tools including microscopy, rapid diagnostic tests (RDTs), and molecular methods highlighting use cases, their advantages, challenges, and limitations for diagnosis.

[1] Malaria Branch, Division of Parasitic Diseases and Malaria, Centers for Disease Control and Prevention, Atlanta, GA.
[2] Oak Ridge Institute for Science and Education (ORISE) Fellowship Program at Centers for Disease Control and Prevention, Atlanta, GA.
* Corresponding author: ynp4@cdc.gov

Microscopy-Based Malaria Diagnosis

Microscopic detection of malaria parasites in blood films stained with Giemsa is regarded as the "gold standard" method for malaria diagnosis by the WHO (WHO 1999). Microscopy is one of the most used methods for diagnosing malaria in the field and is essential for effective disease management and malaria surveillance (Berzosa et al. 2018). It is a cost-effective method that can differentiate the *Plasmodium* species as well as quantify parasite density, which is important for estimating disease severity and monitoring response to treatment. These features make it suitable for use as the standard method in evaluating the efficacy of antimalarial drugs in clinical trials and malaria epidemiological surveys. As microscopy remains the gold standard method for diagnosing malaria in many countries, it is the method against which other diagnostic tests are evaluated (Tangpukdee et al. 2009).

Microscopy-based diagnosis requires laboratory infrastructure that includes clean water, quality reagents, electricity or a good light source, and a binocular microscope capable of 1000X immersion oil magnification (Ojurongbe et al. 2013). In addition, a highly skilled microscopist is required to accurately identify the different life-cycle stages of the parasite in the smear and to distinguish the malaria parasite species. Therefore, the quality of microscopy depends on the existence and appropriate use of laboratory reagents and supplies as well as competent microscopists using a well-functioning microscope.

WHO recommends Giemsa staining for screening blood smears for malaria parasites. This staining technique was introduced in 1904 by Gustav Giemsa (Fleischer 2004). Giemsa stain is a mixture of acidic and basic stains (Eosin, Methylene Blue, and Azure), which optimizes visualization and distinction of the parasite and host cell features that are necessary for *Plasmodium species* identification. On Giemsa-stained blood smears, RBCs are pale red, parasite nuclear material stains red to purple-red while the cytoplasm stains blue. Schüffner's dots (morphologic features that appear as dots in infected erythrocytes that are specific to *Plasmodium ovale* and *Plasmodium vivax*) and other inclusions in the RBCs, stain red or pink and can be identified using Giemsa stain. Complete staining of the smear may be achieved within 20–30 minutes using a 5% Giemsa solution or up to 45–60 minutes with a 2.5% solution. For fast turnaround results, a 10% Giemsa solution can stain parasites in smears in about 10 minutes.

Other stains such as Wright's stain, which is a methanol-based staining that contains a mixture of Eosin and Methylene blue, can be used for staining malaria parasites in smears in approximately 3–5 minutes. With this stain, the malaria parasite cytoplasm appears pale blue, and the nuclear material stains red. However, Wright's stain is not optimal for blood parasites because Schüffner's dots and other inclusions in the RBCs usually do not stain or stain very pale. Wright's stain can be used if rapid results are needed but should be followed up with a confirmatory Giemsa stain when possible so that Schüffner's dots can be clearly identified, aiding in species identification (Garcia 2006).

Fresh blood from finger sticks is most commonly used to prepare malaria smears for microscopy. Blood collected with ethylenediaminetetraacetic acid (EDTA) anticoagulant is also acceptable but delays of an hour or more in preparing the smear may result in changes in parasite morphology and staining characteristics, which could decrease the accuracy of parasite detection and species identification (Garcia 2006). To identify the *Plasmodium species* and determine parasitemia, it is recommended that both thick and thin blood films be prepared for the examination. The thick and thin film can be made on the same slide to facilitate detection and species identification promptly and save on laboratory supplies. The thick blood film is prepared with two or three drops of blood and spread to make an even circular or rectangular 1 cm-wide film, generating several layers of erythrocytes (Figure 1).

Because thick films use a larger volume of blood, they are more useful for screening malaria parasites when parasitemia is expected to be low as well as detecting mixed infections in which one of the infecting species often occurs at a lower density. Thick smears require lysis of RBCs and therefore not ideal for species identification since the appearance of the RBC or the parasite in the RBC can be used to distinguish species.

The thin film is more appropriate for identifying *Plasmodium species* because preparation maintains RBCs in the smear and therefore allows identification of species-specific characteristics at different stages of the parasite's life cycle within the RBCs such as stippling (i.e., spots, dots, or clefts, representing the effect that the parasite has on the host cell, which is emphasized by Giemsa stain), malaria pigment (a granular by-product of parasite growth), as well as size and shape alterations of the RBC induced by the parasite. A summary of the key characteristics of the different malaria parasites is found in Figures 2 and 3 and Table 1.

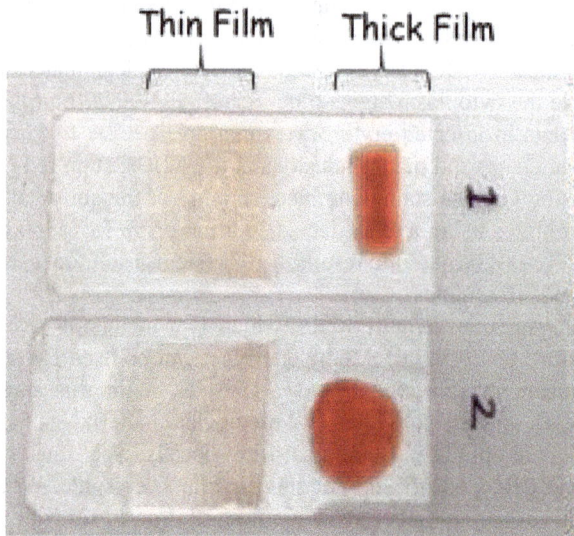

Figure 1. Thick and thin blood films on the same slide.
A circular or rectangular thick and thin smear can be made by adding 3–5 µL and 1–2 µL of blood, respectively.
Source: Malaria Laboratory Research and Development Team, CDC.

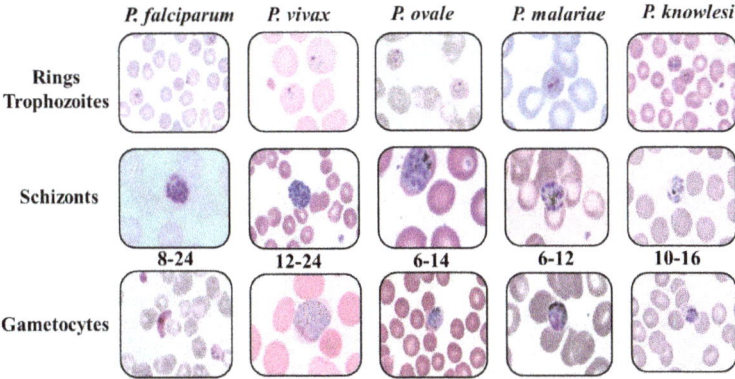

Figure 2. Malaria species and stages identification in thin smears.
Source: Division of Parasitic Disease, DPDx /CDC; numbers below the second row represent the range of merozoites within schizonts of specific *Plasmodium* species that can aid in species identification.

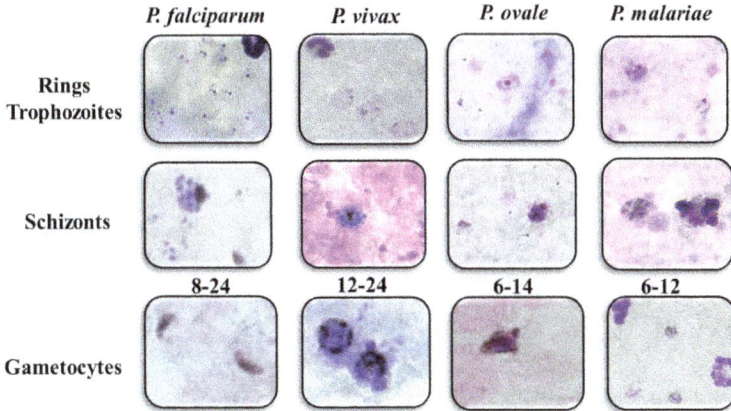

Figure 3. Malaria species and stages identification in thick smears.
Source: Division of Parasitic Disease, DPDx/CDC and WHO 2016*. The numbers below the second row represent the range of merozoites within schizonts of specific *Plasmodium* species that can aid in species identification. *Reference listed in the reference section.

Although microscopic diagnosis has many advantages for the management of malaria, there are some disadvantages to this method. It is labor-intensive and requires considerable expertise, particularly to accurately identify species at low parasitemia or in mixed malarial infections. At low compared to high parasite densities, microscopy has relatively low sensitivity.

An expert microscopist (WHO Level 1 certification) can typically detect as few as five parasites/µL, but this level of sensitivity is difficult to achieve in the clinical settings in endemic countries, where the workload is high, and time spent on a single slide is limited (WHO 2016). It has been estimated that a detection threshold of between 50–100 parasites/µL is operationally more practical in the field (Payne 1988, Tangpukdee et al. 2009).

Table 1. Key characteristics of different *Plasmodium* species.

Plasmodium species	Trophozoite	Schizont	Gametocytes
Plasmodium falciparum	**Size:** small to medium; ring common form; multiple infection of RBC; chromatin with one or two dots and delicate cytoplasm.	**Size:** small, compact; mature forms: 8-24 merozoites in compact cluster; dark pigment.	**Shape:** crescent or sausage shape; chromatin in a single mass (macrogametocyte) or diffuse (microgametocyte); dark pigment mass.
Plasmodium vivax	**Size:** small to large: rings usually thicker, with a single larger chromatin dot; developing trophozoites usually amoeboid in appearance..	**Size:** large; mature schizonts usually contain 12-24 merozoites; mature schizonts have coalesced pigment; Infected RBCs may be enlarged. Schüffner's dots may be present.	**Shape:** round to oval and usually fill host RBCs; chromatin: single, well defined; pigment is usually fine and evenly dispersed. Schüffner's dots may be seen
Plasmodium ovale	**Size:** may be smaller *than P. vivax*; trophozoites may start to become amoeboid, but not to the degree of *P. vivax*; elongation and fimbriation common be seen.	**Size:** round: mature schizonts usually have merozoites 6-14. Schüffner's dots may be seen; enlarged, but usually not as much as with *P. vivax*.	**Shape:** round to oval; enlarged, but not usually as big as *P. vivax* (1-1.25x normal RBC); pigment usually more coarse *than P. vivax*. Schüffner's dots may be seen.
Plasmodium malariae	**Size:** small; ring to rounded, compact form; elongate as they develop; may see 'basket' or 'band' forms; chromatin: single, large, may see 'bird's eye' forms; cytoplasm regular and dense.	**Size:** small, compact; mature schizonts have 6-12 merozoites; often in rosette-shaped patterns; pigment usually coalesced and centrally-located.	**Shape:** round compact; may be smaller than normal RBC; pigment usually coarse chromatin: single, well defined.
Plasmodium knowlesi	**Size:** : small to medium; Early ring-form trophozoites are similar to *P. falciparum*. rings may show double chromatin dots. Appliqué forms may appear, as well as rectangular rings harboring one or more accessory chromatin dots.	**Size:** small, compact. Sinton and Mulligan's stippling may be observed. 10-16 merozoites can be seen. The matures schizont fills the host RBC and the pigment collects into one or a few masses.	**Shape:** round compact; mature macrogametocytes are usually spherical and fill the host RBC. The cytoplasm stains blue and the nucleus stains red. The microgametocyte is smaller than the macrogametocyte. The cytoplasm usually stains a pale pink while the nucleus stains a darker red.

The reliable use of microscopic diagnosis for case management requires a well-developed quality management system that can be implemented across the health care system. However, this has been challenging in many endemic countries with limited resources. Therefore, in areas where good quality microscopy cannot be established or maintained, such as in remote areas, the use of malaria RDTs is recommended (WHO 2021a).

Malaria RDTs

Malaria RDTs are immunochromatographic tests that work by detecting specific malaria parasite antigens in a finger-prick blood specimen of an infected person. The development of RDTs began in the 1990s with the simplest and earliest version of an RDT being a dipstick. The time-to-results for many RDTs is between 20–30 minutes, and they are easy to perform with little technical training required to interpret the results, making RDTs viable options for use in field settings (WHO 2003).

The typical features of an RDT are presented in Figures 4A and 4B. RDTs use monoclonal antibodies against malaria antigen targets conjugated to gold particles in

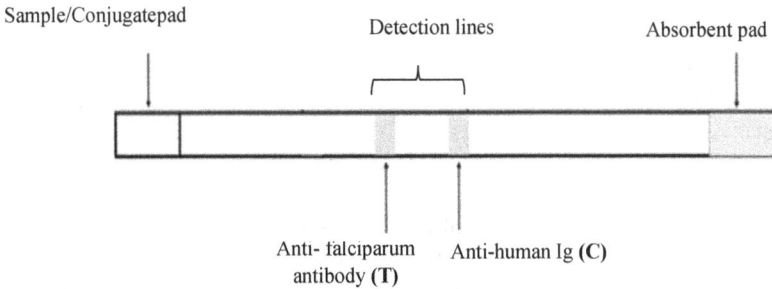

Figure 4A. Schematic diagram of typical features of a malaria RDT.

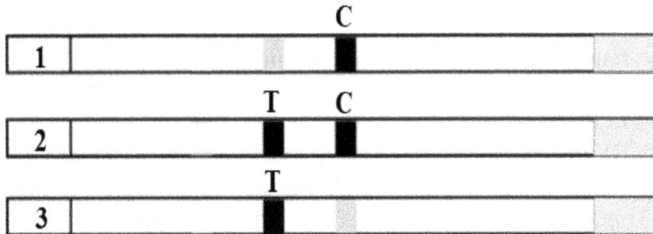

Figure 4B. Schematic diagram of examples of RDT results and interpretation.
1. Negative Result Control Line "C" appears in the results window.
2. Positive Result: Control Line "C"; Test line "T" appears in results window.
3. Invalid Result Control Line "C" does not appear in the results window The test is still classified as invalid irrespective of the appearance of the "T" line.

a pad (conjugate pad) adjacent to a sample pad. A second or third capture monoclonal antibody (forming a test band) is immobilized on a nitrocellulose strip. On addition of a positive sample to the sample well of a test followed by the addition of buffer, which lyses RBCs in the sample, parasite antigen (from blood) and antibody (from the conjugate pad) form an antigen/antibody complex that migrates in a liquid phase along the nitrocellulose strip, allowing the labeled antigen/antibody complex to be captured by the immobilized monoclonal antibody and thus producing a visible colored line (test line). A control line made of labeled anti-human immunoglobulin (Ig) captured on the nitrocellulose strip is incorporated to indicate adequate sample migration along the nitrocellulose strip. The test is considered valid only when this control line appears.

Malaria Antigens Used in the Current RDTs

There are three main Plasmodium antigens targeted by current RDTs: *P. falciparum*-specific histidine-rich protein-2 (HRP2), *Plasmodium* lactate dehydrogenase (pLDH), and aldolase (Barber et al. 2013). HRP2 is a water-soluble protein produced primarily by asexual blood-stage parasites and young gametocytes of only *P. falciparum* parasites (Rock et al. 1987). Therefore, HRP2-based RDTs are specific for the diagnosis of *P. falciparum* malaria. They are the most used RDTs mainly because *P. falciparum* is the most common species in sub-Saharan Africa where the malaria burden is the highest. They are also the most sensitive when compared to pLDH and aldolase-based RDTs because abundant quantities of HRP2 are produced by the parasite. Most of the pLDH and aldolase-based RDTs diagnose malaria at the genus level (pan-specific) because these antigens are highly conserved across the species of human malaria parasites (WHO 2004). Although most pLDH-based RDTs are pan-specific, commercial RDTs are now available that detect *P. falciparum* and *P. vivax*-specific LDH. Some RDTs combine two or more of these antigens, e.g., HRP2 and a pan-aldolase or pLDH specific to detect *P. falciparum* and non-*falciparum* infections. The availability of reliable commercial RDTs created a new momentum for evidence-based treatment as WHO revised its guidelines in 2010 advising treatment of malaria cases based on parasite-based diagnosis rather than symptoms. RDTs are now extensively used in Africa and in other regions in health centers where microscopy cannot be supported and by community health workers without the requisite training to perform microscopy. Globally, approximately 2.7 billion malaria RDTs were sold between 2010 and 2019 (WHO 2021c).

In order to ensure that quality RDTs are available for routine care, the WHO Global Malaria Programme 2008 established a quality assurance program for commercial RDTs in collaboration with Special Programme for Research and Training in Tropical Diseases (TDR), the Foundation for Innovative New Diagnostics (FIND), the U.S. Centers for Disease Control and Prevention (CDC), and other partners. This product evaluation program compares the performance of all RDT products submitted by manufacturers using a panel of well-characterized clinical samples assembled in a specimen bank established for this purpose. All the products are tested for their performance against a panel of parasite samples diluted to a low (200 parasites/µL)µL and a high (2,000 parasites/µL) parasite density; µLA panel detection score is determined for each test in an algorithm that accounts for inter- and intra-lot variation. The results from this evaluation along with procurement guidelines have been published annually since 2009 by the WHO (WHO 2018).

RDTs have some advantages over microscopy as a diagnostic tool, especially outside a laboratory setting. RDTs are simpler to perform with all items needed to obtain a result available in a kit and not requiring laboratory infrastructure, extraneous reagents, or electricity. Although storage in cool (20–25°C) conditions is preferred, most RDTs have been manufactured to withstand higher temperatures and can be shipped and stored at temperatures between 30 and 40°C. It is easy to train staff, including community-level volunteer workers, to perform this test. The test can be completed in less than 30 minutes with results available immediately for clinicians. The availability of many high-quality commercial RDTs has made it possible for the WHO to recommend RDTs as one of the primary diagnostic tools, along with microscopy, for case management. However, RDTs have limitations; they are only qualitative and therefore not suitable for detailed investigations such as treatment efficacy (Bell and Peeling 2006). The species-level diagnosis using RDTs is limited as non-falciparum parasites are identified only at the genus level except for in cases where tests detect *P. vivax*-specific LDH. The HRP2 protein persists for weeks after parasites are cleared following treatment and therefore can provide a false-positive diagnosis (Iqbal et al. 2004). In addition, recently it has been determined that *P. falciparum* parasites in some malaria-endemic countries have genes encoding

HRP2 and the paralogue HRP3 (*hrp2* and *hrp3*) deleted and therefore produce false-negative results on HRP2-based RDTs. Currently, the WHO recommends a switch from HRP2 to alternate target based RDT when a local prevalence of false negative RDTs exceeds 5% due to *pfhrp2* gene deletion among sysmptomatic cases (WHO 2019a). The current WHO RDT evaluation sets performance criteria at 200 parasite/μL because most malaria cases are typically characterized by densities higher than that threshold. However, a small proportion of cases present with low parasite densities, and RDT sensitivity is lower at such densities making it possible that some clinical cases with low-density parasitemia could be missed when RDTs are used (Bell et al. 2005, Cunningham et al. 2019). Given these limitations, there is a need for developing next generation RDTs with improved sensitivity and using target antigens other than HRP2. However, RDTs have been developed to identify clinical malaria cases typically associated with parasite densities higher than 200 parasite/μL.

Molecular Malaria Diagnostics

Nucleic acid-based tests (molecular tests) use various types of amplification techniques to detect parasite DNA (or RNA) usually from whole blood samples. Different types of malaria molecular tests have been developed which include conventional gel-based PCR assays, various types of real-time quantitative PCR (Roth et al. 2016), and non-PCR amplification assays such as the loop-mediated isothermal amplification (LAMP) that require single temperature (isothermal) heating rather than multiple thermal cycles (Lucchi et al. 2018). Molecular diagnosis is not typically used for routine diagnosis in endemic country health facilities as it is expensive, requires longer time-to-results and sophisticated laboratory support as well as higher levels of technical skills. However, molecular diagnosis is adopted in reference laboratories in developed countries for reconfirmation of malaria infection and species identification after initial testing by microscopy or RDTs. Most of the molecular tests for malaria parasite detection are used in research and surveillance studies for improving the sensitivity of parasite detection threshold and in vaccine trial settings for early detection of parasitemia in volunteers for early treatment. Here, we highlight various molecular diagnostic tests that have been developed and used in various contexts.

One of the first malaria PCR tests was based on the amplification of the *Plasmodium* 18S ribosomal RNA target, which typically exists in 5–8 copies depending on the species (Snounou and Singh 2002). To improve the sensitivity of the molecular tests, many researchers have utilized genome targets that are present in multiple copies such as the mitochondrial genome, the chromosomal sub-telomeric targets, telomere-associated repetitive element 2 (TARE-2), and var gene acidic terminal sequence (varATS) (Haanshuus et al. 2019). Many of the malaria molecular tests have been shown to have high (~ 90%) sensitivity and specificity (Roth et al. 2016). Although it is generally accepted that PCR-based tests are more sensitive than microscopy and RDTs until 2014, there was no defined parasite density threshold for an acceptable detection limit of malaria molecular test. In 2014, the WHO Evidence Review Group consultation on Malaria Diagnosis in Low Transmission settings recommended that molecular tests be able to detect a parasite density of at least two parasites/µL to be considered a "significant improvement" over expert microscopy (WHO 2014). This recommendation is for molecular tests used in surveillance studies and not for clinical management. Several molecular tests described to date have limits of detection equal to or less than two parasites/µl.

Brief Overview of Current Malaria Molecular Diagnostics

Gel-based PCR Tests

Both single-step and nested gel-based PCRs have been described for malaria parasite detection. The nested PCR described by Snounou et al., has been one of the most sensitive methods for many years since its development (Snounou and Singh 2002). The procedure consists of two rounds of PCR amplification in which the first genus-specific round of PCR detects any *Plasmodium* DNA, and the second PCRs amplify species-specific regions from the first-round PCR products. This necessitates the running of at least five rounds of PCR assays if detection of the four human infecting species (excluding *P. knowlesi*) is required: a genus PCR followed by four species-specific PCRs. The results from gel-based PCR tests require that the final PCR products are visualized on an agarose gel to qualitatively obtain positive or negative results. Alternative single-step gel-based PCR assays have been developed in place of the two-step nested PCR test (Demas et al. 2011); however, the nested PCR test has been demonstrated to be more sensitive (LoD of approximately 0.4 parasite/µL of blood) and ideal for the detection of mixed infections (Mixson-Hayden et al. 2010).

Real-time PCR

Real-time PCR assays allow quantification of parasite density based on the detection of a fluorescent signal emitted during the DNA amplification and measured, in real-time, by a thermal cycler combined with a fluorescence reader. Different fluorescence dyes have been utilized in real-time PCR assays: non-specific DNA intercalating dyes, such as SYBR Green dye, molecular probes such as TaqMan probes (Rougemont et al. 2004), and self-quenching fluorescence-labeled primers such as the Photoinduced electron transfer (PET)-PCR (Lucchi et al. 2014). Although intercalating dyes are easier and cheaper to use, these assays are not amenable to multiplexing allowing for the detection of mixed-species infections in fewer PCR tests. In contrast, the more commonly used probe-based detection tests are conducive to multiplexing and are widely used in research studies and diagnostic tests (Roth et al. 2016). Molecular probes are also utilized in real-time Quantitative Nucleic Acid Sequence Based Amplification (real-time QT-NASBA), an assay that amplifies parasite ribosomal RNA. As ribosomal RNA is more abundant in the parasite genome than DNA, QT-NASBA can detect lower parasite densities than DNA-based real-time PCR (Schneider et al. 2005). However, despite the wide variety of real-time PCR assays available, a combination of the need for sophisticated equipment, high cost, special handling of reagents, and longer turnaround times hinder their widespread adoption.

LAMP Assays

As recently reviewed (Lucchi et al. 2018) regarding the advent of isothermal tests, such as the LAMP-based tests, presented an opportunity to develop molecular tests for clinical diagnosis in point-of-care settings as well as for use under field environments. LAMP is a nucleic acid amplification technique that utilizes isothermal reaction conditions, multiple primer sets, and a polymerase with strand displacement capabilities that allow for DNA amplification without the need for thermal cycling. The pioneer LAMP assays detected the formation of magnesium pyrophosphate, a visible precipitate by-product of the amplification, as an indicator of a positive sample (Khairnar et al. 2009). Adaptations of LAMP include the use of fluorescence dyes to allow for real-time LAMP detection (Real Amp) and a variety of colorimetric LAMP assays that use color change as a readout (Lucchi et al. 2018). In addition, high-throughput LAMP platforms have been described that allow for large-scale surveillance studies (Britton et al. 2015). Many of the malaria LAMP assays have similar sensitivities compared to PCR (96–98%) which makes LAMP assays a viable alternative molecular test for malaria parasite detection (Lucchi et al. 2018).

Potential Roles for Molecular Tests in Malaria Diagnosis

Both microscopy and conventional RDTs continue to be the tests of choice for the clinical management of microscopically detectable levels of infection associated with acute malaria illness. Malaria molecular tests will likely play a significant role in enabling the detection of low-density infections that are beyond the limits of the detection of RDTs and microscopy in research settings. They also have potential applications in the clinical diagnosis in developed non-endemic countries and focused investigations in elimination settings, such as detect-and-treat approaches, gametocyte detection, and controlled human malaria infection used in vaccine development (Aydin-Schmidt et al. 2014, Cook et al. 2015, Morris et al. 2015, Mwingira et al. 2014). In addition, molecular tests will be used in research activities as reference tests when the evaluation of a new test is needed and as confirmatory tests in reference laboratories. The availability of cost-effective and easy to perform molecular assays can provide a test of choice for case management in facilities that lack skilled microscopists or quality microscopes or in regions where the use of HRP2-based RDTs is inappropriate due to the high prevalence of *hrp2/3* deletions, if alternative RDTs are not available. Commercially available malaria molecular tests, including the LAMP tests, can be utilized as a confirmatory test, especially in non-malaria-endemic countries where imported malaria cases require diagnostic confirmation.

Strengths and Limitations of Malaria Molecular Tests

Molecular tests have revolutionized pathogen detection and identification by offering high sensitivity and specificity. Malaria molecular tests allow for the accurate identification of the infecting species and detection of parasite densities that are well below the limits of detection of both microscopy and RDTs. As described earlier in this chapter, some situations require the use of very sensitive tests. However, the cost, time-to-results, technical support, and training required for most molecular tests pose challenges to their implementation in many malaria-endemic countries where testing is done close to the point of care including within communities by village health workers. A comparison between malaria diagnostic tests is summarized in Table 2.

Table 2. Comparison of test parameters between microscopy, RDTs, and molecular assays for the diagnosis of malaria.

Parameter/consideration	Microscopy	RDTs	Molecular		
			Nested PCR	Real-time PCR	Isothermal amplification
Limits of detection (parasites/μL)	4–100	> 100	1–10	0.01–40	1–100
Sensitivity, by reference test (%)					
Microscopy	–	86.5–97.2	95.7[1]	99.41	96.7
RDT		–			
PCR	86.2–88	83.7–85.2			
Specificity, by reference test (%)					
Microscopy	–	71.0–91.7	91.7	90.88	91.7
RDT		-			
PCR	99.6–100	99.3			
Time to obtain results	< 3 hours	20–30 minutes	> 8 hours	3–4 hours	1–2 hours
Start-up costs for equipment (USD, $)*		None	3,000–8,000	15,000–> 40,000	6,344[#]
Cost per patient/sample (USD, $)**	0.32–1.27	0.60–1.20	3.67	5–10	2.66–5.05
Training and skill level requirements	Medium	Low	High	High	Medium
Quantitative results provided	Yes	No	No	Yes	No

References: (Hopkins et al. 2008, Khairnar et al. 2009, Lucchi et al. 2010, McMorrow et al. 2011, Payne 1988, Shillcutt et al. 2008, Stauffer et al. 2009, WHO 1988).

* Refers to the cost of buying the equipment as listed by various major suppliers in the USA; note that the cost will vary greatly depending on specifications.

Refers to the price we paid for the equipment.

** Cost includes all the necessary reagents and consumables; it does not include personnel cost; note that the cost will vary greatly depending on specifications.

In summary, molecular tests, especially the simpler tests such as the LAMP assays, provide alternative accurate, and sensitive options for the detection of malaria parasites in some select settings and particular use cases. The optimal molecular test(s) will require consideration of the acceptable balance between the analytical sensitivity required, cost, and the turnaround time needed for the interventions that can be administered based on test results. There is a need for highly sensitive point-of-care diagnostic tools with LoDs below that for current PoC tests as well as high-throughput tools for surveillance; all these considerations will direct the ultimate utility of malaria molecular tests.

Conclusion

The multiple methods for malaria diagnosis have use cases in which one or the other is advantageous. Microscopy and RDTs continue to remain primary diagnostic tests for case management in most countries. Other tests may be applied for diagnostic confirmation in reference laboratories, surveillance, or research and such tests described in this chapter can all be improved to make them more sensitive, specific, and cost-effective. Deploying the tests to maximize their usefulness, therefore, requires an in-depth understanding of the tests, their advantages as well as limitations.

Acknowledgments

The authors would like to thank the DPDx team for reviewing this manuscript and also for providing the malaria parasite figures.

Financial support: Not applicable.

Disclaimer: This Book Chapter has the objective to provide an overview of malaria diagnosis tools' strengths and limitations. The content in this report does not necessarily represent the official position of the Centers for Disease Control and Prevention.

References

Aydin-Schmidt, B., W. Xu, I. J. González, S. D. Polley, D. Bell, D. Shakely et al. (2014). Loop mediated isothermal amplification (LAMP) accurately detects malaria DNA from filter paper blood samples of low density parasitaemias. PloS One 9(8): e103905.

Barber, B. E., T. William, M. J. Grigg, K. Piera, T. W. Yeo, N. M. Anstey et al. (2013). Evaluation of the sensitivity of a pLDH-based and an aldolase-based rapid diagnostic test for diagnosis of uncomplicated and severe malaria caused by PCR-confirmed *Plasmodium knowlesi, Plasmodium falciparum*, and *Plasmodium vivax*. Journal of Clinical Microbiology 51(4): 1118–1123.

Bell, D. and R. W. Peeling. (2006). Evaluation of rapid diagnostic tests: Malaria. Nature Reviews Microbiology 4(9): S34–S38.

Bell, D. R., D. W. Wilson and L. B. Martin. (2005). False-positive results of a *Plasmodium falciparum* histidine-rich protein 2–detecting malaria rapid diagnostic test due to high sensitivity in a community with fluctuating low parasite density. The American Journal of Tropical Medicine and Hygiene 73(1): 199–203.

Berzosa, P., A. de Lucio, M. Romay-Barja, Z. Herrador, V. González, L. García et al. (2018). Comparison of three diagnostic methods (microscopy, RDT, and PCR) for the detection of malaria parasites in representative samples from Equatorial Guinea. Malaria Journal 17(1): 1–12.

Britton, S., Q. Cheng, C. J. Sutherland and J. S. McCarthy. (2015). A simple, high-throughput, colourimetric, field applicable loop-mediated isothermal amplification (HtLAMP) assay for malaria elimination. Malaria Journal 14(1): 1–12.

Cook, J., B. Aydin-Schmidt, I. J. González, D. Bell, E. Edlund, M. Nassor et al. (2015). Loop-mediated isothermal amplification (LAMP) for point-of-care detection of asymptomatic low-density malaria parasite carriers in Zanzibar. Malaria Journal 14(1): 1–6.

Cunningham, J., S. Jones, M. L. Gatton, J. W. Barnwell, Q. Cheng, P. L. Chiodini et al. (2019). A review of the WHO malaria rapid diagnostic test product testing programme (2008–2018): Performance, procurement and policy. Malaria Journal 18(1): 1–15.

Demas, A., J. Oberstaller, J. DeBarry, N. W. Lucchi, G. Srinivasamoorthy, D. Sumari et al. (2011). Applied genomics: Data mining reveals species-specific malaria diagnostic targets more sensitive than 18S rRNA. Journal of Clinical Microbiology 49(7): 2411–2418.

Fleischer, B. (2004). 100 years ago: Giemsa's solution for staining of plasmodia. Tropical Medicine and International Health 9(7): 755–756.

Garcia, L. S. (2006). Diagnostic Medical Parasitology: American Society for Microbiology Press.

Haanshuus, C. G., K. Mørch, B. Blomberg, G. E. A. Strøm, N. Langeland, K. Hanevik et al.(2019). Assessment of malaria real-time PCR methods and application with focus on low-level parasitaemia. PloS One 14(7): e0218982.

Hopkins, H., L. Bebell, W. Kambale, C. Dokomajilar, P. J. Rosenthal, G. Dorsey et al. (2008). Rapid diagnostic tests for malaria at sites of varying transmission intensity in Uganda. The Journal of Infectious Diseases 197(4): 510–518.

Iqbal, J., A. Siddique, M. Jameel and P. R. Hira. (2004). Persistent histidine-rich protein 2, parasite lactate dehydrogenase, and panmalarial antigen reactivity after clearance of Plasmodium falciparum monoinfection. Journal of Clinical Microbiology 42(9): 4237–4241.

Khairnar, K., D. Martin, R. Lau, F. Ralevski and D. R. Pillai. (2009). Multiplex real-time quantitative PCR, microscopy and rapid diagnostic immuno-chromatographic tests for the detection of *Plasmodium* spp: Performance, limit of detection analysis and quality assurance. Malaria Journal 8(1): 1–17.

Lucchi, N. W., A. Demas, J. Narayanan, D. Sumari, A. Kabanywanyi, S. P. Kachur et al. (2010). Real-time fluorescence loop mediated isothermal amplification for the diagnosis of malaria. PloS One 5(10): e13733.

Lucchi, N. W., M. A. Karell, I. Journel, E. Rogier, I. Goldman, D. Ljolje et al. (2014). PET-PCR method for the molecular detection of malaria parasites in a national malaria surveillance study in Haiti, 2011. Malaria Journal 13(1): 1–5.

Lucchi, N. W., D. Ndiaye, S. Britton and V. Udhayakumar. (2018). Expanding the malaria molecular diagnostic options: opportunities and challenges for loop-mediated isothermal amplification tests for malaria control and elimination. Expert Review of Molecular Diagnostics 18(2): 195–203.

McMorrow, M., M. Aidoo and S. Kachur. (2011). Malaria rapid diagnostic tests in elimination settings— can they find the last parasite? Clinical Microbiology and Infection 17(11): 1624–1631.

Mixson-Hayden, T., N. W. Lucchi and V. Udhayakumar. (2010). Evaluation of three PCR-based diagnostic assays for detecting mixed Plasmodium infection. BMC Research Notes 3(1): 1–7.

Morris, U., M. Khamis, B. Aydin-Schmidt, A. K. Abass, M. I. Msellem, M. H. Nassor et al. (2015). Field deployment of loop-mediated isothermal amplification for centralized mass-screening of asymptomatic malaria in Zanzibar: A pre-elimination setting. Malaria Journal 14(1): 1–6.

Mwingira, F., B. Genton, A. -N. M. Kabanywanyi and I. Felger. (2014). Comparison of detection methods to estimate asexual Plasmodium falciparum parasite prevalence and gametocyte carriage in a community survey in Tanzania. Malaria Journal 13(1): 1–8.

Ojurongbe, O., O. O. Adegbosin, S. S. Taiwo, O. A. T. Alli, O. A. Olowe, T. A. Ojurongbe et al. (2013). Assessment of clinical diagnosis, microscopy, rapid diagnostic tests, and polymerase chain reaction in the diagnosis of Plasmodium falciparum in Nigeria. Malaria Research and Treatment, 2013.

Payne, D. (1988). Use and limitations of light microscopy for diagnosing malaria at the primary health care level. Bulletin of the World Health Organization 66(5): 621.

Rock, E., K. Marsh, A. Saul, T. Wellems, D. W. Taylor, W. Maloy et al. (1987). Comparative analysis of the Plasmodium falciparum histidine-rich proteins HRP-I, HRP-II and HRP-III in malaria parasites of diverse origin. Parasitology 95(2): 209–227.

Roth, J. M., D. A. Korevaar, M. M. Leeflang and P. F. Mens. (2016). Molecular malaria diagnostics: A systematic review and meta-analysis. Critical Reviews in Clinical Laboratory Sciences 53(2): 87–105.

Rougemont, M., M. Van Saanen, R. Sahli, H. P. Hinrikson, J. Bille and K. Jaton. (2004). Detection of four Plasmodium species in blood from humans by 18S rRNA gene subunit-based and species-specific real-time PCR assays. Journal of Clinical Microbiology 42(12): 5636–5643.

Schneider, P., L. Wolters, G. Schoone, H. Schallig, P. Sillekens, R. Hermsen et al. (2005). Real-time nucleic acid sequence-based amplification is more convenient than real-time PCR for quantification of Plasmodium falciparum. Journal of Clinical Microbiology 43(1): 402–405.

Shillcutt, S., C. Morel, C. Goodman, P. Coleman, D. Bell, C. J. Whitty et al. (2008). Cost-effectiveness of malaria diagnostic methods in sub-Saharan Africa in an era of combination therapy. Bulletin of the World Health Organization 86: 101–110.

Snounou, G. and B. Singh. (2002). Nested PCR analysis of Plasmodium parasites. In Malaria Methods and Protocols (pp. 189–203): Springer.

Stauffer, W. M., C. P. Cartwright, D. A. Olson, B. A. Juni, C. M. Taylor, S. H. Bowers et al. (2009). Diagnostic performance of rapid diagnostic tests versus blood smears for malaria in US clinical practice. Clinical Infectious Diseases 49(6): 908–913.

Tangpukdee, N., C. Duangdee, P. Wilairatana and S. Krudsood. (2009). Malaria diagnosis: A brief review. The Korean Journal of Parasitology, 47(2): 93.

WHO. (1988). Malaria diagnosis: Memorandum from a WHO meeting. Bulletin of the World Health Organization (WHO) 66(5): 575–594.

WHO. (1999). New Perspectives Malaria Diagnosis. Report of a Joint WHO/USAID Informal Consultation. Retrieved from https://www.who.int/tdr/publications/documents/malaria-diagnosis.pdf.

WHO. (2003). Malaria Rapid Diagnosis Making it Work. Retrieved from https://www.who.int/malaria/publications/atoz/rdt2.pdf?ua=1.

WHO. (2004). Malaria Rapid Diagnostic Tests. Retrieved from https://apps.who.int/iris/bitstream/handle/10665/206940/9290610883_en.pdf?sequence=2&isAllowed=y.

WHO. (2014). WHO Evidence Review Group on Malaria Diagnosis in Low Transmission Settings. Malaria Policy Advisory Committee Meeting 12-14 March 2014, WHO HQ, Geneva. Retrieved from https://www.who.int/malaria/mpac/mpac_mar2014_diagnosis_low_transmission_settings_report.pdf?ua=1.

WHO. (2016). Malaria Microscopy Quality Assurance Manual-version 2: World Health Organization.

WHO. (2018). Malaria rapid diagnostic test performance: Results of WHO product testing of malaria RDTs: round 8 (2016–2018).

WHO. (2019a). Response plan to pfhrp2 gene deletions. Retrieved from https://www.who.int/publications/i/item/WHO-CDS-GMP-2019.02.

WHO. (2019b). World Malaria Report 2019. Retrieved from https://www.who.int/publications/i/item/9789241565721.

WHO. (2021a). Global Malaria Programme. Retrieved from https://www.who.int/teams/global-malaria-programme/case-management/diagnosis/.

WHO. (2021b). Malaria Key facts. Retrieved from https://www.who.int/news-room/fact-sheets/detail/malaria.

WHO. (2021c). Statement by the Malaria Policy Advisory Group on the urgent need to address the high prevalence of pfhrp2/3 gene deletions in the Horn of Africa and beyond. Retrieved from https://www.who.int/news/item/28–05–2021-statement-by-the-malaria-policy-advisory-group-on-the-urgent-need-to-address-the-high-prevalence-of-pfhrp2–3-gene-deletions-in-the-horn-of-africa-and-beyond.

Chapter 4

Advances in the Diagnosis of Filarial Nematodes

Arwa Elaagip[1] and *Tarig Higazi*[2,*]

Introduction

The phylum Nematoda (roundworms) includes many successful tissue-dwelling parasites of major public health and socio-economic importance. Filarial nematodes belong to the superfamily Filarioidea, and many filarial worms cause chronic and profoundly debilitating diseases in both humans and animals (Tritten et al. 2014). Human filarial nematodes include *Wuchereria bancrofti*, *Brugia malayi*, *Brugia timori*, *Loa loa*, *Onchocerca volvulus*, *Mansonella perstans*, *Mansonella ozzardi*, and *Mansonella streptocerca* (Mathison et al. 2019) (Table 1).

Filarial nematodes cause a variety of clinical manifestations in the human host, ranging from asymptomatic infection to lymphedema (*W. bancrofti* and *Brugia* spp.), dermatitis, and subcutaneous nodules (*O. volvulus*), and ocular involvement (*L. loa* and *O. volvulus*) (Bennuru et al. 2018). Infections of many filarial nematodes such as *W. bancrofti*, *Brugia* species (lymphatic filariasis or LF), and *O. volvulus* (onchocerciasis or River blindness) are considered major neglected tropical diseases in the tropics with tremendous health and socio-economic consequences that affect the poorest communities in developing countries (Ricciardi and Ndao 2014). Other filarial parasite species from the genus *Mansonella* that produce chronic human microfilaremia: *M. ozzardi*, *M. perstans*, and *M. streptocerca* cause mansonellosis in Africa, the Caribbean, and South and Central America. However, the disease is typically either asymptomatic or associated with mild pathologies, and it is not considered a major public health threat (Ta-Tang et al. 2021). A complicating feature of *Mansonella* infections, however, is that their geographic distribution overlap with that of other filarial diseases that may have similar clinical manifestations.

---

[1] Department of Parasitology and Medical Entomology, Faculty of Medical Laboratory Sciences, University of Khartoum, Khartoum, Sudan.
[2] Ohio University, 1425 Newark Rd, Zanesville OH 43701, USA.
* Corresponding author: higazi@ohio.edu

Table 1. Human filarial parasites: A summary of location in host, clinical symptoms, disease vectors, anddiagnostic methods.

Parasite/Disease	Location of Adults/ Microfilariae	Clinical Symptoms	Arthropod Vectors	Diagnostic Methods	References
Brugia malayi and *B. timori*/ Lymphatic Filariasis LF; also known as Elephantiasis	Lymphatics/Blood	Lymphoedema, swollen legs, thick skin	Mosquitoes: *Anopheles*, *Mansonia*[1]	Microscopy and concentration technique Ultrasonography Enzyme-linked immunosorbent assay (ELISA) *Brugia* Rapid™ antibody-detection test Alere™ Filaria Test Strip (FTS) ICT SD BIOLIN LF IgG4 test SD BIOLIN Onchocerciasis/LF IgG4 Biplex test Diagnostic test (RDT) PCR and RT-PCR LAMP	WHO 1997, CLSI 2000, Dreyer et al. 1998, Lammie et al. 2004, Rahmah et al. 2003, Weil et al. 2013, Rahumatullah et al. 2019, Kamatchi et al. 2016, Buchan and Ledeboer 2014, Drame et al. 2014, Laney et al. 2008, Poole et al. 2017, Nancy et al. 2021
Wuchereria bancrofti/ Lymphatic Filariasis LF; also known as Elephantiasis	Lymphatics/Blood	Lymphoedema, swollen legs, thick skin, hydrocele	Mosquitoes: *Culex*, *Anopheles*, *Aedes*	Microscopy and Knott's concentration technique Ultrasonography Filariasis Cellab ELISA Tropbio Og4C3 Filariasis Ag ELISA Alere™ FTS SD BIOLIN LF IgG4 test SD BIOLIN Onchocerciasis/LF IgG4 Biplex test LIPS ELISA PCR/RT-PCR LAMP	WHO 1997, CLSI 2000, Dreyer et al. 1998, Joseph et al. 2011, PATH 2017, Chandrashekar et al. 1994, Hamlin et al. 2012, Masson et al. 2017, Weil et al. 1997, Rahumatullah et al. 2019, Rahman et al. 2019, Kamatchi et al. 2016, Takagi et al. 2011, Laney et al. 2010, Poole et al. 2017, Nancy et al. 2021

Table 1 contd.....

Disease	Location	Symptoms	Vector	Diagnostic techniques	References
Loa loa/ Loaiasis also known as African eye worm	Subcutaneous tissue/Blood	Dermatitis, itchy skin, adult worms in conjunctivitis	Deer flies: *Chrysops* sp.	Microscopy and concentration technique; Direct exam of the eye; Mobile phone-based video-microscopy; LIPS; LFA; PCR + real-time PCR; LAMP	Harnett et al. 1998, D'Ambrosio et al. 2015, Herzog-Neto et al. 2014, Burbelo et al. 2008, Pedram et al. 2017, Drame et al. 2017, Drame et al. 2014, Alhassan et al. 2015
Onchocerca volvulus/ Onchcocerciasis also known as River Blindness	Subcutaneous tissue/skin	Dermatitis, itchy skin, depigmentation, blindness	Black flies: *Simulium* sp.	Microscopy and concentration technique; Skin snips biopsies; Slit-lamp eye examination; Nodule palpation; Anti-helminthic DEC patch; Ultrasonography; ELISA e.g. Ov-16 assay; LIPS; AMRAD ICT; SD BIOLIN onchocerciasis IgG4 rapid test; SD BIOLIN Onchocerciasis/LF IgG4 Biplex test; PCR e.g. O-150 assay; Real-time PCR; MicroRNA (miRNA); LAMP	WHO 1997, Herzog-Neto et al. 2014, Toé et al. 2000, Ngoumou and Walsh 1993, Mand et al. 2005, Harentt et al. 1998, Lobos et al. 1990, Umasch et al. 2018, Nde et al. 2002, Burbelo et al. 2008, Weil et al. 2000, Meredith et al. 1991, Toé et al. 1994, Lloyd et al. 2015, Thiele et al. 2016, Tritten et al. 2014, Poole et al. 2017, Nancy et al. 2021
Mansonella streptocerca and *M. ozzardi*/ Mansonellosis	Subcutaneous tissue/Skin[2] and blood	Generally asymptomatic, Dermatitis and itchy skin[3]	Biting midges: *Culicoides* sp. Black flies[4]: *Simulium* sp.	Microscopy and concentration technique; Skin snips biopsies; Nested PCR	WHO 1997; CLSI 2000; Joseph et al. 2011; Fischer et al. 1996; Morales-Hojas et al. 2001
Mansonella perstans/ Mansonellosis	Body cavity/Blood	Generally asymptomatic	Biting midges: *Culicoides* spp.	Microscopy and concentration technique; Nested PCR	WHO 1997, Joseph et al. 2011, Jiménez et al. 2011

[1] Mosquito vector for *Brugia malayi* only.
[2] Microfilariae of *Mansonella streptocerca* only.
[3] Symptoms for *M. ozzardi* only.
[4] For *M. streptocerca* only.

Filarial parasites are highly prevalent in regions of Africa, Asia, South and Central America, and the Yemen peninsula, and contribute to a total of 120 million infections worldwide (Vanhamme et al. 2020). The global disease burden of human onchocerciasis was recently estimated at 20.9 million infected people (99% of them living in sub-Saharan Africa) with 90 million at risk (James et al. 2018) and the World Health Organization (WHO) has extended its efforts to eliminate the disease to all endemic African countries through mass drug administration (MDA) at the community level with the goal of eliminating 80% of the disease in sub-Saharan Africa by 2025. Lymphatic filariasis accounted for an estimated 50 million cases (as of 2018), while 893 million people in 50 countries worldwide remain threatened by infection and require preventive chemotherapy (WHO 2020). The WHO has initiated a global program [Global Program to Eliminate Lymphatic Filariasis (GPELF)] to eliminate LF as a public health problem based on MDA, and the target year to achieve this objective has recently been set to 2030 instead of 2020. These worldwide ongoing programs have significantly reduced the burden of filarial infections worldwide.

Biology and Life Cycle of Filarial Nematodes

All human filarial nematodes have similar patterns to their life cycles, and it is helpful to have an understanding of these patterns to appreciate several key diagnostic aspects of infection. Adult worms reside in various tissues of the definitive host, including the lymphatics (*W. bancrofti, Brugia* spp.) and subcutaneous tissue (*L. loa, O. volvulus*) (Foster et al. 2013) while adults and larvae of some species may migrate to the eyes (*L. loa, O. volvulus*). Mated females release microfilariae (mf, L1 larva) into the blood or surrounding subcutaneous tissue, where they are picked up by an appropriate insect vector while taking a blood meal. A variety of blood-feeding flies serve as vectors of filarial nematodes, including mosquitoes (*W. bancrofti* and *Brugia* spp.), black flies (*O. volvulus*), and deer flies (*L. loa*) (Table 1). Microfilariae penetrate the midgut of the vector and migrate to the musculature where they develop into infectious L3 (third-stage, or filariform) larvae. The L3 larvae migrate to the fly's mouthparts and infect a new host when the vector takes a blood meal (Mathison et al. 2019).

Host immunological reactions encapsulate adult female *O. volvulus* in fibrous nodules which are palpable when present over bony structures. A major cause of *O. volvulus* pathology is the hosts' reactions upon the death of microfilariae which manifests primarily as itching, skin lesions and depigmentation, and visual impairment that can progress to blindness in older individuals (Remme et al. 2007). The majority of LF, also known as elephantiasis, infections are due to *W. bancrofti*. These filarial parasites that live in the lymphatic tissue and release their microfilaria in the blood with predicted periodicity, can disrupt lymphatic function and lead to long-term disability due to lymphedema (most commonly swollen lower limbs) and scrotal hydrocele (Taylor et al. 2010). Clinical symptoms due to *L. loa* infection are generally mild and include angioedema known as Calabar edema believed to be caused by the migration of adult worm in the skin and ocular passage of the adult worm (also known as an eye worm) under the conjunctiva (Akue et al. 2018) (Table 1).

Diagnosis of Filarial Nematodes

Accurate and sensitive detection of filarial nematodes is essential for the treatment, implementation, and evaluation of MDA and surveillance programs. Determining the infection levels in vector populations is also important for assessing transmission, deciding when drug treatments may be terminated, and monitoring recrudescence (Poole et al. 2017). In addition, mixed infections with more than one filarial nematode can be common in areas of endemicity. In Africa, for instance, mixed infections usually involve *M. perstans* and/or another species. It is important to assess each patient for potential co-infections based on their geographic exposures, as the presence of more than one filarial species may present a diagnostic challenge; when *L. loa* is present, it may change the therapeutic options. Patients with high levels of *L. loa* microfilaremia are at risk of severe and often fatal, neurologic manifestations following ivermectin or diethylcarbamazine (DEC) administration; thus, these drugs should not be administered for therapy of other filarial infections in the presence of *L. loa* co-infection (Mathison et al. 2019).

Several methods exist for diagnosing filarial infections (Table 2). Microscopy-based parasitological diagnosis (reviewed in Mathison et al. 2019) has been the gold standard for the detection of filarial parasites for a long time with several limitations, such as the low sensitivity, laboriousness, requirement of expertise to perform, lack of throughput capability, and inconvenience for patients. For these reasons, considerable work has been done to develop and expand the use of advanced forms of diagnosis, in particular immunoassays and molecular-based assays for detecting parasite DNA (Harnett et al. 1998, Ricciardi and Ndao 2014, Poole et al. 2019). Immunoassays have been used to complement microscopy for many years. These assays rely on antigen or antibody detection from the provided patient samples (Table 1). Rapid diagnostic tests (RDTs) have recently become some of the most popular serology-based assays (Houze et al. 2013, Hawes et al. 2014) in the detection of parasitic infections due to their potential to be used in field settings, however, cross-reactivity issues have been reported (Poole et al. 2017). More recently, there has been a focus on the development of molecular diagnostic techniques (Ndao 2009, Muldrew 2009). Nucleic acid-based molecular assays (Table 2) offer high levels of specificity and sensitivity and can be used to detect infection in both humans and vectors (Poole et al. 2017), in addition to the detection of simultaneous infections with multiple parasites (Shokoples et al. 2009). Furthermore, new and innovative diagnostic tools are constantly being tested (Ricciardi and Ndao 2014).

Traditional/Standard Diagnosis

Traditionally, diagnosis of filarial parasitic infections is based on morphological identification of mf in skin biopsies (onchocerciasis) and blood samples (lymphatic filariasis and loiasis), as well as insect vectors using light microscopy. The slit-lamp eye examination is used for the identification of *O. volvulus* mf in patients with eye disease. Direct examination of the eye and palpation of skin nodules formed by the host can also be helpful in the identification of *L. loa* and *O. volvulus* adult parasites

Table 2. Characteristics of current methods used for diagnosis of filarial infections.

Method	Major Advantages	Major Disadvantages	Suitability for Clinical Setting/ Elimination Programs	Comments
Parasitological	Low cost, suitable for poor endemic countries	Require some training, laborious and low sensitivity in treated and amicrofilaremic individuals, and specific time for sample collection	Yes/No	The historic gold standard, a minimal role in monitoring elimination programs
Immunological	Based on antigen or antibody capture, feasible pool and high throughput screening, rapid format and point-of-care available	No distinction between present and past infection, limited specificity (cross-reaction)	Limited/Yes[1]	Antigen detection is the current gold standard for LF, which WHO recommended for children
Nucleic acid-based				WHO recommended
PCR	High sensitivity and specificity, amenable to pool screening and multiplexing	Require training, reagents, equipment, and purified DNA, sensitive to inhibitors in the sample	Limited/Yes[1]	Amenable to improvement, suitable for insect vectors
LAMP	No major equipment, can be a single step, can use semi-purified DNA, can be multiplexed, can be used in the field, near point-of-care	Complex primer/ probe design, some tests need multiple enzymes, require DNA extraction	Limited/Yes[1]	Most recent and advanced, amenable to improvement

[1] Diagnostic value based on sensitivity and specificity.

respectively. While morphological interpretation is a valuable technique, it requires substantial expertise as well as being time-consuming, and subjective. Issues with sensitivity, specificity, and inefficiency in the detection of low infection densities are also seen with these techniques (Table 2). Because mf prevalence decreases in response to MDA, screening blood pools has become a necessary and cost-effective procedure. However, this method is more likely to produce false-negative results in low mf carriers that may still be infectious to competent insect vectors. In addition, the major drawback that all parasitological strategies share is that they cannot detect infection until many months or even more than one year after the infection has been initiated (Ramzy 2002). This will lead to the absence or delay in therapeutic intervention for infected individuals, which are unwelcome implications for disease transmission and monitoring of MDA and insecticide-based control programs. Despite these limitations, parasitological diagnosis remains a popular method due to its low cost and suitability for laboratories with limited resources.

Microscopic Detection of Microfilariae

Microscopy remains the cornerstone of diagnostic laboratory testing for filarial parasites. The microscopic examination of thick and thin peripheral blood smears stained with Giemsa or other appropriate stains is used for the detection of many parasitic infections, including the filarial nematodes species (i.e., *Brugia*, *Mansonella*, and *Wuchereria*) (CLSI 2000). Examination of blood smears is less sensitive but acceptable and has better sensitivity than a biopsy and histological evaluation (Dietrich et al. 2019).

Proper collection and processing of blood specimens are essential for a reliable diagnosis. The mf of some species of filarial nematodes exhibit periodicity in which they circulate in the blood predominately at certain times of the day. The time of circulation corresponds with the primary times that the insect vector takes its blood meal; it is important to obtain blood specimens during these periods. *Wuchereria bancrofti* and the *Brugia* species exhibit nocturnal periodicity, *L. loa* exhibits diurnal periodicity, and *Mansonella* sp. do not exhibit specific periodicity (Mathison et al. 2019). Mf can be detected from either venous blood or finger-prick blood. The commonly used diagnostic methods for the detection of mf include the thick smear, three-line thick smear, Knott's concentration technique, and membrane filtration (Joseph et al. 2011).

Morphological identification of microfilariae (reviewed in Mathison et al. 2019) is used to separate sympatric closely related species. For example, *B. malayi* can be separated from *W. bancrofti* by the length of the headspace and characteristics of the tail nuclei or the color of the sheath. In rare cases, mf may be identified in other body fluids, e.g., urine, sputum, and hydrocele fluid (Anderson et al. 1975, Verma and Vij 2011). Trained ophthalmologists may also detect onchocercal eye disease through observation of mf in the eye by slit-lamp exam (Herzog-Neto et al. 2014).

Special attention needs to be given to the diagnosis of *L. loa* in areas where *O. volvulus* is co-endemic in Central Africa. To this end, a novel system has been developed using a mobile phone-based video microscope that automatically quantifies *L. loa* microfilariae in whole blood loaded directly into a small glass capillary from a finger prick without the need for conventional sample preparation or staining. This point-of-care method has been validated and successfully used under field conditions (D'Ambrrosio et al. 2015).

The notable exception to the use of blood specimens is in the diagnosis of onchocerciasis and *M. streptocerca* infection, which involves an examination of skin snips or nodules. In the skin snip test, a small snipped piece of skin is incubated in saline followed by microscopic identification of the emerging mf. It remains the gold standard for the diagnosis of onchocerciasis and can be used for the detection of *M. streptocerca*. A sclerocorneal biopsy may also be used to obtain diagnostic skin specimens (WHO 1997, Ash and Orihel 2007). This test is specific but poorly sensitive, particularly if the intensity of infection within a community is low (Taylor et al. 1987, Chandrashekar et al. 1994, Udall 2007). This is probably one of the reasons why it still falls short of assessing control programs. It is also invasive and therefore associated with potential infection problems (Vanhamme et al. 2020). Skin samples can be further analyzed by PCR or qPCR for enhanced sensitivity (Patton et al. 2018).

Skin snips should be thin, including just the epidermis and superficial dermis, and collected with minimal bleeding to avoid contamination of the specimen with peripherally circulating mf (particularly in areas where multiple infections are common). The skin snips are generally collected from several sites on the body to maximize detection sensitivity; common locations include the lower extremities and the skin over the iliac crest and scapula. Surveys have demonstrated that when the microfilarial density is high, two snips can be adequate; but if the density is low, using six snips at multiple sites improves the sensitivity. Mf in skin snips does not exhibit periodicity and thus can be obtained at any time (Mathison et al. 2019). In areas of co-endemicity, *O. volvulus* mf in skin snips need to be differentiated from the smaller *M. streptocerca*.

A non-invasive alternative method to skin snipping is the anti-helminthic DEC patch test based upon the observation that DEC elicits a localized rash within 24–48 hours to the skin of microfilaremia individuals infected with *O. volvulus*. However, inconsistencies in specificity and sensitivity (Toé et al. 2000) and its impractical application in the field have led to its less popular use.

Detection of Adult Worms

Ultrasound detection of motile adult filarial worms in major lower extremity lymphatics (lymphatic filariasis) or subcutaneous and deep nodules (onchocerciasis) is another valuable diagnostic method (Dreyer et al. 1998, Mand et al. 2006). Palpation of subcutaneous nodules of *O. volvulus* is recommended by WHO for pre-MDA rapid epidemiology mapping of the disease (Ngoumou and Walsh 1993). The diagnostic value of nodule palpation, however, seems to be reliable only in highly endemic areas due to high intra- and inter-individual variability and considerable false-positive diagnoses (Duerr et al. 2008). *Loa loa* adult worms can sometimes be observed in the sub-conjunctival space of the eye, thus allowing for a presumptive diagnosis (Dietrich et al. 2019). Ultrasonography provides a non-invasive method for the detection of hard-to-detect adult worms in deep nodules and lymphatic vessels. However, it does need sophisticated technical knowledge and sensitive/expensive equipment that limits its application in the field. Other valuable diagnostic methods include surgical recovery of adult worms from a subcutaneous nodule.

Detection of Infective Larvae in Vector Flies

Detection of infective L3 larvae in the vector flies has major advantages when used to monitor disease transmission during and after elimination programs as it provides the most timely and accurate measure of transmission or its cessation. Traditionally, the detection of *O. volvulus* infective larvae in vectors has been accomplished through the dissection of vector black flies and identification of the infective L3 larvae. However, there are some disadvantages associated with this method. First, in the face of an effective control or elimination program, flies carrying infective larvae become increasingly rare. This means that large numbers of flies need to be examined to detect the rare infective flies, which makes the skillful process highly laborious and expensive. Second, *Simulium damnosum s.l.*, the most important black fly vector throughout Africa, is known also to serve as the vector of several zoonotic *Onchocerca* species whose larvae are morphologically difficult or impossible to distinguish from *O. volvulus*, confounding accurate measurement of the prevalence of the human parasite infective flies. Molecular methods involving polymerase chain reaction (PCR) amplification of *O. volvulus*-specific DNA sequences in DNA prepared from pools of flies or individual larvae have been developed to overcome these difficulties (Zimmerman et al. 1992, Yamèogo et al. 1999). Similar protocols are available for screening mosquito vectors of lymphatic filariasis (Rao et al. 2006a).

Immunological Diagnosis

An alternative to the definitive identification of parasites in host tissues is immunological assays for detecting antibodies and circulating parasite antigens in patients' blood specimens (Tables 1 and 2). This involves the development of immunoassays [e.g., Enzyme-linked immunosorbent assay (ELISA)] employing recombinant antigens for the detection of parasite-specific antibodies (e.g., *O. volvulus* infection) and immunoassays to measure circulating parasite antigens (e.g., *W. bancrofti* infection).

Antibody-Based Tests

Serologic assays for the detection of antibodies are usually available as adjunctive methods for the diagnosis of a number of filarial infections (Fink et al. 2011). ELISA has been the most popular test for the detection of parasite-specific antibodies in patients' sera. However, the detection of these antibodies can be an indicator that an individual has been recently infected with a specific parasite but not a current infection due to the persistence of antibodies in these individuals. The extensive cross-reactivity between filarial parasites precluded the use of whole parasite extracts in antibody-based assays (Harnett et al. 1998). The use of recombinant antigens has become the mainstream antibody detection in patient sera (Pastor et al. 2021).

The best example of a successful antibody-based filarial immunoassay comes from *O. volvulus* infections. Several *O. volvulus* antigens have been characterized for vaccines and diagnostic purposes. The use of Ov-16 as a possible marker for infection began with Lobos and his colleagues in 1990 when they screened cDNA expression libraries from mf-producing female *O. volvulus* worms using affinity-purified antibodies from West African onchocerciasis patients. In this study, with the aid of immunoelectron microscopy, the 16 kDa *O. volvulus* antigen protein was localized in the hypodermis, cuticle, and uterus and has been found in all stages of the parasite. Lobos and his colleagues proposed the antigen to be an early marker of infection. So far, no functional studies have been carried out on the Ov-16 antigen, but analysis indicates it is a phosphatidylethanolamine-binding protein (Vanhamme et al. 2020).

Screening of several low molecular weight *O. volvulus* protein fractions as antigens in serological assays resulted in the selection of Ov-16 as the best candidate. The assay targets the detection of IgG4 antibodies to the antigen in an ELISA with a reported sensitivity and specificity of 96% (Lobos et al. 1990). The Ov-16 assay has evolved over the years and becomes more amenable to field conditions, including the use of dried blood dots as input sample type, minimum refrigeration requirement, and relatively low cost. Ov-16 antibody detection for onchocerciasis is widely available and used primarily for research purposes and monitoring of elimination programs (Unnasch et al. 2018). It is usually used in children ≤ 10 yrs old who would have remained naive to exposure if the transmission had been suppressed, and their test results serve as a surrogate measure of exposure incidence in the population. Due to its reliability and robustness and suitability for endemic regions, the WHO currently recommends the use of the Ov-16 assay for demonstrating the interruption of transmission and assessing the elimination of oncochocersis (WHO 2016). Ov-16 assay remains the most common test for *O. volvulus* exposure despite various other types of assays that have been developed, including Ov-20 and Ov-33 (Nde et al. 2002), a cocktail of four recombinant antigens Ov-FAR-1, Ov-API-1, Ov-MSA-1, and Ov-CPI-1 used with a luciferase immunoprecipitation system (LIPS) (Burbelo et al. 2008), and many others (McNulty et al. 2015, Unnasch et al. 2018, Vanhamme et al. 2020).

The Ov-16 antigen was adapted into a rapid format card test by AMRAD ICT (Australia) with a 90% sensitivity (Weil et al. 1997) which ultimately led to the development of two RDTs incorporating the Ov-16 antigen which is now commercially available. One is a single *O. volvulus* IgG4 rapid test and the other is combined with the *W. bancrofti* antigen Wb123 with 81.1% and 99–100% specificity for the single and biplex tests, respectively (PATH 2017). It is expected that the new Ov-16-containing RDTs for anti-Ov-16 serology will be rapidly incorporated into field studies and surveillance activities (Dieye et al. 2017).

Bancroftian and *Brugia*n lymphatic filariasis can also be diagnosed by antibody-based ELISA using the Bm14 and BmR1 antigens (Chandrashekar et al. 1994, Lammie et al. 2004). These assays, which detect IgG4 in exposed individuals' blood, reported 91–45% and 96–100% sensitivities for *W. bancrofti* and *B. malayi*, respectively, but they exhibit some cross-reactivity with antigens of *O. volvulus* and *L. loa*. The Wb123, an antigen from *W. bancrofti* L3 larvae, is another target that has the advantage of detecting exposure to infection much earlier than adult-specific circulating antigens and is a favorable feature for screening children in posttreatment campaigns. The Wb123 is highly sensitive (98–100%) for *W. bancrofti* and its specificity is improved to 94–100% with the detection of IgG4 rather than with IgG (84 to 100%). This specificity improvement was primarily attributed to IgG4 not cross-reacting with *L. loa* and *O. volvulus*, which was seen when detecting IgG. The Wb123 assay is available in LIPS, ELISA, and more recently low-flow immunochromatography test (ICT) format. The Wb123 is the target antigen used in commercially available assays and is effective for the diagnosis and evaluation of elimination programs in areas of endemicity (Steel et al. 2013). For *Brugia* sp., WHO recommends the use of the *Brugia* Rapid™ antibody-detection test (Reszon Diagnostics International, Subang Java, Selangor, Malaysia) that uses a recombinant *B. malayi* antigen *Bm*R1 and has been previously evaluated for sensitivity and specificity (Rahmah et al. 2003).

Most recently, an antibody-based assay using a chimeric antigen containing multi-B-cell epitopes from antigens highly expressed in different stages of *W. bancrofti* has been developed to detect LF infection and its transmission. It showed high sensitivity and specificity with both IgG1 and IgG4 and good potential in detecting active LF infection and in assessing its transmission in endemic communities (Yasin et al. 2020).

The development of immunoassays for the detection of *L. loa* has been guided by the issue of severe responses to anti-filarial therapies in areas of co-endemicity of loiasis with onchocerciasis and lymphatic filariasis. The LIPS assay developed based on IgG4 subclass antibodies to a recombinant *L. loa* SXP-1 antigen reported 56% sensitivity and 98% specificity with some cross-reactivity to *O. volvulus*. A LIPS and quick LIPS (QLIPS) format of the antigen seems to increase both sensitivity and specificity (Burbelo et al. 2008). The most promising assay has been a lateral flow assay (LFA) with the same recombinant antigen that showed the sensitivity of up to 94% and 100% specificity (Pedram et al. 2017).

Antigen-Based Tests

Detection of circulating filarial antigens in sera of infected individuals is one of the precise methods to identify this infection. Good diagnostic tests for detecting and quantifying circulating filarial antigens in humans have been developed for bancroftian filariasis and it is the gold standard defined by WHO for diagnosing lymphatic filariasis (Melrose 2004). These tests are sensitive and specific and do not require the presence of circulating mf. The blood sample from a finger prick can be taken at any time and can detect both microfilaremic and amicrofilaremic cases. Additionally, the tests can provide an indication of adult parasite infection intensity.

Out of eight commercial tests in use, there are two established antigen detection tests for LF patient diagnosis derived from antibodies raised against protein extracts from filarial worms that do not cause human LF. The first is an ELISA test based on the recombinant antibody Og4C3 (Cellabs Pty Ltd., New South Wales, Australia), the first commercialized test to detect circulating *W. bancrofti* antigen in serum, plasma, or hydrocele fluid. The test showed high diagnostic sensitivity and was reported not to cross-react with other helminthic infections and is suitable for field application in endemic countries (Hamlin et al. 2012, Masson et al. 2017). The other antigen detection test is a point-of-care lateral flow cassette test, called the Alere

Filaria Test Strip (FTS) (Abbot, Scarborough, ME), which is a modified version of Alere BinaxNOW® Filariasis (Alere, Scarborough, ME) card ICT (Weil et al. 1997). Because of its field applicability and high diagnostic value, it is one of the tools used by the GPELF in bancroftian filariasis areas. The rapid test is easy to perform and requires no equipment. However, cross-reactivity with *L. loa* and *M. perstans* infections has been reported (Wanji et al. 2015, 2016).

A recently reported recombinant monoclonal antibody (5B) specific to the filarial antigen BmSXP has been used, together with a polyclonal antibody, in an ELISA to detect circulating antigens in sera of bancroftian filariasis patients. It showed excellent sensitivity and specificity and no cross-reactivity to related infections. The ELISA was also able to detect *W. bancrofti* antigens in eluted from dried blood samples, albeit with reduced OD values (Rahumatullah et al. 2019). In addition, *Wuchereria bancrofi* SXP1 ELISA was successfully used to detect the circulating filarial antigen in the urine of school children and proved to be a new effective surveillance system to identify hidden LF transmission foci (Rahman et al. 2019).

In an effort to develop a single detection system to identify circulating filarial antigens in both *W. bancrofti* and *B. malayi* infections based on WbSXP1, a single-chain fragment variable (scFv) was constructed with Vk-linker-VH from the monoclonal antibody 2E12E3, which was raised against rWbSXP1 to produce an entirely functional antigen-binding fragment (Kamatchi et al. 2016). More recently, a simple procedure was developed to create diverse libraries of scFv based on a single DNA framework with all the requisites for an *in vitro* protein synthesis. This evolutionary method coupled with ribosome display has facilitated and improved the reactivity of the ScFv without diminishing the specificity (Mahalakshmi et al. 2019) and indicated that antibody engineering could be used to explore mutagenic studies that can remarkably increase the affinity and sensitivity of antigen detection.

The need for antigen-based immunoassays for point-of-care quantification of *L. loa* microfilariae has led scientists to use transcriptomic approaches with bioinformatics analysis to identify specific putative proteins with potential value as biomarkers of *L. loa* infection. Antigen capture immunoassays were developed to quantify a couple of these proteins in individual serum samples. One of these quantifiable circulating biomarkers showed high specificity, particularly with a monoclonal antibody-based immunoassay, and positively correlated to the mf densities in the corresponding blood samples. It is expected that this promising biomarker will be used in a quantitative point-of-care immunoassay for the detection of *L. loa* and the determination of its mf densities (Drame et al. 2014).

Molecular Diagnosis of Filarial Nematodes

Nucleic acid-based molecular assays offer higher sensitivity than parasitological or immunological methods and can be used to detect infection in both humans and vectors (Tables 1 and 2), as well as to monitor the development of drug-resistant parasite strains (Poole et al. 2017). Molecular assays are not routinely available for the diagnosis of filariasis in most clinical or reference labs but may be available at specialized research centers and public health labs. Several assays have been developed for the detection of filarial parasites that are primarily for research or epidemiologic investigations. These assays mainly use PCR or real-time PCR in the laboratory as well as loop-mediated isothermal amplification (LAMP) (Table 1). Real-time PCR is of benefit to laboratories in developed countries that have adequate laboratory infrastructure and for which cost is less of a prohibitive metric, while LAMP assays are an attractive option for developing countries due to the lower cost of reagents (compared to real-time PCR) and potential for near point-of-care application.

PCR and PCR-Based Assays

PCR-based methods have been used for more than 30 years in research laboratories, however, the requirement for trained personnel and relatively expensive equipment limit their suitability for field use (Poole et al. 2017) (Table 2). PCR assays are available for the detection of all filarial parasites, but they are not commonly used for routine clinical diagnosis.

Onchocerca volvulus was one of the first filarial parasites targeted by molecular assays. The target of the original DNA amplification assay for *O. volvulus* was a tandemly repeated sequence present in the *O. volvulus* genome with a unit length of ~ 150 bp, designated the O-150 repeat. This O-150 repeat family was found to be present in animal *Onchocerca* species but not in other human filarial parasites (Meredith et al. 1991). The repeat family was found to have genus, species, and strain-specific repeat units, that allow for the development of species and strain-specific probes that could be used to classify the amplicons generated from PCR amplification of the O-150 repeat (Toé et al. 1994). The O-150 assay currently in use is designed to specifically identify the parasite DNA in human skin snips or black fly vector DNA extracts by detecting biotin-labeled PCR products, which is captured on a streptavidin-coated microtitre ELISA plate through hybridization to fluorescein-labeled *O. volvulus*-specific probes followed by colorimetric detection (Nutman et al. 1994).

The most direct measure of the status of transmission of onchocerciasis is to measure infectivity in the black fly vector population itself. This has traditionally been done through individual black fly dissections with all of its limitations. A solution to the inability of vector dissection to accurately describe transmission was to develop a specific PCR and techniques to overcome the cost and time implications of having to test 6000 black flies (the required number for verification of interruption of transmission) individually. The O-150 assay has been adapted to provide a reliable and more sensitive and specific alternative to replace black fly dissection (Katholi et al. 1995). This PCR method distinguishes *O. volvulus* from zoonotic *Onchocerca* present in black fly vectors, thereby improving the accuracy of the transmission estimates; more importantly, the PCR assay can be applied to screening black fly pools and is capable of detecting a single infected fly in a pool of up to100 flies. The O-150 PCR is not quantitative but it uses probability distribution estimates to calculate the probability estimate of the number of infected flies in a pool, given the proportion of negative and positive pools and the number of flies contained in each pool. An associated software named PoolScreen calculates the prevalence of infectious flies and associated confidence intervals from the proportion of positive pools, the pool size, and the number of pools screened (Katholi et al. 1995). The O-150 assay has been validated through several field studies in Africa (Yamèogo et al. 1999) and Latin America (Rodriguez-Pérez et al. 1999) and it is currently recommended by WHO as the major assay to provide evidence of *O. volvulus* interruption of transmission (WHO 2016). The O-150 PCR assay has subsequently been widely applied to collect entomological data verifying the elimination of transmission of *O. volvulus* in Mexico (Rodriguez-Pérez et al. 2015), Guatemala (Richards et al. 2015), and Sudan (Zarroug et al. 2016). Using oligonucleotide capture of *O. volvulus* genomic DNA capture during black fly DNA extraction in the current version of the O-150 assay allows for the screening of up to 200 flies per pool and a significant reduction in the cost and time of the assay (Gopal et al. 2012). The O-150 assay is also been used to verify mf positivity of skin snips as it replaces the microscopic examination of the snip with the detection of amplified parasite DNA. As a result, the amplification of *O. volvulus* parasite DNA from skin snips has become the accepted standard for the diagnosis of patent *O. volvulus* infection in humans (Unnasch et al. 2018).

Real-time PCR assays have also been developed for the amplification of *O. volvulus* DNA (Lloyd et al. 2015, Thiele et al. 2016), decreasing the limit of detection of these assays to less than a single parasite and permitting rapid colorimetric detection of the amplified products (Poole et al. 2017). These assays employ a Taqman qPCR targeting the O-150 repeat and the conserved ITS1 and 5.8S regions of the rDNA gene.

DNA-based techniques, including PCR, have also been developed to diagnose and differentiate lymphatic filarial parasites in humans and mosquito vectors (reviewed in McNulty et al. 2013) and to assist in monitoring disease transmission for GPELF. Assays developed to detect filarial nematode DNA have historically targeted repeated species-specific sequences in parasite genomes. The *Hha*I repeat present in *B. malayi* and *B. pahangi* was the first sequence employed for this purpose. Probes designed to target this sequence successfully hybridized to and detected DNA from *Brugia* species but not *W. bancrofti* DNA (McReynolds et al. 1986). Later, genus-specific conventional and real-time PCR assays for *Brugia* and *Wucheraria* were designed and implemented based on the *Hha*I repeat (Rao et al. 2006a, 2006b). The *Hha*I repeat family has been the primary target for parasite detection in humans and mosquitoes since its identification due to its superior sensitivity related to the high copy number and nucleotide identity of the *Hha*I repeats. *Hha*I real-time PCR has recently been proven to have higher sensitivity than antibody tests for the detection of pre-patent and amicrofilaremic patients (Albers et al. 2014). Another repeat family, the long dispersed repeat (LDR1), which contains the *Ssp*I repeat, has been used as a specific target for *W. bancrofti* (Fischer et al. 1996). Subsequent assays were designed to amplify species-specific conserved DNA sequences (e.g., glutathione peroxidase, cytochrome oxidase I, and ITS1) and distinguish them based on restriction fragment length polymorphism of PCR products (PCR-RLFP) (Nuchprayoon et al. 2005, Thanomsub et al. 2000). To evaluate disease transmission in mosquitoes, recent reports employed reverse transcriptase PCR (RT-PCR) assays to target L3 collagen and cuticulin mRNA of *B. malayi* and *W. bancrofti* respectively (Laney et al. 2008, 2010). Sequencing data have also been used to devise a single-step PCR assay targeting part of the abundant larval transcript-2 (alt-2) gene that shows a significant size difference between *B. malayi* and *W. bancrofti* due to increased numbers of tandem repeats in the target sequence (Sakthidevi et al. 2010). It is worth mentioning that no comprehensive comparative analyses have been performed to determine which of these LF biomarkers perform best in PCR. WHO does not recommend specific PCR assay for verification of LF transmission for GPELF.

Multiple PCR assays, including nested and real-time PCR, have also been described for *L. loa* based on *Loa* interspersed repeat, ITS1, and 15r3 of *Loa* allergen (Alhassan et al. 2015). These and other *L. loa*-specific molecular assays have the potential of being used as a species-specific diagnostic tool for infection in endemic areas with concurrent filarial infections. For instance, a nested-PCR assay targeting the ITS1, the internal transcribed spacer 1 region has been developed to differentiate *M. perstans*, *L. loa*, and *W. bancrofti* in areas where they are co-endemic (Jiménez et al. 2011). In addition, nested-PCR assays targeting species-specific 5S rRNA and ITS2 spacer regions were reported to distinguish *O. volvulus* skin snip mf from *M. streptocerca* and *M. ozzardi*, respectively (Fischer et al. 1996, Morales-Hojas et al. 2001).

A novel approach using RNA for diagnosis and understanding of the host-parasite interaction in filarial infection has been reported. This study investigated the presence of circulating microRNAs (miRNA) released by filarial nematodes into the host bloodstream. miRNA targets were identified by miRNA deep-sequencing combined with bioinformatics using sera from *O. volvulus* and *D. immitis* (dog heartworm) infected samples. Stem-loop RT-qPCR assays were then used to detect the presence of target miRNA in infected dog sera. However, absolute miRNA copy numbers were not significantly correlated with microfilaraemia for either parasite. This report demonstrated the presence of filarial miRNAs in host blood and suggest that they are suitable targets for detection by RT-qPCR (Tritten et al. 2014). Circulating miRNAs have also been described from *O. volvulus*, *Brugia pahangi*, *L. loa*, and *O. ochengi* (Tritten et al. 2014) setting the stage for a future for RNA-based detection for filarial diagnostics.

Loop-Mediated Isothermal Amplification (LAMP)

LAMP is one of several recently developed isothermal amplification techniques used for DNA and RNA. As it became the most widely adopted molecular method, it has recently been used in the detection of filarial parasites and other infectious agents (Buchan and Ledeboer 2014) and commercial kits are available for several parasitic infections. LAMP is a single-step reaction that can amplify a few copies of the target up to 109 copies in less than one hour even when large amounts of non-target DNA are present. It uses 4–6 primers to recognize 6–8 distinct regions of target DNA. A strand displaying DNA polymerase initiate synthesis, and two of the primers form loop structures to facilitate subsequent rounds of amplification. In addition, the Bst DNA polymerases used in LAMP are more tolerant to inhibitors commonly found in clinical specimens and insects (Table 2). Determination of amplification is based on simple visual detection of turbidity produced by the precipitation of magnesium pyrophosphate; fluorescence via an intercalating dye or through a color change of metal-sensitive indicators. This lack of post-amplification processing offers a considerable advantage over PCR (Notomi et al. 2015).

LAMP assays displaying equal or higher levels of specificity and sensitivity of PCR have been described for various filarial nematodes including *B. malayi*, *L. loa* (Drame et al. 2014), *O. volvulus* (Alhassan et al. 2014, 2016), and *W. bancrofti* (Takagi et al. 2011). These assays can be performed using a simple electric device such as a heat block or water bath set at a single constant temperature. The robustness and simplicity of these assays indicate that they may be a useful field tool for surveillance in endemic countries.

More recently, LAMP assays using a non-instrumented nucleic acid amplification (NINA) heater have been described which greatly facilitate rapid and simple pathogen detection in rural settings. Colorimetric NINA-LAMP assays targeting *B. malayi*, *O. volvulus*, and *W. bancrofti* exhibit species-specificity with high sensitivity, detecting DNA equivalent to 1/10–1/5000th of one mf with reaction times of 40–70 minutes depending on whether a single copy gene [glutathione S-transferase 1a (GST1a, *O. volvulus*) or repetitive DNA (*Hha*1, *B. malayi* and LDR, *W. bancrofti*)] was employed as a biomarker. The NINA heater can be used to detect multiple infections simultaneously. The accuracy, simplicity, and versatility of the technology suggest that colorimetric NINA-LAMP assays are ideally suited for monitoring the success of filariasis elimination programs (Poole et al. 2017). Optimized assays were then evaluated further using clinical samples (*W. bancrofti* infected blood) or infected insects (*O. volvulus* infected black flies or *B. malayi* infected mosquitoes) (Takagi et al. 2011). A LAMP assay based on GST1 has recently been reported to easily distinguish between *O. volvulus* and the zoonotic *O. ochengi* DNA. Most recently, a point-of-care LAMP has been optimized for the detection of *W. bancrofti* in human blood (Nancy et al. 2021).

Role of Diagnosis in Elimination Programs and Future Needs

The advances in the diagnosis of filarial infections have been guided by intensified global efforts to eliminate onchocerciasis and lymphatic filariasis. Current control and elimination programs are largely based on annual or semi-annual mass drug distribution (MDA) of the microfilaricidal ivermectin (Mectizan, Merck) for onchocerciasis and a combination of albendazole and ivermectin (where onchocerciasis is co-endemic) or diethylcarbamazine citrate (where onchocerciasis is not present) for lymphatic filariasis. Diagnosis of these filarial infections was needed to map endemic areas at the onset of these programs. As these MDA programs progress, accurate diagnostic tools suitable for field use are paramount for careful monitoring of infection levels in human populations and vectors, measuring MDA success, guiding decisions to stop

MDA, and certifying elimination. For instance, highly sensitive methods are required to detect low mf densities in skin or blood, amicrofilaremic infections, and low-level L3 larvae in vectors, which are often the outcome of MDA programs in progress (Rebollo and Bockarie 2013). Stringent specificity is also required to differentiate the closely related filarial parasites, especially where loiasis is endemic, because of ivermectin's serious or fatal side effects in patients co-infected with *L. loa.*

The current diagnostic tools described here (Tables 1 and 2), when applicable, have served well for verifying suppression and interruption of transmission of *O. volvulus*, *W. bancrofti*, and *Brugia* sp. in most countries where interruption of transmission has been achieved. However, there are several tools that could accelerate and augment existing elimination programs as well as incidences of recrudescence of infection. Specificity of diagnostic assays is very essential, especially when used for stopping MDA decisions or verification of elimination. Single antigen-antibody tests cannot usually provide a very high degree of specificity without scarifying significant loss of sensitivity. The future solution could come from an independent confirmatory test using an alternative target or biomolecule. Both tests should show a positive outcome to declare a positive human or vector sample. An attractive assay would use two independent parasite antigens as two lines in an RDT, which could allow the tailoring of the test to provide the highest sensitivity in one line of the test and the highest specificity in the second line. PCR assays, which are highly sensitive and specific, could also use an independent PCR assay targeting a second genomic sequence to overcome the issue of false-positive signals. Further studies are needed to develop and select which combination of tests would result in the highest combined sensitivity and specificity for verifying elimination (Unnasch et al. 2018). The extensive genomic and expressed sequence tag (EST) data from filarial and other nematodes, available in NEM-BASE4 (Elsworth et al. 2011), together with transcriptome studies on different developmental stages (Choi et al. 2011) may be used to identify new biomarkers for improved diagnosis of filarial infection.

The ability to detect RNA and specific metabolites produced by filarial worms has distinct advantages because both fecund, species- and stage-specific detection becomes feasible. RNA-based diagnosis will help to determine if positive testing is the result of adult worms not responding to drug treatment or is due to recent infection with larval stages that would indicate the active transmission or recrudescence of transmission. The detection of miRNA or specific metabolites produced by adult females in the blood of infected individuals will also identify people infected with fecund adult females (Alhassan et al 2014, Unnasch et al 2018). Such diagnostic assays may directly detect potentially fertile female parasites in the human population that could pose a risk for recrudescence after MDA and provide the opportunity to detect and treat people who harbor adult worm infections. In terms of technology, the future seems to side with isothermal nucleic acid-based detection technologies with a particular focus on those suitable for the field in low-resource settings. LAMP currently appears to be at the forefront of all isothermal amplification assays and has the potential to be easily adapted to detect multiple neglected tropical diseases (Avendaño and Patarroyo 2020).

References

Akue, J., E. Eyang-Assengone and R. Dieki. (2018). *Loa loa* infection detection using biomarkers: Current perspectives. Research and Reports in Tropical Medicine 9: 43–48.

Albers, A., E. Sartono, S. Wahyuni, M. Yazdanbakhsh, R. Maizels, U. Klarmann-Schulz et al. (2014). Real-time PCR detection of the HhaI tandem DNA repeat in pre- and post-patent *Brugia malayi* infections: A study in Indonesian transmigrants. Parasites & Vectors 7: 146.

Alhassan, A., B. Makepeace, E. LaCourse, M. Osei-Atweneboana and C. Carlow. (2014). A simple isothermal DNA amplification method to screen black flies for *Onchocerca volvulus* infection. PLoS ONE 9(10): e108927.

Alhassan, A., M. Osei-Atweneboana, F. KyeremehKwadwo, C. Poole, Z. Li, E. Tettevi et al. (2016). Comparison of a new visual isothermal nucleic acid amplification test with PCR and skin snip analysis for diagnosis of onchocerciasis in humans. Molecular and Biochemical Parasitology 210: 10–12.

Alhassan, A., Z. Li, C. Poole and C. Carlow. (2015). Expanding the MDx toolbox for filarial diagnosis and surveillance. Trends in Parasitology 31(8): 391–400.

Anderson, R., D. Thomas, A. MacRae and A. Buck. (1975). Onchocerciasis: Prevalence of microfilaruria and other manifestations in village of Cameroon. The American Journal of Tropical Medicine and Hygiene 24(1): 66–70.

Ash, L. and T. Orihel. (2007). Atlas of Human Parasitology, 5th ed. ASCP Press, Chicago, IL.

Avendaño, C. and M. Patarroyo. (2020). Loop-mediated isothermal amplification as point-of-care diagnosis for neglected parasitic infections. Int. J. Mol. Sci. 21(21): 7981.

Bennuru, S., E. O'Connell, P. Drame and T. Nutman. (2018). Mining filarial genomes for diagnostic and therapeutic targets. Trends Parasitol. 34(1): 80–90.

Buchan, B. and N. Ledeboer. (2014). Emerging technologies for the clinical microbiology laboratory. Clinical Microbiology Reviews 27(4): 783–822.

Burbelo, P., R. Ramanathan, A. Klion, M. Iadarola and T. Nutman. (2008). Rapid, novel, specific, high-throughput assay for diagnosis of *Loa loa* infection. Journal of Clinical Microbiology 46(7): 2298–2304.

Chandrashekar, R., K. Curtis, R. Ramzy, F. Liftis, B. Li and G. Weil. (1994). Molecular cloning of *Brugia malayi* antigens for diagnosis of lymphatic filariasis. Molecular and Biochemical Parasitology 64: 261–271.

Choi, Y., E. Ghedin, M. Berriman, J. McQuillan, N. Holroyd, G. Mayhew et al. (2011). A deep sequencing approach to comparatively analyze the transcriptome of lifecycle stages of the filarial worm, *Brugia malayi*. PLoS Negl. Trop. Dis. 5(12): e1409.

CLSI (formerly NCCLS). (2000). Laboratory diagnosis of blood-borne parasitic diseases: Approved guideline. CLSI document M15-A. Wayne, PA: CLSI.

D'Ambrrosio, M., M. Bakalar, S. Bennuru, C. Reber, A. Skandarajah, I. Nilsson et al. (2015). Point-of-care quantification of blood-borne filarial parasites with a mobile phone microscope. Science Translational Medicine 7(286): 286re4.

Dietrich, C., N. Chaubal, A. Hoerauf, K. Kling, M. Piontek, L. Steffgen et al. (2019). Review of dancing parasites in lymphatic filariasis. Ultrasound Int. Open. 5: E65–E74.

Dieye, Y., H. Storey, K. Barrett, E. Gerth-Guyette, L. Di Giorgio, A. Golden et al. (2017). Feasibility of utilizing the SD BIOLINE Onchocerciasis IgG4 rapid test in onchocerciasis surveillance in Senegal. PLoS Neglected Tropical Diseases 11(10): e0005884.

Drame, P., D. Fink, J. Kamgno, J. Herrick and T. Nutman. (2014). Loop-mediated isothermal amplification for rapid and semi-quantitative detection of *Loa loa* infection. J. Clin. Microbiol. 52: 2071–2077.

Dreyer, G., A. Santos, J. Noroes, F. Amaral and D. Addiss. (1998). Ultrasonographic detection of living adult *Wuchereria bancrofti* using a 3.5-MHz transducer. The American Journal of Tropical Medicine and Hygiene 59(3): 399–403.

Duerr, H., G. Raddatz and M. Eichner. (2008). Diagnostic value of nodule palpation in onchocerciasis. Transactions of the Royal Society of Tropical Medicine and Hygiene 102(2): 148–154.

Elsworth, B., J. Wasmuth and M. Blaxter. (2011). NEMBASE4: The nematode transcriptome resource. International Journal for Parasitology 41(8): 881–894.

Fink, D., G. Fahle, S. Fischer, D. Fedorko and T. Nutman. (2011). Molecular parasitologic diagnosis: Enhanced diagnostic sensitivity for filarial infections in mobile populations. Journal of Clinical Microbiology 49(1): 42–47.

Fischer, P., T. Rubaale, S. Meredith and D. Büttner. (1996). Sensitivity of a polymerase chain reaction-based assay to detect *Onchocerca volvulus* DNA in skin biopsies. Parasitol. Res. 82(5): 395–401.

Foster, J., A. Hoerauf, B. Slatko and M. Taylor. (2013). The Wolbachia bacterial endosymbionts of filarial nematodes. pp. 308–336. *In*: Kennedy, M. W. and W. Harnett. (eds.). Parasitic Nematodes: Molecular Biology, Biochemistry and Immunology, 2nd ed. CABI, Wallingford, United Kingdom.

Gopal, H., H. Hassan, M. Rodríguez-Pérez, L. Toé, S. Lustigman and T. Unnasch. (2012). Oligonucleotide based magnetic bead capture of *Onchocerca volvulus* DNA for PCR pool screening of vector black flies. PLoS Neglected Tropical Diseases 6(6): e1712.

Hamlin, K., D. Moss, J. Priest, J. Roberts, J. Kubofcik, K. Gass et al. (2012). Longitudinal monitoring of the development of antifilarial antibodies and acquisition of *Wuchereria bancrofti* in a highly endemic area of Haiti. PLoS Neglected Tropical Diseases 6(12): e1941.

Harnett, W., J. Bradley and T. Garate. (1998). Molecular and immunodiagnosis of human filarial nematode infections. Parasitology 117: S59–S71.

Hawkes, M., A. Conroy, R. Opoka, S. Namasopo, W. Liles, C. John et al. (2014). Use of a three-band HRP2/pLDH combination rapid diagnostic test increases diagnostic specificity for falciparum malaria in Ugandan children. Malar. J. 13: 43.

Herzog-Neto, G., K. Jaegger, E. Nascimento, V. Marchon-Silva, D. Banic and M. Maia-Herzog. (2014). Ocular onchocerciasis in the Yanomami communities from Brazilian Amazon: Effects on intraocular pressure. The American Journal of Tropical Medicine and Hygiene 90(1): 96–98.

Houze, S., I. Boutron, A. Marmorat, M. Dalichampt, C. Choquet, I. Poilane et al. (2013). Performance of rapid diagnostic tests for imported malaria in clinical practice: Results of a national multicenter study. PLoS One 8: e75486.

James, S., D. Abate, K. Abate, S. Abay, C. Abbafati, N. Abbasi et al. (2018). Global, regional, and national incidence, prevalence, and years lived with disability for 354 diseases and injuries for 195 countries and territories, 1990–2017: A systematic analysis for the global burden of disease study 2017. Lancet 392: 1789–1858.

Jiménez, M., L. González, C. Carranza, B. Bailo, A. Pérez-Ayala, A. Muro et al. (2011). Detection and discrimination of *Loa loa*, *Mansonella* perstans and *Wuchereria bancrofti* by PCR-RFLP and nested-PCR of ribosomal DNA ITS1 region. Experimental Parasitology 127(1): 282–286.

Joseph, H., F. Maiava, T. Naseri, U. Silva, P. Lammie and W. Melrose. (2011). Epidemiological assessment of continuing transmission of lymphatic filariasis in Samoa. Annals of Tropical Medicine and Parasitology 105(8): 567–578.

Kamatchi, R., J. Charumathi, R. Ravishankaran, P. Kaliraj and S. Meenakshisundaram. (2016). Construction and bacterial expression of a recombinant single-chain antibody fragment against *Wuchereria bancrofti* SXP-1 antigen for the diagnosis of lymphatic filariasis. Journal of Helminthology 90(1): 74–80.

Katholi, C., L. Toé, A. Merriweather and T. Unnasch. (1995). Determining the prevalence of *Onchocerca volvulus* infection in vector populations by polymerase chain reaction screening of pools of black flies. J. Infect. Dis. 172: 1414–1417.

Lammie, P., G. Weil, R. Noordin, P. Kaliraj, C. Steel, D. Goodman et al. (2004). Recombinant antigen-based antibody assays for the diagnosis and surveillance of lymphatic filariasis—a multicenter trial. Filaria Journal 3(1): 9.

Laney, S., C. Buttaro, S. Visconti, N. Pilotte, R. Ramzy, G. Weil et al. (2008). A reverse transcriptase-PCR assay for detecting filarial infective larvae in mosquitoes. PLoS Neglected Tropical Diseases 2(6): e251.

Laney, S., R. Ramzy, H. Helmy, H. Farid, A. Ashour, G. Weil et al. (2010). Detection of *Wuchereria bancrofti* L3 larvae in mosquitoes: A reverse transcriptase PCR assay evaluating infection and infectivity. PLoS Neglected Tropical Diseases 4(2): e602.

Lloyd, M., R. Gilbert, N. Taha, G. Weil, A. Meite, I. Kouakou et al. (2015). Conventional parasitology and DNA-based diagnostic methods for onchocerciasis elimination programmes. Acta Tropica. 146: 114–118.

Lobos, E., M. Altmann, G. Mengod, N. Weiss, W. Rudin and M. Karam. (1990). Identification of an *Onchocerca volvulus* cDNA encoding a low-molecular-weight antigen uniquely recognized by onchocerciasis patient sera. Mol. Biochem. Parasitol. 39: 135–145.

Mahalakshmi, N., R. Ravishankaran, R. Kamatchi, N. Sangith, P. Kaliraj and S. Meenakshisundaram. (2019). Molecular evolution of single chain fragment variable (scFv) for diagnosis of lymphatic filariasis. Molecular Biology Reports 46: 5409–5418.

Mand, S., T. Supali, J. Djuardi, S. Kar, B. Ravindran and A. Hoerauf. (2006). Detection of adult *Brugia malayi* filariae by ultrasonography in humans in India and Indonesia. Tropical Medicine and International Health 11(9): 1375–1381.

Masson, J., J. Douglass, M. Roineau, K. Aye, K. Htwe, J. Warner et al. (2017). Relative performance and predictive values of plasma and dried blood spots with filter paper sampling techniques and dilutions of the lymphatic filariasis Og4C3 Antigen ELISA for samples from Myanmar. Tropical Medicine and Infectious Disease 2(2): 7.

Mathison, B., M. Couturier and B. Pritt. (2019). Diagnostic identification and differentiation of microfilariae. J. Clin. Microbiol. 57: e00706–19.

McNulty, S., M. Mitreva, G. Weil and P. Fischer. (2013). Inter and intra-specific diversity of parasites that cause lymphatic filariasis. Infection, Genetics and Evolution. Journal of Molecular Epidemiology and Evolutionary Genetics in Infectious Diseases 14: 137–146.

McNulty, S., B. Rosa, P. Fischer, J. Rumsey, P. Erdmann-Gilmore, K. Curtis et al. (2015). An integrated multiomics approach to identify candidate antigens for serodiagnosis of human onchocerciasis. Molecular and Cellular Proteomics 14(12): 3224–3233.

McReynolds, L., S. DeSimone and S. Williams. (1986). Cloning and comparison of repeated DNA sequences from the human filarial parasite *Brugia malayi* and the animal parasite *Brugia pahangi*. Proc. Natl. Acad. Sci. U.S.A. 83: 797–801.

Melrose, W., D. Durrheim and G. Burgess. (2004). Update on immunological tests for lymphatic filariasis. Trends Parasitol. 20(6): 255–257.

Meredith, S., G. Lando, A. Gbakima, P. Zimmerman and T. Unnasch. (1991). *Onchocerca volvulus*: Application of the polymerase chain reaction to identification and strain differentiation of the parasite. Exp Parasitol. 73: 335–344.

Morales-Hojas, R., R. Post, A. Shelley, M. Maia-Herzog, S. Coscarón and R. Cheke. (2001). Characterisation of nuclear ribosomal DNA sequences from *Onchocerca volvulus* and *Mansonella ozzardi* (Nematoda: Filarioidea) and development of a PCR-based method for their detection in skin biopsies. International Journal for Parasitology 31(2): 169–177.

Muldrew, K. (2009). Molecular diagnostics of infectious diseases. Curr. Opin. Pediatr. 21: 102–111.

Nancy, K., W. Lillian and M. Wilkinson. (2021). Optimization of a loop-mediated isothermal amplification assay as a point-of-care tool for the detection of *Wuchereria bancrofti* in human blood in Tana River Delta, Kenya. J. Parasitol. Res. 2021: 1–9.

Ndao, M. (2009). Diagnosis of parasitic diseases: old and new approaches. Interdiscip. Perspect. Infect. Dis. 2009: 1–15.

Nde, P., T. Pogonka, J. Bradley, V. Titanji and R. Lucius. (2002). Sensitive and specific serodiagnosis of onchocerciasis with recombinant hybrid proteins. Am. J. Trop. Med. Hyg. 66: 566–571.

Ngoumou, P. and J. Walsh. (1993). A manual for rapid epidemiological mapping of onchocerciasis (No. TDR/TDE/ONCHO/93.4. Unpublished). World Health Organization, Geneva, Switzerland.

Notomi, T., Y. Mori, N. Tomita and H. Kanda. (2015). Loop-mediated isothermal amplification (LAMP): Principle, features, and future prospects. Journal of Microbiology (Seoul, Korea) 53(1): 1–5.

Nuchprayoon, S., A. Junpee, Y. Poovorawan and A. Scott. (2005). Detection and differentiation of filarial parasites by universal primers and polymerase chain reaction-restriction fragment length polymorphism analysis. The American Journal of Tropical Medicine and Hygiene 73(5): 895–900.

Nutman, T., P. Zimmerman, J. Kubofcik and D. Kostyu. (1994). A universally applicable diagnostic approach to filarial and other infections. Parasitol. Today 10: 239–243.

Pastor, A., M. Silva, W. Dos Santos, T. Rego, E. Brandão, O. de-Melo-Neto et al. (2021). Recombinant antigens used as diagnostic tools for lymphatic filariasis. Parasites & Vectors 14(1): 474.

PATH. (2017). SD BIOLINE Lymphatic Filariasis IgG4 rapid test procedure.

Patton, J., S. Bennuru, M. Eberhard, J. Hess, A. Torigian, S. Lustigman et al. (2018). Development of *Onchocerca volvulus* in humanized NSG mice and detection of parasite biomarkers in urine and serum. PLoS Negl. Trop. Dis. 12(12): e0006977.

Pedram, B., V. Pasquetto, P. Drame, Y. Ji, M. Gonzalez-Moa, R. Baldwin et al. (2017). A novel rapid test for detecting antibody responses to *Loa loa* infections. PLoS Neglected Tropical Diseases 11(7): e0005741.

Poole, C., Z. Li, A. Alhassan, D. Guelig, S. Diesburg, N. Tanner et al. (2017). Colorimetric tests for diagnosis of filarial infection and vector surveillance using non-instrumented nucleic acid loop-mediated isothermal amplification (NINA-LAMP). PLoS ONE 12(2): e0169011.

Poole, C., L. Sinha, L. Ettwiller, L. Apone, K. McKay, V. Panchapakesa et al. (2019). *In silico* identification of novel biomarkers and development of new rapid diagnostic tests for the filarial parasites *Mansonella* perstans and *Mansonella ozzardi*. Scientific Reports 9(1): 10275.

Rahmah, N., R. Shenoy, T. Nutman, N. Weiss, K. Gilmour, R. Maizels et al. (2003). Multicentre laboratory evaluation of *Brugia* Rapid dipstick test for detection of brugian filariasis. Trop. Med. Int. Heal. 8: 895–900.

Rahman, M., T. Yahathugodaa, B. Tojob, P. Premaratnec, F. Nagaokad, H. Takagid et al. (2019). A surveillance system for lymphatic filariasis after its elimination in Sri Lanka. Parasitology International 68: 73–78.

Rahumatullah, A., T. Lim, M. Yunus and R. Noordin. (2019). Development of an antigen detection ELISA for bancroftian filariasis using BmSXP-specific recombinant monoclonal antibody. The American Journal of Tropical Medicine and Hygiene 101(2): 436–440.

Ramzy, R. (2002). Recent advances in molecular diagnostic techniques for human lymphatic filariasis and their use in epidemiological research. Transactions of The Royal Society of Tropical Medicine and Hygiene 96(supplement 1): S1/225–S1/229.

Rao, R., L. Atkinson, R. Ramzy, H. Helmy, H. Farid, M. Bockarie et al. (2006a). A real-time PCR-based assay for detection of *Wuchereria bancrofti* DNA in blood and mosquitoes. Am. J. Trop. Med. Hyg. 74(5): 826–832.

Rao, R., G. Weil, K. Fischer, T. Supali and P. Fischer. (2006b). Detection of *Brugia* parasite DNA in human blood by real-time PCR. J. Clin. Microbiol. 44(11): 3887–3893.

Rebollo, M. and M. Bockarie. (2013). Toward the elimination of lymphatic filariasis by 2020: Treatment update and impact assessment for the endgame. Expert. Rev. Anti. Infect. Ther. 11(7): 723–731.

Remme, J., U. Amazigo, D. Engels, A. Barryson and L. Yameogo. (2007). Efficacy of ivermectin against *Onchocerca volvulus* in Ghana. Lancet (London, England) 370(9593): 1123–1125.

Ricciardi, A. and M. Ndao. (2014). Diagnosis of parasitic infections: What's going on? Journal of Biomolecular Screening, 1–16.

Richards, F., N. Rizzo, C. Diaz Espinoza, Z. Monroy, C. Crovella Valdez, R. de Cabrera et al. (2015). One hundred years after its discovery in Guatemala by Rodolfo Robles, *Onchocerca volvulus* transmission has been eliminated from the Central Endemic Zone. The American Journal of Tropical Medicine and Hygiene 93(6): 1295–1304.

Rodríguez-Pérez, M., R. Danis-Lozano, M. Rodríguez, T. Unnasch and J. Bradley. (1999). Detection of *Onchocerca volvulus* infection in Simulium ochraceum sensu lato: Comparison of a PCR assay and fly dissection in a Mexican hypoendemic community. Parasitology 119(Pt 6): 613–619.

Rodríguez-Pérez, M., N. Fernández-Santos, M. Orozco-Algarra, J. Rodríguez-Atanacio, A. Domínguez-Vázquez, K. Rodríguez-Morales et al. (2015). Elimination of onchocerciasis from Mexico. PLoS Neglected Tropical Diseases 9(7): e0003922.

Sakthidevi, M., V. Murugan, S. Hoti and P. Kaliraj. (2010). Lymphatic filarial species differentiation using evolutionarily modified tandem repeats: Generation of new genetic markers. Infection, Genetics and Evolution: Journal of Molecular Epidemiology and Evolutionary Genetics in Infectious Diseases 10(4): 591–594.

Shokoples, S., M. Ndao, K. Kowalewska-Grochowska and S. Yanow. (2009). Multiplexed real-time PCR assay for discrimination of Plasmodium species with improved sensitivity for mixed infections. J. Clin. Microbiol. 47: 975–980.

Steel, C., A. Golden, J. Kubofcik, N. LaRue, T. de Los Santos, G. Domingo et al. (2013). Rapid Wuchereria bancrofti-specific antigen Wb123-based IgG4 immunoassays as tools for surveillance following mass drug administration programs on lymphatic filariasis. Clinical and Vaccine Immunology 20(8): 1155–1161.

Takagi, H., M. Itoh, S. Kasai, T. Yahathugoda, M. Weerasooriya and E. Kimura. (2011). Development of loop-mediated isothermal amplification method for detecting *Wuchereria bancrofti* DNA in human blood and vector mosquitoes. Parasitology International 60(4): 493–497.

Ta-Tang, T., S. Luz, J. Crainey and J. Rubio. (2021). An overview of the management of mansonellosis. Research and Reports in Tropical Medicine 12: 93–105.

Taylor, H., L. Keyvan, H. Newland, A. White and B. Green. (1987). Sensitivity of skin snips in the diagnosis of onchocerciasis. Tropical Medicine and Parasitology 38: 145–147.

Taylor, M., A. Hoerauf and M. Bockarie. (2010). Lymphatic filariasis and onchocerciasis. Lancet 376(9747): 1175–1185.

Thanomsub, B., K. Chansiri, N. Sarataphan and S. Phantana. (2000). Differential diagnosis of human lymphatic filariasis using PCR-RFLP. Molecular and Cellular Probes 14(1): 41–46.

Thiele, E., V. Cama, T. Lakwo, S. Mekasha, F. Abanyie, M. Sleshi et al. (2016). Detection of *Onchocerca volvulus* in skin snips by microscopy and real-time polymerase chain reaction: Implications for monitoring and evaluation activities. The American Journal of Tropical Medicine and Hygiene 94(4): 906–911.

Toé, L., A. Merriweather and T. Unnasch. (1994). DNA probe-based classification of Simulium damnosum s. l.-borne and human-derived filarial parasites in the onchocerciasis control program area. The American Journal of Tropical Medicine and Hygiene 51(5): 676–683.

Toé, L., A. Adjami, B. Boatin, C. Back, E. Alley, N. Dembélé et al. (2000). Topical application of diethylcarbamazine to detect onchocerciasis recrudescence in West Africa. Transactions of the Royal Society of Tropical Medicine and Hygiene 94(5): 519–525.

Tritten, L., E. Burkman, A. Moorhead, M. Satti, J. Geary, C. Mackenzie et al. (2014). Detection of circulating parasite-derived microRNAs in filarial infections. PLoS Negl. Trop. Dis. 8(7): e2971.

Udall, D. (2007). Recent updates on onchocerciasis: Diagnosis and treatment. CID 44(1): 53–60.

Unnasch, T., A. Golden, V. Cama and P. Cantey. (2018). Diagnostics for onchocerciasis in the era of elimination. International Health 10(suppl.1): i20–i26.

Vanhamme, L., J. Souopgui, S. Ghogomu and F. Njume. (2020). The functional parasitic worm secretome: Mapping the place of *Onchocerca volvulus* excretory secretory products. Pathogens 9: 0975.

Verma, R. and M. Vij. (2011). Microfilariae of *Wuchereria bancrofti* in urine: An uncommon finding. Diagnostic Cytopathology 39(11): 847–848.

Wanji, S., N. Amvongo-Adjia, B. Koudou, A. Njouendou, P. Chounna Ndongmo, J. Kengne-Ouafo et al. (2015). Cross-reactivity of filariasis ICT cards in areas of contrasting endemicity of *Loa loa* and *Mansonella* perstans in Cameroon: Implications for shrinking of the lymphatic filariasis map in the Central African region. PLoS Neglected Tropical Diseases 9(11): e0004184.

Wanji, S., N. Amvongo-Adjia, A. Njouendou, J. Kengne-Ouafo, W. Ndongmo, F. Fombad et al. (2016). Further evidence of the cross-reactivity of the Binax NOW® Filariasis ICT cards to non-*Wuchereria bancrofti* filariae: Experimental studies with *Loa loa* and Onchocerca ochengi. Parasites & Vectors 9: 267.

Weil, G., P. Lammie and N. Weiss. (1997). The ICT filariasis test: A rapid-format antigen test for diagnosis of bancroftian filariasis. Parasitology Today (Personal ed.) 13(10): 401–404.

World Health Organization (WHO). (1997). Bench Aids for the Diagnosis of Filarial Infections. Geneva, Switzerland.

World Health Organization (WHO). (2016). Guidelines for stopping Mass Drug Administration and verifying elimination of human onchocerciasis: Criteria and procedures. WHO document WHO/HTM/NTD/PCT/2016.1. Geneva, Switzerland.

World Health Organization (WHO). (2020). Lymphatic filariasis. World Health Organization fact sheet of 2nd March 2020. Geneva, Switzerland.

Yaméogo, L., L. Toé, J. Hougard, B. Boatin and T. Unnasch. (1999). Pool screen polymerase chain reaction for estimating the prevalence of *Onchocerca volvulus* infection in Simulium damnosum sensu lato: Results of a field trial in an area subject to successful vector control. The American Journal of Tropical Medicine and Hygiene 60(1): 124–128.

Yasin, N., H. Sugerappa Laxmanappa, U. Muddapur, J. Cheruvathur, S. Uday Prakash and H. Venkataramaiah Thulasiram. (2020). Design, expression, and evaluation of novel multiepitope chimeric antigen of *Wuchereria bancrofti* for the diagnosis of lymphatic filariasis—A structure-based strategy. International Immunopharmacology 83: 106431.

Zarroug, I., K. Hashim, W. ElMubark, Z. Shumo, K. Salih, N. ElNojomi et al. (2016). The first confirmed elimination of an onchocerciasis focus in Africa: Abu Hamed, Sudan. Am. J. Trop. Med. Hyg. 95(5): 1037–1040.

Zimmerman, P., K. Dadzie, G. De Sole, J. Remme, E. Alley and T. Unnasch. (1992). *Onchocerca volvulus* DNA probe classification correlates with epidemiologic patterns of blindness. The Journal of Infectious Diseases 165(5): 964–968.

Chapter 5

Diagnosis and Treatment of Acute Lung Injury

Understanding the Molecular Mechanisms

Kaiser M. Bijli

Introduction

Diseases of the Respiratory system (airways and the lungs) are one of the most common medical conditions affecting humans around the world. Being directly connected to the environmental air, the lungs are exposed to foreign agents both infectious and non-infectious. Bacteria, viruses, fungi, etc., are common infectious agents, whereas non-infectious agents such as pollen, cigarette smoke, air pollutants, like CO_2, CO, SO_2, etc., and hypoxic conditions at high altitudes are other causative factors that cause acute or chronic lung diseases. The current chapter will start with an introductory overview of different types of diseases of the respiratory system, followed by basics and current diagnostic approaches for Acute Respiratory Distress Syndrome and Acute Lung Injury, its associated pathophysiology, molecular mechanisms, and finally current therapeutic approaches that are being followed in the management of Acute Lung Injury.

Brief Overview of Lung Diseases/Conditions

Diseases of the lungs, both non-infectious and infectious, can affect different parts of the respiratory system. The trachea (windpipe) branches into the lung as tubes called bronchi, which in turn branch into smaller tubes called bronchioles throughout both the lungs. The bronchioles further branch into small clusters of air sacs called alveoli

National Center for Immunization and Respiratory Diseases, Centers for Disease Control & Prevention, 1600 Clifton Road, Atlanta, GA 30329, USA.
Email: kbijli@cdc.gov

that constitute a major part of the lungs. Lung diseases can be classified into two types, those that affect the airways and those that affect the alveoli.

Lung Diseases/Conditions Affecting the Airways

Asthma

The pathology of asthma is associated with constant inflammation of the airways causing wheezing and shortness of breath. The lining of the air passages swells and the muscles surrounding the airways become tight, thus reducing the amount of air that can pass through the airway. Pollutants and allergens derived from pollens, fungal spores, house dust mites, certain foods, etc., can cause asthma. Bronchial asthma is a common immune-mediated disorder characterized by reversible airway inflammation, mucus production, and variable airflow obstruction with airway hyperresponsiveness. Allergen exposure results in the activation of numerous cells of the immune system of which dendritic cells (DCs), Th2 (T-helper 2) lymphocytes, and mast cells are of paramount importance. Immunoglobulin E (IgE) antibodies are also central players in the allergic response in which their cross-linking by allergen on the mast cell surface release histamine granules and thereby causes allergic inflammation (Buc et al. 2009, Maddox and Schwartz 2002).

Chronic Obstructive Pulmonary Disease (COPD)

This type of lung condition is associated with difficulty in breathing especially when air is exhaled out of the lungs. Both smoking and exposure to air pollution cause COPD. Two types of COPD have been described based on associated pathology. First is "chronic bronchitis," which involves enhanced inflammation of the bronchial tubes in the lungs. This results in coughing and the release of unusually high amounts of mucus also referred to as "wet cough." These conditions result in a narrowing of the airways and thereby difficulty in breathing. This condition is categorized as chronic when it persists for several months to two years. Second is "Emphysema," which is another chronic medical condition in which the air sacs (alveoli) in the lungs get damaged and thereby lose elasticity due to destruction of parenchymal cells. The required elasticity is important for proper inflation of alveoli and the delivery of oxygen from the lungs into the blood. However, due to loss of elasticity, air is entrapped into the lungs, causing shortness of breath and difficulty in exhaling air out of the lungs (Baraldo et al. 2012, Rabe and Watz 2017).

Acute Bronchitis

This is a sudden and quick inflammation of bronchioles, most commonly caused by infection with contagious viruses, especially common cold and flu viruses, but it can also be caused due to bacterial infection. The infection starts with nose and progresses through sinuses, throat, and reaches the bronchiolar lining. Swelling occurs due to inflammation of the bronchiolar lining, resulting in mucus production. The swelling also results in narrowing of the airways, causing difficulty in breathing (Lugo and Nahata 1993, Kinkade and Long 2016, Wilson and Rayner 1995).

Cystic Fibrosis

Cystic Fibrosis is an autosomal recessive genetic disorder due to mutation in both copies of Cystic Fibrosis Transmembrane Conductance Regulator (CFTR) gene. Cystic fibrosis lung disease is characterized by persistent bacterial infection that is usually acquired in childhood and maintained throughout the patient's life. It is associated with reduced ability of a person to clear thick mucus due to failure of innate immune response in the airways. This reduced mucus clearance causes susceptibility to bacterial infections, most commonly by *Staphylococcus aureus*, *Heamophilus influenzae*, *Pseudomonas aeroginosa*, and fungal infections such as bronchopulmonary aspergillosis caused by *Aspergillus fumigatus*. The CFTR gene mutation can also impact other systems in the body that includes hepatic, gastrointestinal tract, and endocrine system (Clunes and Boucher 2008, Konrad et al. 2020).

Lung Diseases Affecting the Air Sacs (Alveoli)

Pneumonia

An infection of the alveoli is usually caused by bacteria, viruses, or fungi including the coronavirus that causes COVID-19. Due to infection, the alveoli get inflamed and accumulated with resulting fluid or pus formation. This causes cough, fever, chills, and trouble breathing.

(i) Bacterial Pneumonia: The most common bacteria that falls in this category is *Streptococcus pneumoniae* which causes pneumococcal pneumonia. Bacterial pneumonia can also manifest as an opportunistic infection after a viral infection, such as cold or flu. Bacterial pneumonia often affects just one part or lobe of a lung, which is also referred to as lobar pneumonia. People recovering from surgery, people with respiratory disease or viral infection, and people who have a weakened immune system are at the greatest risk for bacterial pneumonia (Kim et al. 2017). Other forms of pneumonia caused by bacteria are atypical (different from that caused by Streptococcus pneumoniae) and often mild in nature. These are caused by *Mycoplasma pneumoniae*, *Chlamydophila pneumoniae*, and *Legionella pneumophila* (Shim 2020).

(ii) Viral Pneumonia: Viruses that infect the upper respiratory tract can also cause pneumonia. The influenza virus is the most common cause of viral pneumonia in adults. while Respiratory Syncytial Virus (RSV) is the most common cause of viral pneumonia in young children. The duration of viral pneumonia is generally shorter than bacterial pneumonia. However, pneumonia caused by the influenza virus may get severe and can sometimes be fatal. The virus invades the lungs and multiplies, although physical signs of pulmonary edema (accumulation of fluid in the lung tissue) are generally not visible. This pneumonia can result in serious complications in people who have pre-existing heart or lung disease. Opportunistic infection by bacteria could further complicate viral pneumonias, resulting in all the typical symptoms associated with bacterial pneumonia (Bakaletz 2017, Oliva and Terrier 2021).

(iii) Fungal Pneumonia: It is most common in people who are exposed to large doses of certain fungi from contaminated soil or bird droppings and in people with chronic health problems or weakened immune systems. *Pneumocystis pneumonia* is a serious fungal infection caused by *Pneumocystis jirovecii*, which infects people who have weak immune systems due to HIV/AIDS or long-term use of immunosuppressants, such as those used in the management of organ transplant rejection (Weyant et al. 2021). *Coccidioidomycosis*, also known as Valley fever, is an infection caused by inhaling spores of the fungus *Coccidioides*, which is found in the soil. This infection is not contagious, and the symptoms are minimal with no treatment required. In extreme cases, once inhaled, the *Coccidioides* fungus can multiply and spread in the body, leading to the worsening of the disease. The time from exposure to the development of symptoms may take several weeks. Because the fungus is inhaled, the disease typically affects the lung (Gabe et al. 2017, Kimes et al 2020). *Histoplasmosis* is caused by breathing fungal spores from soil that has been contaminated by bird or bat droppings. It is not contagious, and most of these infections have mild or no symptoms that do not require treatment. Patients with weakened immune systems or underlying respiratory disease are more likely to develop a severe form of histoplasmosis that may become chronic or even life-threatening. Once inhaled, if the person has a healthy immune system, the fungus can cause mild symptoms such as lung infection or pneumonia. However, in immunocompromised patients, the disease can spread throughout the body, including the mouth, liver, central nervous system, skin, and adrenal glands, which is also known as "disseminated histoplasmosis," that can be extremely dangerous and fatal if left untreated (Tobon and Gómez 2021). *Cryptococcosis* is another fungal infection caused by spore inhalation of *Cryptococcus neoformans* and *Cryptococcus gattii* that are present in soil contaminated with bird droppings. Pulmonary cryptococcosis is an important opportunistic invasive mycosis that is mostly prevalent in immunocompromised patients such as those who have advanced HIV/AIDS. Pulmonary cryptococcosis is still underdiagnosed due to limitations in diagnostic tools. Clinically, it can mimic lung cancer, pulmonary tuberculosis, bacterial pneumonia, and other pulmonary mycoses. Cryptococcosis usually affects the lungs or the central nervous system (the brain and spinal cord), but it can also affect other parts of the body such as skin, prostrate and bones. Infection of brain by this fungus is referred to as cryptococcal meningitis. Most cases of *C. neoformans* infection occur in people who have weakened immune systems, particularly those who have advanced HIV/AIDS (Brizendine et al. 2011, Setianingrum et al. 2019).

Tuberculosis

Tuberculosis (TB) is an airborne bacterial infection caused by the organism *Mycobacterium tuberculosis*, which primarily affects the lungs, although other organs and tissues may also be affected. The disease spreads form person to person when an infected individual coughs or sneezes out the bacteria, which gets aerosolized and can be inhaled by others. Upon inhalation, the bacterium lodges into the lung tissue.

Healthy individuals may contract latent TB, but the disease can acquire an active form if the immune system becomes weak, in which case TB may develop within days or weeks after the infection. In active TB, bacteria multiply and attack the lungs from which they can migrate through the blood or lymphatic system to different parts of the body, such as the lymph nodes, bones, kidney, brain, spine, and even the skin thus affecting other organs (Moule and Cirillo 2020, Ryndak and Laal 2019).

Lung Cancer

Smoking is a leading cause of lung cancer worldwide in both active and passive smokers (people exposed to secondhand smoke). Cigarette smoke has carcinogens that can damage the lung cells causing morphological changes in the lung tissue almost immediately. The body's immune system may facilitate repair of the damage caused initially. However, each repeated exposure, causes increasing damage to the cells that may eventually lead to cancer. Moreover, immunocompromised individuals such as those with HIV infection face greater risk of lung cancer exacerbation (Sigel et al. 2016). Two general types of lung cancer include "small cell lung carcinoma," which predominantly occurs in heavy smokers, and "non-small cell lung carcinoma," which is a broad term for different types of lung cancers, including adenocarcinoma, squamous cell carcinoma, and large cell carcinoma. Regardless of cancer type, shortness of breath occurs when cancer progresses to block major airways and also due to associated pulmonary edema. Bleeding in the airway results in hemoptysis (coughing of blood) and pleural effusion in which case fluid accumulates in the space surrounding the affected lung in the chest cavity (pleural space), causing shortness of breath and lastly metastasis in which lung cancer spreads to other parts of the body, such as the brain and the bones (Gershman et al. 2019, Miles and Islam 2019).

Pneumoconiosis

This is an inflammatory condition caused mostly due to occupational exposure of the lungs to dust, asbestos, silicone, and other such agents. The primary pneumoconioses are asbestosis, silicosis, and coal workers' pneumoconiosis, also known as black lung, caused by inhalation of asbestos fibers, silica dust, and coal mine dust, respectively. While these conditions take many years to develop and manifest, rapid progressive forms do occur, especially in silicosis, which can cause lung collapse and premature death. Symptoms of pneumoconiosis includes shortness of breath, persistent cough, and fatigue. The size of the particles determines where in the lungs the disease/inflammation will occur. Large particles are mostly caught in the bronchi (upper airways) where clearance mechanisms effectively help their entrapment in the mucus and their eventual expulsion by the action of cilia (tiny hair-like structures) on the lung cells that constantly beat in the upward direction to remove foreign particles away from the lungs. Intermediate-size particles (2–10 microns size) land mostly in bronchioles. Combination of both mucus and ciliary action in bronchioles can sometimes remove the particles. However, small particles (size less than 2 microns in diameter) tend to accumulate in alveoli, where they bypass normal clearance mechanisms and are thereby engulfed and phagocytosed (eaten) by immune cells called macrophages (alveolar macrophages) that reside in the alveoli. Pulmonary fibrosis is one of the major effects of pneumoconiosis (Fujimura 2000, Barber and Fishwick 2016).

Pulmonary Edema

Pulmonary edema, also termed "wet lung," is a condition in which the lungs fill with fluid due to leaks from the small blood vessels, present inside the lung, into the alveoli and surrounding areas. It is a pathological condition that can be associated with any type of lung disease or related disorder depending on disease severity. The body struggles to get enough oxygen, causing shortness of breath. One of the most common cause of pulmonary edema is congestive heart failure (CHF) in which the heart is no longer able to pump blood properly throughout the body, thereby generating a backup pressure in the small blood vessels surrounding the alveoli that in turn cause a leakage of blood vessels. The accumulation of fluid in alveoli prevents transport of oxygen into the bloodstream, thus depriving the rest of the body with oxygen. Other common medical conditions that can cause pulmonary edema include heart attack, damaged heart valves, sudden high blood pressure, pneumonia, kidney failure, lung damage caused by severe infection, severe sepsis (infection of the blood), or blood poisoning caused by infection. External factors that cause pulmonary edema include drug overdose, lung damage caused by inhalation of toxins, severe trauma, or drowning. Symptoms of pulmonary edema include shortness of breath when being physically active and difficulty in breathing when lying down, wheezing, waking up at night due to breathlessness that disappears when a person sits in an upright position, rapid weight gain, especially in the legs and swelling in the lower part of the body. Pulmonary edema can also be caused due to altitude sickness or the absence of enough oxygen in the air (hypoxia) at high altitudes. This can result in headaches, irregular and rapid heartbeat, shortness of breath after exertion and during rest, coughing, fever, and difficulty walking uphill and on flat surfaces (Murray 2011, Matthay et al. 2019).

Pulmonary edema is a major component associated with the pathophysiology of Acute Lung Injury and Acute Respiratory Distress Syndrome. The remaining part of this book chapter will focus on the pathophysiology, molecular mechanisms, and therapeutic implications of Acute Lung Injury.

Acute Respiratory Distress Syndrome

Causes

Acute Respiratory Distress Syndrome (ARDS) was first described in 1967 as a severe form of cascading events following Acute Lung Injury (ALI), which frequently results in significant morbidity and death. Approximately 150,000 individuals are diagnosed with ARDS in the United States each year. Mortality due to ARDS has remained at approximately 40% for the past two decades (Phua et al. 2009). ARDS can develop as a manifestation of disease severity, most commonly associated with bacterial or viral pneumonia, primary graft dysfunction following lung transplantation, high-altitude pulmonary edema, and drug-induced lung injury.

ARDS can also be caused by sepsis as well as infection of other non-pulmonary tissues/organs, such as urinary tract, peritoneum, aspiration of gastric or oral, and esophageal contents and major physical trauma, such as blunt or penetrating injuries or burns. Less common scenarios associated with ARDS development include inflammation of pancreas (acute pancreatitis), transfusion of red blood cells and/or platelets or frozen plasma (transfusion-associated acute lung injury/TRALI), drug overdose with various agents, water inhalation due to drowning, hemorrhagic shock or reperfusion injury, and smoke inhalation (often associated with cutaneous burn injuries). Current treatment for ARDS is primarily focused on treatment of underlying conditions that includes mechanical ventilation and corticosteroid administration (Acute Respiratory Distress Syndrome Network et al. 2000).

Biomarkers in the Diagnosis and Disease Progression in ARDS/ALI

Years of basic and clinical research have led to the identification of numerous biomarkers that have profoundly facilitated the diagnosis, as well as the determination of disease severity and mortality associated with ARDS/ALI.

Markers of Respiratory Epithelial Cells

These include surfactant proteins (SP), vascular endothelial growth factor (VEGF), Krebs von den Lungen-6 (KL-6) protein, and Soluble Receptor for Advanced Glycation End-products (sRAGE). Levels of SP are elevated in ARDS. For example, SP-B can cross damaged alveolocapillary membranes and leak into the blood (Doyle et al. 1997, Greene et al. 1999). Also, blood SP-D levels have been shown to correlate with ARDS mortality (Ware et al. 2010, Eisner et al. 2003). KL-6 levels have been correlated with ARDS mortality as opposed to ARDS development (Sato et al. 2004). A meta-analysis of plasma biomarkers for ARDS found KL-6, lactate dehydrogenase, sRAGE, and von Willebrand factor to be associated with ARDS diagnosis in at-risk populations (Terpstra et al. 2014). In one study, VEGF was shown to correlate with severity of illness (Koh et al. 2008). The alveolar epithelial type II cells in the lung express RAGE in very high amounts (Shirasawa et al. 2004). Studies have shown that higher levels of RAGE were associated with impaired alveolar fluid clearance in patients with ARDS, correlating with severity of lung epithelial injury (Jabaudon et al. 2015). The plasma levels of RAGE in patients with severe ARDS correlated with mortality in patients with high tidal volume ventilation (Ware and Calfee 2016). In one meta-analysis sRAGE (soluble RAGE) was found to be useful in ARDS diagnosis in a high risk population, but did not correlate with mortality (Terpstra et al. 2014).

Markers of Endothelial Cells

Angiopoietin-2 (Ang-2) is an important biomarker for endothelial dysfunction in sepsis and ALI (Hendrickson and Matthay 2018). Elevated levels of Ang-2 in both ARDS and at-risk patients are predictive of mortality (Agrawal et al.

2013, Xing et al. 2012, Wada et al. 2013) and also correlates with ARDS development in trauma patients (Fremont et al. 2010).

Inflammatory Cytokines

The pro-inflammatory cytokine, IL-8, has been shown in predicting the outcome of ARDS (Ware et al. 2010, Calfee et al. 2011). Another cytokine, IL-18 was found to be increased in patients with ARDS and also associated with mortality (Dolinay et al. 2012). An external validation of biomarkers and a clinical prediction model for hospital mortality in ARDS included SP-D and IL8 in various clinical settings and suggested that these biomarkers may be useful in risk assessment for clinical trial enrollment (Zhao et al. 2017).

Coagulation and Fibrinolysis

The protein, plasminogen activator inhibitor-1 (PAI-1), is an inhibitor of fibrinolysis. Elevated levels of PAI-1 were found in serum of patients with ARDS (Ware et al. 2010, Moalli et al. 1989, Prabhakaran et al. 2003), and also correlated with overall mortality in critically ill patients (Jalkanen et al. 2013).

Pathophysiology

Current research aims to understand the molecular pathophysiology of ALI/ARDS toward developing prognostic molecular biomarkers and molecular-based therapy. Diagnosis of ARDS primarily involves clinical and radiological assessments, but lung biopsy facilitates diagnostic determination in certain situations. While significant amount of progress has been made in the elucidation of ARDS pathophysiology and in predicting patient response, there are currently no viable molecular biomarkers for predicting the severity of ARDS or molecular-based ARDS therapies. Currently, the pro-inflammatory cytokines tumor necrosis factor α (TNF-α), interleukin (IL)–1β, IL-6, IL-8, and IL-18 are among the most promising biomarkers for predicting morbidity and mortality of ARDS. Since ARDS develops within 2 to 5 days of hospitalization (Gajic et al. 2011) in majority of the cases, the development of therapies for interrupting the progression of ALI to ARDS is of significant importance and urgently needed (Ruthman and Festic 2015).

Inflammatory mechanisms in the lung are activated when it is injured by trauma, infection, or due to other existing inflammatory conditions. While the inflammatory response (excessive immune response) can facilitate pathogen clearance, excess inflammation can also contribute to alveolar tissue damage (Imai et al. 2008). Thus, a delicate balance has to exist between inflammation and tissue injury for the injured lung to be recovered. The inflammation-induced damage impacts both endothelial and epithelial cells in the lung alveolus. Endothelial cells make up the walls of blood capillaries that surround the alveoli, whereas the alveolar epithelial cells make up the alveolar wall. Damage to these cells results in permeability and pulmonary edema. Further, leakage of this fluid into the lung interstitium (spaces in between alveoli) and air spaces inside the lungs leads to increased effort in breathing and impaired gas exchange resulting in hypoxemia (reduced oxygen in the blood), reduced CO_2 excretion, and finally acute respiratory failure. In uninjured lungs, the process of active ion transport across the alveolar epithelium creates an osmotic gradient that drives alveolar fluid clearance (AFC) out of the alveoli, thus preventing any pathological complications (Matthay et al. 2002). However, in ARDS, the osmotic gradient is disrupted and AFC is reduced, rendering the removal of edema fluid extremely difficult from the distal airspaces of the lung. Thus, two critical events, epithelial and endothelial damage/ destabilization and associated pathophysiology, play a central role in the ALI and form the hallmark of ARDS (Matthay et al. 2012, Bachofen and Weibel 1982, Fein et al. 1979). The following two sections below describe these aspects in more detail. Figure 1 shows the difference between normal alveoli and alveoli that is injured in ALI and the associated pathological features.

Epithelial Destabilization

The alveolar epithelium (wall lining the alveoli) is made up of two types of epithelial cells, flat-shaped alveolar type I (ATI) cells and cuboidal-shaped alveolar type II (ATII) cells (Figure 1A). Both these cells form a very tight barrier, which not only restricts the passage of even small solutes but also allows easy diffusion of oxygen and carbon dioxide. This barrier is maintained and stabilized by proteins called E-cadherin (epithelial cadherin), which are junctional proteins forming bridge-like structures joining two epithelial cells. Further, under normal conditions, the ATII cells secrete SP that reduce surface tension, enabling the alveoli to remain open for gas exchange. However, both ATI and ATII cells are capable of absorbing excess fluid from the airspaces by vectorial (directional) ion transport, facilitated by sodium channels and Na+/K+-ATPase pumps (Matthay 2014), which then gets cleared by lymphatic system and lung microcirculation. The normal alveolus consists of immune cells called alveolar macrophages but not neutrophils (polymorphonuclear leukocytes). Neutrophils can, however, be rapidly recruited from the circulation during infection. Upon infection, alveolar macrophages, neutrophils, and other immune effector cells, including monocytes and platelets, are critical in defense of the normal lung from pathogens. However, under severe inflammatory conditions, excess neutrophils migrate into the lungs and cause epithelial injury by destabilizing and disrupting intercellular junctions (E-cadherin bridges) and by causing their apoptosis (programmed cell death). This results in disruption of epithelial cell layer leading to increased epithelial permeability and accumulation of edematous fluid in the alveoli (Ginzberg et al. 2004), as shown in Figure 1B. Thus, severity of inflammation dictates the level of barrier integrity and the intactness of ion transport channels in the alveolar epithelial cells required for the resorption of edematous fluid. These events suggest that restoration of epithelial integrity is critical for recovery and survival during ALI.

Endothelial Destabilization

Similar to alveolar epithelial cells, in normal lungs, the integrity of the lung microvascular barrier (walls of blood microvessels surrounding the alveoli)

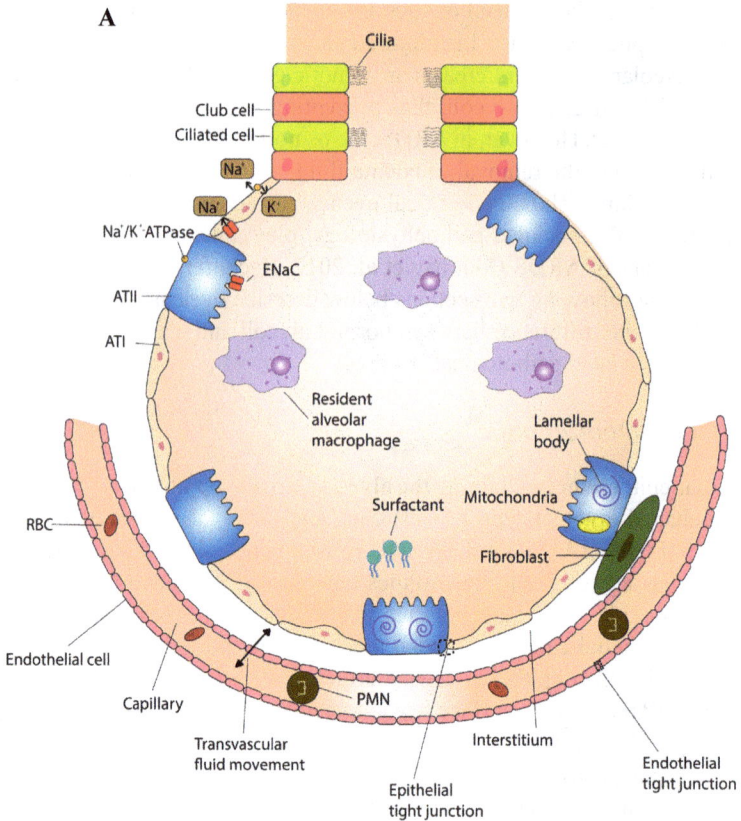

Figure 1A. Schematic diagram of normal alveolus. The alveolar epithelium consists of a continuous monolayer of alveolar type I (ATI) cells (very thin cells that permit gas exchange) and ATII cells (which produce surfactant to enable lung expansion with low surface tension); both cells transport ions and fluid from the alveolus to maintain dry airspaces. The intact alveolar epithelium is linked by intercellular tight junctions made up of E-cadherin (not shown). Tight junctions are responsible for barrier function and regulating the movement of fluid and ions across the epithelium. Endothelial cells regulate the movement of fluid and inflammatory cells into the interstitial space and are connected by intercellular junctions comprising tight junctions and adherens junctions that contain VE-cadherin (not shown). The VE-cadherin mediates cell-cell contact and plays a key role in maintaining barrier integrity. Under normal conditions, transvascular movement of fluid moves water and low- molecular-weight solutes out of the capillary into the interstitial space and then into the lymphatics. The fluid, however, does not cross the epithelial barrier. Resident alveolar macrophages in the airspaces provide host defense. Large numbers of polymorphonuclear leukocytes (PMNs) reside in the alveolar capillaries and can be rapidly mobilized to the airspaces during infection or inflammation. ENaC, epithelial sodium channel; RBC, red blood cell.

is maintained through the stabilization of endothelial cells via bridging by VE-cadherins (Vascular Endothelial Cadherin) that serve as adherens junctional proteins between two endothelial cells. During lung injury, increased concentrations of the pro-coagulant, thrombin, inflammatory cytokines, such as tumor necrosis factor-α (TNF-α), Interleukin-8 (IL-8), Interleukin-6 (IL-6), VEGF, and signals generated from leukocytes destabilize the VE-cadherin bonds, resulting in increased endothelial permeability and accumulation of alveolar fluid (Corada et al. 1999).

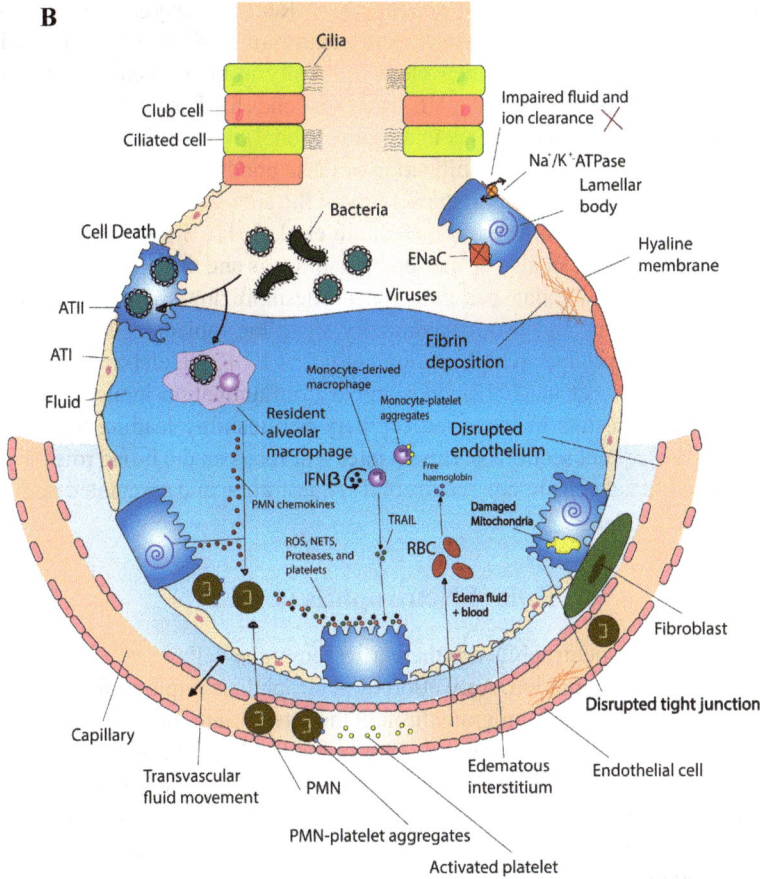

Figure 1B. Schematic diagram of injured alveolus. The alveolar epithelium can be injured by a variety of insults (such as viruses, bacteria, acid, ventilator-associated lung injury, hyperoxia, etc.), either directly or by inducing inflammation, which in turn injures the epithelium. Activation of Toll-like receptors (not shown) on ATII cells and resident macrophages induces the secretion of chemokines, which recruit circulating immune cells into the airspaces. As neutrophils migrate across the epithelium, they release toxic mediators, including proteases, ROS, and neutrophil extracellular traps (NETs), which play an important role in host defense but also cause endothelial and epithelial injury. Monocytes also migrate into the lung and can cause injury, including epithelial cell apoptosis via IFNβ-dependent release of TNF-α-related apoptosis-inducing ligand (TRAIL), which then activates death receptors. Activated platelets form aggregates with polymorphonuclear (PMN) leukocytes, which are involved in the NET formation and monocyte–platelet aggregates. RBCs release cell-free hemoglobin, which exacerbates injury via oxidant-dependent mechanisms. Permeability-promoting agonists destabilize VE-cadherin between endothelial cells resulting in enhanced permeability. Additionally, loss of cell-cell adhesion results in the formation of occasional gaps between endothelial cells. The epithelial injury also involves wounding of its plasma membrane caused by bacterial pore-forming toxins or mechanical stretch and mitochondrial dysfunction. Together, these effects result in endothelial and epithelial permeability, which facilitates the transmigration of leukocytes and the influx of edematous fluid and RBCs. The edematous fluid fills the airspace causing hypoxaemia, resulting in the need for mechanical ventilation. The vascular injury and alveolar edema contribute to the decreased ability to excrete CO_2 (hypercapnia). In turn, both hypoxaemia and hypercapnia impair vectorial sodium transport, reducing alveolar edema clearance, a major pathological condition in ALI/ARDS. ENaC, epithelial sodium channel; IFNβ, Interferon-β.

The destabilization occurs due to generation of Reactive Oxygen Species (ROS) and acidic proteases released from activated neutrophils and leukocytes in the blood circulation and more so due to their close proximity in the malieu surrounding the endothelial cells. The importance of VE-cadherin bonds has been confirmed in mouse models. Alveolar fluid accumulates in a mouse model of lipopolysaccharide (LPS)-induced lung injury. However, stabilization of these bonds by genetic alterations that prevent breakdown or by blocking the activity of the enzyme, VE phosphodiesterase, resulted in reduced edema formation (Schulte et al. 2011, Broermann et al. 2011). Endothelial disruption can also be caused by pathogens and their toxins, endogenous danger-associated molecular patterns, barrier-destabilizing factors generated by alveolar macrophages, and pro-inflammatory signaling molecules such as TNF-α, the inflammasome product IL-1β, angiopoietin 2, VEGF, platelet-activating factor, and others (Matthay et al. 2012). In summary, inflammation-induced damage to lung endothelium results in increased capillary permeability leading to pulmonary edema. The subsequent sections of this chapter will focus on the broad role played by activated endothelial cells in lung neutrophil sequestration and associated underlying molecular mechanisms.

Role if Neutrophils in ALI

During lung injury, neutrophils are the earliest immune cells to be recruited to the site of injury or inflammation. Activation of neutrophils is required for crossing the microvascular barrier and to migrate through the interstitium into the alveolar space. The crossing of neutrophils across the microvascular barrier normally takes place in postcapillary venules in a sequential manner that involves the capture and rolling of these cells on the endothelial cell surface. Rolling is followed by chemokine-dependent activation of integrins on neutrophils, ultimately leading to adhesion on the endothelium. Subsequently, neutrophils transmigrate into the lung tissue as described later in this chapter. This process is described later in this chapter. Neutrophils contain different types of active biochemical components that play crucial roles in the pathology of ALI as described below.

Neutrophil-Derived Granule Proteins

Neutrophils contain four granule subsets that play different roles in their antimicrobial function: azurophilic (also known as primary) granules, specific (also known as secondary), gelatinase granules (also known as tertiary), and secretory vesicles. Granule proteins of neutrophils are synthesized at different stages of myelopoiesis and targeted to granule subsets (Borregaard and Cowland 1997). Each granule subset shows a distinct propensity for release. While secretory vesicles are mobilized following initial neutrophil-to-endothelial cell contact, tertiary granules are released during subsequent neutrophil transendothelial migration. Both primary and secondary granules are discharged once the neutrophil has entered the tissue. All the granules released at later stages mainly contain proteases and antimicrobial polypeptides (Faurschou and Borregaard 2003). An important role for neutrophil-derived granule proteins during the onset of ALI in mice induced by *Streptococcus pyogenes* was shown in which neutrophil depletion completely abolished lung damage in this model. However, injection of the supernatant from activated neutrophils into neutropenic mice restored the deleterious effect of neutrophils, indicating an important role of neutrophil granule proteins in ALI pathology (Soehnlein et al. 2008a).

Neutrophil Elastase

Neutrophil serine proteases play a critical role in regulating immune response against pathogens but also play a major role in inflammation. For example, for levels of serine protease, neutrophil elastase is elevated in the Bronchoalveolar Lavage (BAL) and plasma of patients with ALI and ARDS (Cochrane et al. 1983, Lee et al. 1981, Donnelly et al. 1995) that correlate with severity of lung injury (Zemans et al. 2009). In murine models of ALI, elastase administration induced lung damage (Delacourt et al. 2002, Janusz and Hare 1994, Tremblay et al. 2002), whereas elastase inhibition attenuated the development of ALI (Hagio et al. 2008, Kawabata et al. 2000). Elastase causes increased alveolar permeability by proteolytic cleavage of E-cadherin and VE-cadherin junctional proteins, an event which is also associated with increased transmigration of neutrophils (Ginzberg et al. 2001, Carden et al. 1998).

Matrix Metalloproteinases (MMPs)

These are zinc-dependent endopeptidases produced by a variety of cell types that occupy a central role in normal physiological conditions, such as proliferation, cell motility, remodeling, wound healing, angiogenesis, and key reproductive events. In neutrophils, MMP-2 (gelatinase A) and MMP-9 (gelatinase B) stored in tertiary granules and MMP-8 (collagenase 2) from secondary granules have been shown to play important roles in ALI pathology. Especially, BAL fluid (Delclaux et al. 1997, Ricou et al. 1996, Torii et al. 1997) and plasma (Pugin et al. 1999, Steinberg et al. 2001) of patients with ALI/ARDS displayed elevated levels of MMPs, which correlated with clinical severity (Fligiel et al. 2006). Besides their functions on extracellular matrix (that is, degradation, turnover, and remodeling), MMPs modulate inflammation and neutrophil influx as well as epithelial and endothelial integrity.

Neutrophil-Derived Cationic Polypeptides

Upon activation, neutrophils release a wide array of cationic polypeptides that primarily possess antimicrobial activity. Lactoferrin is one such molecule belonging to the family of iron-binding proteins and is stored in secondary granules of neutrophils and exhibits antibacterial, antiviral, and antifungal activity (Levay and Viljoen 1995). Neutrophils are a major source of lactoferrin. Normal lactoferrin levels in the blood are very low at 1 μg/mL, but in sepsis, these can rise to 200 μg/mL and are likely to be higher at the inflammatory site itself (Li et al. 2006). It acts as a chemoattractant for monocytes promoting inflammation (de la Rosa et al. 2008). Lactoferrin may also induce the production of pro-inflammatory cytokines, such as Macrophage Inflammatory Protein, MIP-1a, and MIP-2 (Actor et al. 2002).

The antimicrobial polypeptide LL-37 is released from secondary granules of neutrophils in its inactive pro-form, hCAP18, which requires proteolytic modification by proteinase-3 for a complete activation. Additionally, LL-37 can promote inflammatory responses by activating monocytes, neutrophils, and T-lymphocytes (Doss et al. 2010, Kai-Larsen and Agerbeth 2008). LL-37 is elevated significantly in the BAL fluids of ARDS patients compared to normal controls (Fahy and Wewers 2005). When instilled into murine lungs, enhanced levels of MCP-1 (Monocyte Chemoattractant Protein-1) and TNF can be retrieved, likely based on the activation of macrophages and epithelial cells (van der Does et al. 2010, Soehnlein and Lindbom 2010). Additionally, LL-37 forms complexes with self-DNA, which potently activate the immune system (Soehnlein and Lindbom 2010). Necrotic cells, which are abundant in ALI, are a common source of such DNA. LL-37 inhibits neutrophil apoptosis (Barlow et al. 2006, Nagaoka et al. 2006), contributing to enhanced accumulation of neutrophils at the site of inflammation.

Defensins

These are arginine-rich cationic peptides that are divided into two subgroups, α-defensins and β-defensins. Human α-defensins 1–4 (HNPs 1–4) are produced principally by neutrophils and stored in azurophilic granules (Tecle et al. 2010). High concentrations of α-defensins have been found in BAL fluids from patients with ARDS correlating with the disease severity (Ashitani et al. 2004). Besides their antimicrobial function, α-defensins act as effectors of inflammatory cytokine production. HNPs activate macrophages to induce the release of TNF-α and interferon (IFN)-γ and promote a phenotypic switch toward a more pro-inflammatory phenotype (Soehnlein et al. 2008b). In ALI, α-defensins also induce IL-8, a chemokine that potently attracts neutrophils (Sakamoto et al. 2005). Moreover, α-defensins increase the permeability of the epithelial monolayer *in vitro* (Aarbiou et al. 2006, Nygaard et al. 1993, Soong et al. 1997, Van et al. 1997).

Azurocidin

It is stored in secretory vesicles and primary granules of neutrophils and is released upon neutrophil adhesion and during neutrophil extravasation (Soehnlein and Lindbom 2009, Soehnlein et al. 2005). Its positive charge allows for immobilization on the endothelial cell surface, where it induces the adhesion of inflammatory monocytes (Soehnlein et al. 2005, Gautam et al. 2001). *In vivo* experiments studying lung damage induced by *S. pyogenes* revealed an important role for neutrophil granule proteins (Soehnlein et al. 2008a, Herwald et al. 2004) in which M1 protein shed from the surface of *S. pyogenes* forms complexes with fibrinogen. These complexes ligate with β2-integrins present on the neutrophil surface and induce neutrophil activation and degranulation causing tissue damage.

Oxidants and ROS

Neutrophils produce vast quantities of reactive oxygen (ROS) and nitrogen (RNS) species like $O_2^{\bullet-}$ and $NO^{\bullet}$ through their oxidant-generating enzyme complexes such as the phagocyte NADPH (Nicotinamide Adenine Dinucleotide Phosphate) oxidase and nitric oxide synthase (NOS), respectively. The membrane-bound multicomponent enzyme complex NADPH oxidase is dormant in resting cells but can be activated rapidly by chemoattractant peptides or chemokines generating high amounts of ROS. The oxidase consists of the catalytic subunit gp91phox (otherwise known as NOX2), the regulatory subunits p22phox, p47phox, p40phox, p67phox, and the small GTPase RAC. Furthermore, the myeloperoxidase, which is found in the neutrophil granules, catalyzes the production of additional ROS species, the hydroxyl radical (•OH), and hypochlorous acid (HOCl). This controlled enzymatic generation of ROS is an integral component of the innate immune system. During ingestion of invading pathogens into phagosomes, ROS generated at the phagosome membrane are released directly into the phagosome thus killing the phagocytosed pathogens.

Exposure of the lung to inhaled or instilled oxidants induces lung injury (Johnson et al. 1981). The pathogenic role of oxidants is reflected by elevated levels of plasma and lung oxidants in patients with ALI/ARDS. Additionally, these levels of oxidants correlate with the severity of the disease. In animal models of ALI, neutrophil-derived ROS and RNS caused lung injury as demonstrated by histological examination and permeability measurements (Auten et al. 2002, Auten et al. 2001). ROS can also disrupt intercellular tight junctions of the endothelium by phosphorylation of focal adhesion kinase (Chiarugi et al. 2003). *In vitro*, ROS induced cell apoptosis and necrosis of ATII cells during oxygen exposure (Roper et al. 2004). *In vivo*, NOX-1–/– mice, but not NOX-2–/– mice, are protected from hyperoxia-induced ALI, suggesting that NADPH oxidase 1 plays a crucial role in this type of ALI (Carnesecchi et al. 2009). Inhibition of NADPH or NOS has decreased sepsis-induced (Wang et al. 1994) and LPS-induced ALI respectively (Kristof et al. 1998).

Role of Endothelial Cells in Neutrophil Transmigration into the Lung

As described earlier, one of the major hallmarks of inflammation is the recruitment of leukocytes, particularly polymorphonuclear leukocytes (PMNs: these include neutrophils, eosinophils, and basophils) to the site of injury or infection. For better clarity and discussion, neutrophils will be referred to as leukocytes in the context of ALI/ARDS. To reach an inflammatory site in the interstitium, the circulating leukocyte must first traverse the endothelial barrier, a process referred to as transendothelial migration (TEM) or diapedesis. The TEM of leukocytes is a complex but highly ordered multi-step process involving sequential activation of adhesive proteins on endothelial cells and their counter receptors on the surface of leukocytes, as depicted in Figure 2. The first step in the TEM process involves the rolling of a leukocyte along the vessel wall during which they make brief adhesive contacts (i.e., ~ 25 ms) with the endothelium (Simon and Goldsmith 2002). The process of rolling begins with the capture of leukocytes from the blood stream by tethering via l-selectin, a constitutively expressed selectin protein on leukocytes

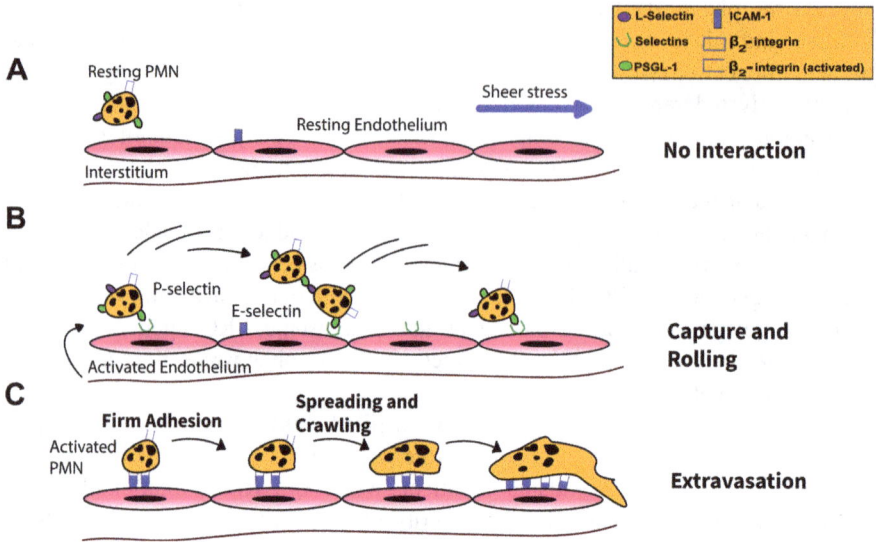

Figure 2. Schematic diagram for transendothelial migration of leukocytes. (A) The resting PMN expresses selectin ligands, but selectins are absent on the resting endothelial cells. Hence, PMN does not interact with the endothelium in the resting stage. (B) Stimulation of the endothelium by pro-inflammatory mediators triggers the expression of selectins on the endothelial cell surface. The tethering of selectins and selectin ligands facilitates primary PMN capture on the endothelium and secondary PMN–PMN recruitment. Tethering transitions to rolling and activation of PMNs which results in the expression of β2-integrins on the PMN surface. (C) The interaction of β2-integrins with ICAM-1 protein expressed on the surface of the activated endothelial cells causes the arrest, followed by spreading and then crawling, and finally trans endothelial migration of PMN into the lung alveolar space and to the site of injury.

that interacts with its glycoprotein ligand expressed on endothelial cells (Abbassi et al. 1991). Rolling is also supported by the binding of endothelial-bound E-selectin and P-selectin to their prototypic ligand, platelet sialoglycoprotein ligand-1 (PSGL-1) on the surface of leukocytes (Jones at al. 1993, Kansas 1996, Lawrence and Springer 1993). The second step, involving the transition from rolling to the arrest of leukocytes, is contingent upon the upregulation of intercellular adhesion molecule-1 (ICAM-1) on the surface of inflamed endothelium (Albelda et al. 1994, Malik and Lo 1996) and the activation of its counter receptor β2-integrins, LFA-1 (Lymphocyte Function Associated Antigen -1), and Mac-1 (Macrophage-1 antigen) on the surface of leukocytes (Diacovo et al. 1996, Diamond et al. 1990, Dustin et al. 1988). Interaction of ICAM-1 with activated β2-integrins ensures a stable shear-resistant adhesion of PMN to the vascular endothelium, enabling PMN to migrate across the endothelial cells into the underlying tissue (Figure 2) (Simon and Green 2005, Smith et al. 1989, Burns et al. 1997, Gopalan et al. 2000).

Intercellular Adhesion Molecule-1

Intercellular Adhesion Molecule-1 (ICAM-1) is a cell surface glycoprotein of 505 amino acids with a molecular weight ranging from 76 to 114 kDa, depending upon the extent of tissue-specific glycosylation. It is a member of the immunoglobulin

Extracellular Domain

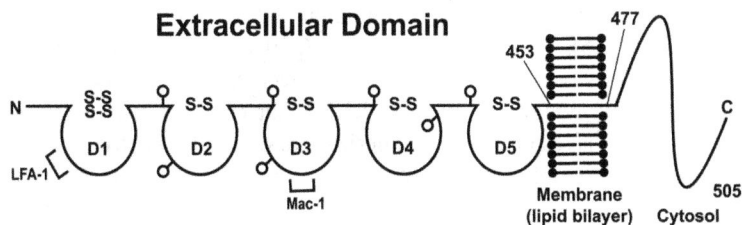

Figure 3. Schematic structure of Intercellular adhesion molecule-1. ICAM-1 contains five extracellular Immunoglobulin-like domains (D1 through D5), a hydrophobic transmembrane domain, and a short cytoplasmic domain. The domains D1 and D3 harbor the binding sites for LFA-1 and Mac-1 that are expressed on activated leukocytes, respectively. S-S represents disulfide bonds that maintain the secondary structure of ICAM-1. The small balloon-like attachments within the structure represent glycosylation (carbohydrate moieties that are tissue-specific). Numbers indicate amino acid residue locations.

superfamily (IgSF) of adhesion molecules and is characterized by the presence of five extracellular Ig-like domains (domains 1–5, D1–5), a hydrophobic transmembrane domain, and a short cytoplasmic domain of 28 amino acids (Figure 3) (Springer 1990, Staunton et al. 1988, Staunton et al. 1989). The binding site for LFA-1 is present in D1 whereas that of Mac-1 maps to D3 of ICAM-1 (Diamond et al. 1990, Diamond et al. 1991, Springer 1990, Staunton et al. 1988).

The extracellular domains of ICAM-1 are essential for the firm adhesion of leukocytes to the endothelium. In addition to the density, the distribution of ICAM-1 on the endothelial cell surface contributes to leukocyte TEM. Engagement of endothelial ICAM-1 with leukocyte β2-integrins alters the distribution dynamics of ICAM-1, leading to its clustering on the endothelial cell surface. Clustering of cell surface ICAM-1 occurs following its engagement with leukocyte β2 integrins and serves to promote leukocyte adhesion to the endothelium and subsequent TEM (Cernuda-Morollon and Ridley 2006, Wojciak–Stothard et al. 1999). The TEM can also be induced by specific antibodies that mimic leukocyte binding to ICAM-1 or exposure of endothelial cells to TNFα (Javaid et al. 2003, Thompson et al. 2002, Wojciak–Stothard et al. 1999). Clustering of constitutively expressed cell surface ICAM-1 plays an important role in mediating the rapid-onset of endothelial adhesivity toward leukocytes (Javaid et al. 2003).

Nuclear Factor-Kappa B: The Master Pro-Inflammatory Regulator

The pro-inflammatory transcription factor, Nuclear Factor-Kappa B, was first discovered in 1986 by Sen and Baltimore (Sen and Baltimore 1986) during studies that were aimed at the identification of proteins that bind to immunoglobulin (Ig) heavy chain and κ light chain enhancers present in the genomic DNA of B lymphocytes. The nuclear factor found to be necessary for the transcription of immunoglobulin kappa light chain in B cells was, therefore, named NF-κB (nuclear factor-κB). Being one of the most intensely studied eukaryotic transcription factors, it plays a pivotal role in controlling varied biological effects ranging from inflammatory, immune, and stress-induced responses to cell fate decisions such as proliferation, differentiation, tumorigenesis, and apoptosis. The mammalian NF-κB family consists of five members: RelA (p65), RelB, c-Rel, NF-κB1 (p50 and its precursor p105), and NF-κB2 (p52 and its precursor p100). All members share a conserved N-terminal 300-amino acid Rel homology domain (RHD) that contains nuclear localization signal (NLS), which is responsible for dimerization, sequence-specific DNA binding, and interaction with inhibitory IκB proteins in the cytoplasm (Figure 4A). A critical feature in RelA, RelB, and c-Rel that distinguishes them from p50 and p52 is the presence of a transactivation domain (TAD) within the carboxy-terminal region of these proteins (Figure 4A).

The diverse biological effects of NF-κB are mediated, in part, by the ability of NF-κB proteins to form numerous homo- and heterodimers that differentially regulate target genes (Bonizzi and Karin 2004). For example, p50 and p52 homodimers serve as repressors, whereas dimers containing RelA or c-Rel are transcriptional activators. Heterodimers of RelB with either p50 or p52 display greater regulatory flexibility and function both as an activator and a repressor (Hayden and Ghosh 2004, Bonizzi and Karin 2004). Activation of specific dimers is mediated by distinct upstream signaling pathways that are activated in a stimulus- and cell-specific manner (Bonizzi and Karin 2004, Senftleben et al. 2001).

The Classical and Alternate Pathways of NF-κB Activation

NF-κB dimers are mostly sequestered in the cytoplasm by IκBs, a family of inhibitory proteins that mask the NLS by virtue of their interaction with RHD. These proteins, which include IκBα, IκBβ, BCL3, IκBε, IκBγ (Figure 4B), and the precursor proteins NF-κB2/p100 and NF-κB1/p105 (Figure 4A), contain five to seven ankyrin repeats that mediate association with the RHD. The presence of these repeats allows the precursors (NF-κB2/p100 and NF-κB1/p105) to also function as IκBs and retain their partners, the Rel proteins, in the cytoplasm (Hayden and Ghosh 2004, Bonizzi and Karin 2004). Crystallographic studies have revealed that IκB proteins mask only the NLS of RelA/p65, whereas the NLS of p50 remain accessible (Hayden and Ghosh 2004, Huxford et al. 1998). The accessibility of the NLS on p50 and the presence of nuclear export signal (NES) on IκBα and RelA/p65 allow constant shuttling of IκBα/NF-κB complexes between the nucleus and the cytoplasm. Despite this dynamic shuttling, the steady-state localization of IκBα/NF-κB is in the cytosol (Hayden and Ghosh 2004, Ghosh and Karin 2002). Following signal-induced degradation of IκBα, which results in the removal of IκB NES and unmasking of RelA/p65 NLS, the steady-state localization is altered and NF-κB becomes predominantly nuclear.

Degradation of IκB is initiated through phosphorylation of IκBs on specific serine residues by a macromolecular cytoplasmic IκB kinase (IKK) complex composed of the catalytic subunits, IKKα and IKKβ and the regulatory subunit NEMO/IKKγ (Figure 4C) (Ghosh and Karin 2002). (In general, phosphorylation of any protein molecule by an enzyme called kinase represents a post-translational modification of that protein molecule, which renders it either active, inactive, or subjects it to degradation or other types of chemical modification depending upon the type of stimuli the cells are challenged with. Kinases could be serine or threonine kinases that

A. Members of NF-κB Family

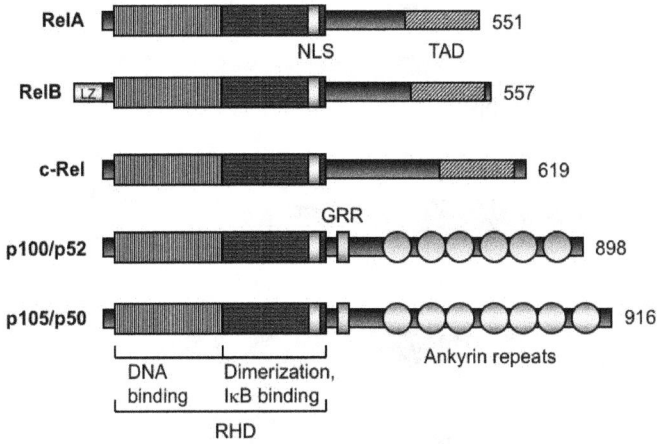

Figure 4A. Schematic representation of NF-κB family members and their regulators. The number of amino acids in each protein is indicated toward the right. (A) The N-terminal region (~ 300 amino acids) of NF-κB proteins has RHD. The RHD contains a DNA-binding domain and dimerization/IκBa binding domains and NLS located on the C-terminal side of the RHD. In addition to RHD, RelA, RelB, and c-Rel contain transactivation domains (TAD). The proteins p105 and p100 contain ankyrin repeats (circles) and a glycine-rich region (GRR). The ankyrin repeats render these proteins inactive and the GRR is required for co-translational processing of p105 to p50 and post-translational processing of p100 to p52 as indicated in (D).

B. Members of IκB Family

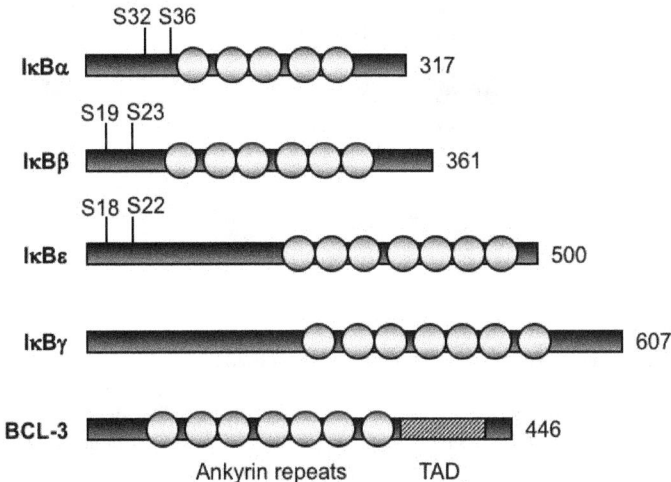

Figure 4B. Members of the IκB family contain ankyrin repeats (circles) that mediate their interaction with RHD. Phosphorylation of indicated serines in these proteins is required for their degradation by the proteasome. Bcl3 by virtue of possessing ankyrin repeats is frequently considered a member of the IκB family. However, Bcl3 also contains a TAD, and therefore complexes resulting from the interaction of Bcl3 with either p50 or p52 are transcriptionally active.

C. Members of IKK family

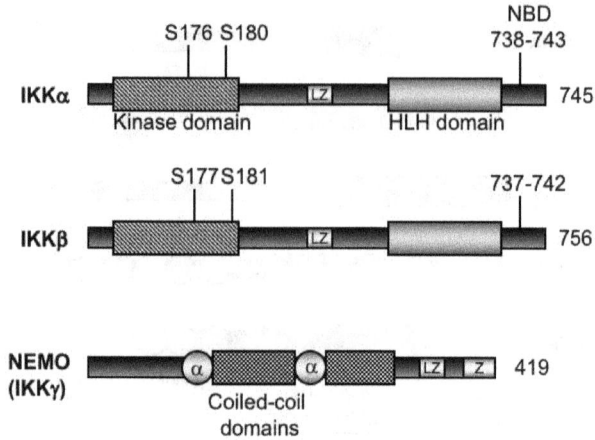

Figure 4C. All three members of the IKK complex possess the LZ motif. Of these, only IKKα and IKKβ possess kinase and HLH domains. Phosphorylation of indicated serines is required for the activation of IKKα and IKKβ. IKKγ (NEMO), which is unrelated to IKKα and IKKβ, possesses a zinc finger domain (Z), coiled-coil domains, and two α-helical (α) domains. These domains are considered to mediate the regulatory function of NEMO and its association with the NEMO binding domain (NBD) of IKK.

D. Processing of p100 to p52

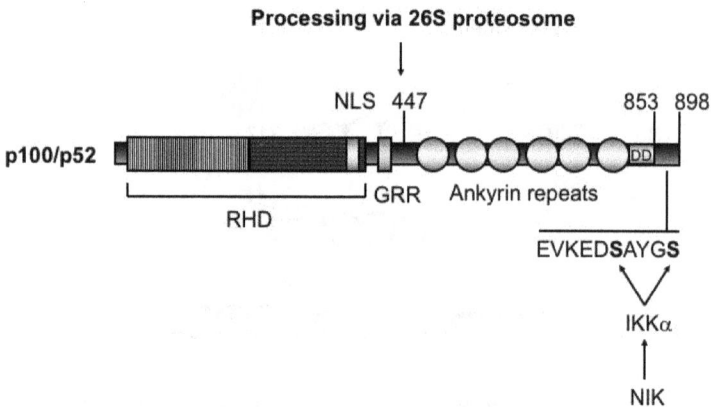

Figure 4D. Processing of p100 to p52. The processing is initiated by the phosphorylation of two serine residues at the C-terminus of p100 by IKKα, secondary to its activation by NF-κB inducing kinase (NIK). The presumed site of the cleavage for p100 (amino acid 447) is indicated. The sequences in GRR prevent further progression of the 26S proteasome, which digests the C-terminal half of p100 following its ubiquitination.

phosphorylate serine or threonine residue(s), respectively, whereas tyrosine kinases cause phosphorylation of tyrosine residue(s) on target proteins). Phosphorylation marks IκBs for polyubiquitination by the E3-SCFβ-TrCP ubiquitin ligase, which in turn targets them to degradation by the 26 S proteasome (Hayden and Ghosh 2004,

Bonizzi and Karin 2004). Degradation of IκB results in translocation of the released NF-κB dimer to the nucleus, where it activates the transcription following its binding to the κB-enhancer consensus sequences (5'-GGGRNYYYCC-3', where R is a purine, Y is a pyrimidine, and N is any nucleotide) in the promoter of target genes.

There are two major signaling pathways by which extracellular stimuli mediate IκB degradation-dependent translocation of dimers to the nucleus. In the classical NF-κB signaling pathway, the key event is the activation of IKKβ induced by pro-inflammatory cytokines and pathogen-associated molecular patterns (PAMPs) following the engagement of different receptors belonging to the tumor necrosis factor receptor (TNFR) and toll-like receptor (TLR)-interleukin-1 receptor (IL-1R) superfamilies (Figure 5A).

Activated IKKβ in association with IKKα and IKKγ catalyzes the phosphorylation of IκBs on two N-terminal serine residues (at sites equivalent to Ser32 and Ser36 of IκBα and Ser19 and Ser23 of IκBβ), polyubiquitination (at sites equivalent to Lys21 and Lys22 of IκBα), and subsequent degradation by the 26 S proteasome. Through this pathway, the liberated NF-κB dimers, generally the prototypical heterodimer p50-p65/RelA, undergo nuclear translocation and DNA binding to

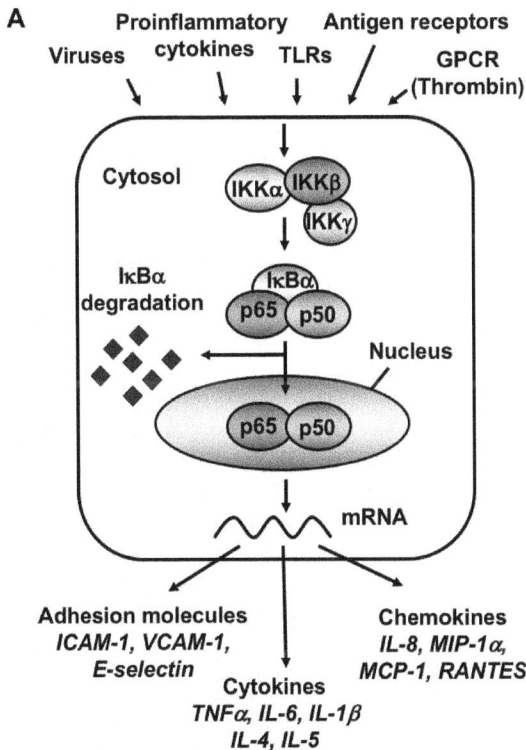

Figure 5A. Pathways of NF-κB activation. The Classical Pathway. This pathway is activated by a host of stimuli including viruses, pro-inflammatory cytokines, antigen receptors TLR, and G-protein coupled receptors (GPCR). This pathway is mediated by IKKβ, which catalyzes the phosphorylation of IκBα leading to its ubiquitination and degradation. The released NF-κB translocates to the nucleus and activates the expression of multiple inflammatory and innate immune genes.

B

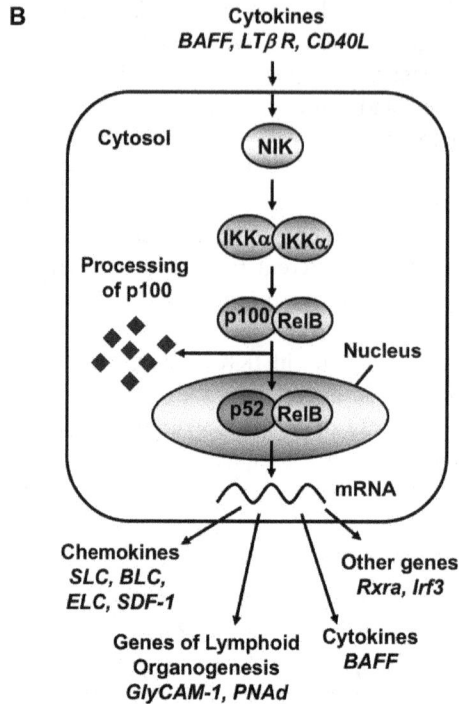

Figure 5B. The Alternate Pathway. This pathway is mediated by IKKα following its activation by NIK in response to cytokines such as LTβR, BAFF, and CD40L. Activation of this pathway leads to phosphorylation and processing of p100, generating p52:RelB heterodimers. Following nuclear translocation, p52:RelB activate the genes mainly involved in the development and maintenance of secondary lymphoid organs. Abbreviations: BAFF, B-cell-activating factor; BLC, B-lymphocyte chemoattractant; ELC, Epstein-Barr virus-induced molecule-1 ligand CC chemokine; GlyCAM, glycosylation-dependent cell adhesion molecule; LTβR, Lymphotoxin-β receptor; PNAd, peripheral lymph node addressin; SLC, secondary lymphoid tissue chemokine; SDF-1, stromal cell-derived factor-1; CD40L, Cluster of Differentiation 40 Ligand.

activate transcription of genes involved in innate immunity and inflammatory responses (Hayden and Ghosh 2004, Bonizzi and Karin 2004, Ghosh and Karin 2002). It should be noted that activated IKKα can also phosphorylate IκBs; however, biochemical and genetic studies indicate that IKKβ is the dominant kinase involved in the phosphorylation of IκB proteins and thus is a crucial regulator of the classical NF-κB pathway (Li et al. 1999, Tanaka et al. 1999).

The alternative NF-κB signaling pathway is another unique pathway that is independent of IKKβ and IKKγ participation but is strictly dependent on IKKα (Figure 5B). The IKKα homodimers selectively phosphorylate the two C-terminal serines of NF-κB2/p100 associated with RelB (Bonizzi and Karin 2004, Senftleben et al. 2001) (Figure 4D). The phosphorylation of these sites is essential for p100 processing to p52. Thus, processing of p100 releases a subset of transcriptionally active NF-κB dimers, consisting mainly of p52 and RelB (Senftleben et al. 2001, Regnier et al. 1997). Processing of p52 is also dependent on ubiquitination and proteasomal degradation of p100 (Xiao et al. 2004). However, unlike complete degradation of IκBs, the phosphorylation-dependent ubiquitination of p100 leads to only degradation of its inhibitory C-terminal half. This releases the p52 polypeptide containing N-terminal RHD associated with RelB and the p52-RelB heterodimer translocate to the nucleus, where it activates the transcription of genes involved in development and maintenance of lymphoid organs (Bonizzi and Karin 2004).

Regulation of I Kappa B Kinase: A Central Event in NF-κB Signaling

Activation of IKK is the central event in the mechanism of NF-κB activation; one possible exception is the casein kinase 2 (CK2), which has been shown to mediate ultraviolet (UV)-induced NF-κB activation by catalyzing the phosphorylation of IκBα at a cluster of C-terminal sites (Kato Jr et al. 2003). The majority of extracellular signals causing activation of NF-κB converge on this high molecular-weight kinase complex, which is composed of at least three subunits: IKKα, IKKβ and IKKγ (Figure 4C). The IKKα and IKKβ are the catalytic subunits and share 52% overall amino acid sequence identity in their primary structures and 65% identity in their catalytic domains (Ghosh and Karin 2002). The characteristic features of these kinases include an N-terminal kinase domain, a C-terminal helix-loop-helix (HLH) domain, and leucine zipper (LZ) domain (Figure 4C). The HLH domain is required for full IKKβ activity as deletion mutants lacking this domain possess diminished kinase activity following overexpression or stimulation (Hayden and Ghosh 2004, Ghosh and Karin 2002). IKKα and IKKβ dimerization is dependent upon LZ domain, which is therefore required for kinase activity (Hayden and Ghosh 2004, Ghosh and Karin 2002). The subunit IKKγ (also termed NEMO, NF-κB Essential Modifier) has no catalytic activity but plays a critical regulatory role in protein-protein interaction by virtue of its long stretches of coiled-coil sequence and C-terminal LZ domain. Gene targeting experiments in mice have shown that the IKK subunits are differentially required for NF-κB activation depending upon the stimulus and the cellular context (Bonizzi and Karin 2004, Hayden and Ghosh 2004, Ghosh and Karin 2002) (Figure 5 A&B).

Activation of the IKK complex involves the phosphorylation of two serine residues in the activation loop within the kinase domain of IKKα (Ser176 and Ser180) or IKKβ (Ser177 and Ser181) (Figure 4C). The NF-κB inducing kinase (NIK), a critical component of the alternative pathway of NF-κB signaling, provides the strongest proof of being an upstream IKK kinase. NIK, a MAPK (Mitogen-Activated Protein Kinase) family member, directly phosphorylates and activates IKKα following activation of the alternative pathway. Despite reports that NIK associates with IKKβ and NEMO and thus participates in classical signaling pathway (Regnier et al. 1997, Bouwmwester et al. 2004), the phenotype of NIK-/- mice, which are severely deficient in lymph node development is consistent with NIK functioning only in the alternative pathway. Under steady-state conditions, NIK is bound to tumor necrosis factor (TNF) receptor-associated factors 2 and 3 (TRAF2/3) and Cellular Inhibitor of Apoptosis Protein 1 and 2 (cIAP1/2), resulting in its ubiquitination and continuous degradation. However, stimulation with cytokines, such as TWEAK

(TNF-like weak inducer of apoptosis), LTα/β (lymphotoxin alpha/beta), or the endotoxin LPS (lipopolysaccharide), and specific binding to their membrane receptors sequesters TRAF2/3, which is then tagged for ubiquitination by cIAP1 and its subsequent degradation thus allowing accumulation of newly synthesized NIK within the cell (Zhang et al. 2017, Bonizzi and Karin 2004, Gilmore 2006). The stabilization and accumulation of NIK are critical for subsequent activation of the non-canonical NF-κB pathway (Qing et al. 2005). Following receptor activation, NIK phosphorylates IKKα at Ser 176 and Ser 180, resulting in its activation and subsequent phosphorylation of p100 (Ling et al. 1998). Phosphorylation of p100 induces its binding to ubiquitin ligase, β-TrCP (beta transducing repeat containing proteins) and induces its partial proteasomal processing to p52 (Heusch et al. 1999, Xiao et al. 2004). This proteasomal processing of p100 removes the C-term ankyrin repeat domain, which otherwise functions similarly to the inhibitory nature of mature IκB proteins, holding the non-canonical transcription factor RelB inactive in the cytoplasm. Thus, after processing, the newly formed p52 binds to RelB forming the p52-RelB complex, which then translocates to the nucleus to regulate transcription (Sun 2012). Although IKKα is the key regulator of p100 phosphorylation and proteolytic processing, NIK functions to activate IKKα and also serves as an adapter protein to recruit IKKα to p100. Ultimately, the NIK-IKKα-p100 complex is required for the generation of mature, transcriptionally active p52 protein (Xiao et al. 2004).

Phosphorylation of RelA/p65

Apart from IκBα degradation and nuclear translocation of NF-κB, the transcriptional activity of NF-κB is also regulated by post-translational modifications, particularly by phosphorylation and acetylation (Chen and Greene 2004, Viatour et al. 2005). Studies have shown that phosphorylation of RelA/p65 at Ser276 and Ser311 in RHD or Ser529 and Ser536 in TAD enhances the transcriptional capacity of NF-κB in the nucleus (Chen and Greene 2004, Viatour et al. 2005). Moreover, phosphorylation of RelA also decreases its affinity for its negative regulator, IκBα (Chen and Greene 2004, Viatour et al. 2005). Unlike IκBα phosphorylation, the RelA phosphorylation site and the kinase involved vary in a stimulus- and cell-specific manner (Chen and Greene 2004, Viatour et al. 2005). For example, phosphorylation of RelA at Ser276 following lipopolysaccharide (LPS) challenge is mediated by the catalytic subunit of protein kinase A (PKAc), whereas TNFα-induced phosphorylation at this residue is catalyzed by mitogen- and stress-activated kinase-1 (MSK-1) (Figure 6). Interestingly, PKAc phosphorylates RelA in the cytoplasm, whereas MSK-1 functions in the nucleus. TNFα also induces phosphorylation of Ser311 within the RHD of RelA and this phosphorylation requires the participation of yet another kinase, PKC-ζ (Protein Kinase C- zeta) (Figure 6). Phosphorylation of Ser529 is mediated by CK2 whereas Ser536 is phosphorylated by IKKα and IKKβ. Other kinases that phosphorylate RelA include glycogen-synthase kinase-3beta (GSK3β), phosphatidylinositol 3-kinase (PI3K) and NF-κB-activating kinase (NAK; also known as TANK biding kinase-1 [TBK-1], and TRAF2-associated kinase [T2K]) (Chen and Greene 2004, Viatour

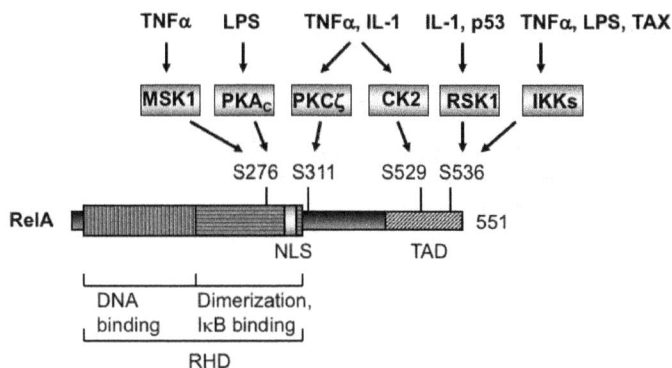

Figure 6. RelA phosphorylation sites. The phosphorylation sites in RelA include Ser276 and Ser311 in RHD, and Ser529 and Ser536 in TAD. These sites are phosphorylated by multiple kinases upon activation by distinct stimuli as indicated. The abbreviated forms are indicated in the main text.

et al. 2005). Given the multiplicity of phosphorylation sites and the kinases involved, it is likely that concurrent phosphorylation of multiple sites has cooperative functional effects on the transcriptional activity of NF-κB.

Phosphorylation of RelA also serves an important function in promoting the recruitment of various transcriptional coactivators. Phosphorylation of RelA at Ser276 by PKAc, MSK1, or at Ser311 by PKC-ζ facilitates the interaction of cAMP-response element binding protein (CREB)/CREB binding protein (CBP) and p300 to RelA (Hayden and Ghosh 2004, Chen and Greene 2004). The RelA-CBP complex effectively displaces the transcriptionally repressive histone deacetylase complexes, especially p50-HDAC1 complexes, which frequently occupy κB enhancers of target genes under unstimulated conditions (Hayden and Ghosh 2004, Chen and Greene 2004, Viatour et al. 2005). Thus, phosphorylation of RelA facilitates its interaction with other components of the basal transcription machinery, thereby controlling the transcriptional responses.

Regulation of Endothelial Inflammation by NF-κB

As emphasized earlier, the expression of adhesion molecules on the endothelial cell surface, the release of pro-inflammatory cytokines and neutrophil transmigration into the lung tissue constitutes an important sequence of events in the pathogenesis of ALI. During inflammation, endothelial cells are exposed to a huge milieu of pro-inflammatory mediators such as thrombin (released during tissue injury and sepsis), TNFα, different pro-inflammatory cytokines, chemokines, endotoxins (lipopolysaccharide released due to bacterial infections and sepsis), components derived from viral infections, etc. While the current literature contains an enormous amount of information on the complex signaling mechanisms in different cell types associated with ALI pathology, given the crucial role played by endothelial cells, the following sections will focus on some of the important findings of the past two decades that led to increased understanding on the mechanisms of NF-κB activation and inflammatory gene expression using different endothelial cell models.

Regulation of ICAM-1 by NF-κB

The human ICAM-1 gene is located on chromosome 19 and comprises seven exons and six introns with each of the five Ig (Immunoglobulin)-like domains encoded by a separate exon (Roebuck and Finnegan 1999). Expression of ICAM-1 gene in endothelial cells can be induced by a variety of mediators including thrombin, TNFα, IL-1β, LPS, phorbol esters (Phorbol Myristic Acid), VEGF, sheer stress, oxidants, infectious agents, and high glucose (Roebuck and Finnegan 1999, Burns et al. 1999, Harcourt et al. 1999, Kim et al. 2001, Lane et al. 1990, Minami and Aird 2005, Quagliaro et al. 2005, Rahman et al. 1999a, Rahman et al. 1999b, Vielma et al. 2003, Wu and Aird 2005). ICAM-1 expression is regulated mainly at the level of transcription (Collins et al 1995; Degitz et al. 1991; Voraberger et al. 1991; Wawryk et al. 1991). Analysis of the 5' flanking region of ICAM-1 gene revealed that ICAM-1 promoter contains binding sites for several transcription factors including two NF-κB sites; an upstream NF-κB site (-533 bases from translation start site), and a downstream NF-κB site (-223 bases from translation start site) (Voraberger et al. 1991) (Figure 7). Site-directed mutagenesis of this region indicated that activation of the downstream NF-κB site is essential for ICAM-1 transcription (Collins et al. 1995, Ledebur and Parks 1995, Rahman et al. 1999a). Gel supershift assays demonstrated that ICAM-1 expression requires NF-κB p65 (RelA/p65) binding to the downstream NF-κB site of the ICAM-1 promoter (Ledebur and Parks 1995, Rahman et al. 1999a).

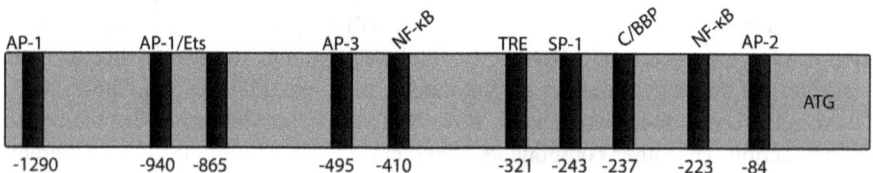

Figure 7. Structure of ICAM-1 promoter. The rectangles indicate the location of the potential binding sites for transcription factors AP-1, AP-2, and AP-3 (Activating Protein-1, -2, and -3), Ets, NF-κB, TRE (tetradecanoyl phorbol acetate responsive element), Sp-1 (promoter selective-1), C/EBP (CAAT enhancer binding protein). The codon ATG indicates the translation start site.

Activation of Endothelial NF-κB by Serine and Tyrosine Phosphorylation

The pathogenesis of ALI involves bidirectional cooperation and close interaction between inflammatory and coagulation pathways. A key molecule linking coagulation and inflammation is the pro-coagulant thrombin, a serine protease, the concentration of which is elevated in plasma and bronchoalveolar lavage fluids of patients with ALI and ARDS.

An important function of cAMP (cyclic Adenosine Monophosphate) is to serve as a messenger to activate protein kinase A (Taylor et al. 1990), which has been implicated in the regulation of numerous genes through phosphorylation and activation of the CREB protein (Daniel et al. 1998). Earlier studies had shown that cAMP regulates the activation of NF-κB in a cell-specific manner. In the promyelocytic cell line HL-60, elevated cAMP levels induced NF-κB activation

(Serkkola and Hurme 1993), and in contrast, exposure of endothelial cells to cAMP prevented NF-κB activation (Ollivier et al. 1996). Studies aimed at identifying the mechanisms of thrombin-induced NF-κB activation and ICAM-1 expression using human umbilical vein endothelial cells (HUVEC) as a model system revealed that elevation of cAMP levels by pretreatment of cells with drugs such as forskolin or dibutyryl cAMP prevented thrombin-induced ICAM-1 expression (Rahman et al. 2004). Investigation of underlying mechanisms revealed that elevated cAMP inhibited thrombin-induced phosphorylation (activation) of p38 MAP kinase (known to cause RelA/p65 phosphorylation), which in turn resulted in inhibition of phosphorylation of RelA/p65 at serine 536 (RelA/p65 is a p65/p65 homodimer of NF-κB that is predominantly activated by thrombin stimulation in endothelial cells). This suggested that thrombin induces ICAM-1 expression in endothelial cells by enhancing the transcriptional activation of RelA/p65 through its serine phosphorylation by p38 MAP Kinase. The elevated levels of cAMP, however, failed to inhibit other events of the NF-κB activation pathway including thrombin-induced IκBα degradation or DNA-binding activity of NF-κB. These data suggest that reduced intracellular cAMP concentration in endothelial cells favors thrombin-induced p38 MAP Kinase activation-dependent phosphorylation of RelA/p65 [transcriptional activation] bound to ICAM-1 promoter, thus promoting inflammatory phenotype in these cells. These observations support the fact that an increase in cellular cAMP levels induced by pharmacological agents pentoxifylline, rolipram, and amrinone suppresses the expression of pro-inflammatory genes and is beneficial in inflammatory conditions such as autoimmune encephalomyelitis and acute cardiac allograft rejection (Han et al. 1990, Hirozane et al. 1995, Sommer et al. 1995). Thus, the above findings provide a basis for the mechanism of the anti-inflammatory action of cAMP, which may have implications in novel therapeutics targeting p38 MAPK.

In addition to serine/threonine kinases, tyrosine kinases, particularly members of the Src oncogene family, are implicated in NF-κB activation (Fan et al. 2003, Huang et al. 2003, Imbert et al. 1996, Mahabeleshwar and Kundu 2003, Waris et al. 2003). Depending on the cell types and stimulus used, c-Src or other members of the Src family are engaged to activate NF-κB via tyrosine phosphorylation of IKKβ or IκBα (Fan et al. 2003, Huang et al. 2003, Imbert et al. 1996, Mahabeleshwar and Kundu 2003, Waris et al. 2003). The c-Src requires its autophosphorylation at Tyr416 for full activation. Studies in HUVEC revealed that pharmacological inhibition of tyrosine kinases using stilbene heterocyclic compounds, such as genistein, herbimycin (general tyrosine kinase inhibitors), and PP2 (c-Src inhibitor) or ablation of c-Src protein via RNA silencing approach prevented thrombin-induced ICAM-1 expression by causing inhibition of NF-κB transcriptional activity (Bijli et al. 2007). The tyrosine kinase inhibition, however, had no impact on IκBα phosphorylation/degradation, RelA/p65 Ser 536 phosphorylation, and NF-κB DNA binding nor was any NF-κB dimer exchange observed. Huang et al. have demonstrated that c-Src signals TNFα-induced ICAM-1 expression by a mechanism involving tyrosine phosphorylation-dependent activation of IKKβ in A549, a lung airway epithelial cell line. Activated IKKβ in turn phosphorylates IκBα on Ser32 and Ser36 to induce its degradation and consequently translocation of NF-κB to the nucleus. Other studies have shown that c-Src controls

NF-κB activation through tyrosine phosphorylation of IκBα at Tyr42 by a pathway that is independent of the IKK complex. Phosphorylation of IκBα at Tyr42 causes it to dissociate from NF-κB and thus facilitates nuclear localization of NF-κB in the absence of ubiquitin-dependent degradation of IκBα (Fan et al. 2003, Imbert et al. 1996, Mahabeleshwar and Kundu 2003). Interestingly, in HUVEC, c-Src appeared to physically associate with RelA/p65 and cause its direct tyrosine phosphorylation upon thrombin stimulation. These data implicate a novel role of c-Src in directly activating NF-κB by causing its tyrosine phosphorylation and thereby ICAM-1 expression in endothelial cells (Bijli et al. 2007).

In a very similar study, inhibition of Syk tyrosine kinase (spleen-rich tyrosine kinase), a member of the ZAP family of non-receptor tyrosine kinases, also prevented thrombin-induced NF-κB transcriptional activity and ICAM-1 expression in HUVEC that was independent of IκBα phosphorylation/degradation, RelA/p65 Ser536 phosphorylation and NF-κB DNA binding (Bijli et al. 2008). Similar to c-Src, activated Syk was also found to associate with and cause tyrosine phosphorylation of RelA/p65 upon thrombin stimulation (Bijli et al. 2008). The above role of Syk in promoting NF-κB activation-dependent inflammatory response is consistent with the described role of Syk in regulating NF-κB-dependent responses in immune cells. For example, treatment of fibronectin-adhered neutrophils with TNF-α, IL-8, and granulocyte-macrophage colony-stimulating factor (GMCSF) results in NF-κB activation in a Syk-dependent manner (Kettritz et al. 2004). Syk also plays a role in mediating H2O2- and TNF-α-induced NF-κB activation in Jurkat cells and thereby protecting them from undergoing apoptosis (Takada et al. 2003, Takada and Aggarwal 2004). In addition to immune cells, activation of Syk is implicated in β1 integrin signaling and TNF-α-induced expression of NF-κB-dependent genes, ICAM-1 and IL-6, in airway epithelial cells (Ulanova et al. 2005). Although these studies demonstrated the role of Syk in activating IKK to facilitate IκBα phosphorylation/degradation-dependent activation of NF-κB, the critical role of c-Src and Syk in activating NF-κB via its tyrosine phosphorylation in HUVEC is a novel observation and suggests that c-Src and Syk likely coordinate with each other in NF-κB activation. Although it is still unclear which tyrosine residues in NF-κB are phosphorylated by c-Src and Syk, the similarity of the kinetics of thrombin-induced tyrosine phosphorylation with IκBα degradation (both peaking at 1-hour post-thrombin challenge) suggested that degradation of IκBα (that is bound to RelA/p65 in the cytoplasm) exposes critical tyrosine residues on RelA/p65 for phosphorylation by c-Src and Syk in the RHD. Analysis by UniProtKB/Swiss-Prot, a protein sequence database, of RelA/p65 has revealed the presence of five potential residues (Tyr20, Tyr150, Tyr257, Tyr306, and Tyr360) for tyrosine phosphorylation. Given that these residues are present within or near the RHD (part of RelA/p65 that binds to IκBα in the cytoplasm), it is likely that in the absence of IκBα degradation, these residues are not accessible for phosphorylation by the bound c-Src/Syk (Bijli et al. 2007). Thus IKKβ-dependent degradation of IκBα by thrombin may result in the unmasking of these residues, rendering them accessible for phosphorylation by c-Src/Syk, thereby causing transcriptional activation of NF-κB.

Proline-rich tyrosine kinase 2 (Pyk2), also known as calcium-dependent tyrosine kinase, is a non-receptor tyrosine kinase and a member of the focal adhesion kinase family. It is expressed in various cell types, including neuronal cells and fibroblasts, but is abundant in cells of hematopoietic origin, especially B lymphocytes and monocytes/macrophages (Lev et al. 1995, Okigaki et al. 2003, Avraham et al. 2000). Pyk2 is also present in different types of endothelial cells and has been implicated in various signaling pathways (Keogh et al. 2002, Cheng et al. 2002). Apart from ICAM-1, other key targets of NF-κB in endothelial cells include vascular cell adhesion molecule (VCAM)-1 and monocyte chemoattractant protein (MCP)-1. VCAM-1 is an inducible adhesive protein that interacts with its counter receptor, very late antigen-4 (VLA-4) present in the circulating monocytes and lymphocytes (Chuluyan et al. 1995). MCP-1 is a secreted protein that specifically attracts monocytes to the site of inflammation (Boring et al. 1997). Thus, the coordinate action of VCAM-1 and MCP-1 serves to promote the adhesion of monocytes to the vascular endothelium and subsequently their TEM to the peripheral tissues, resulting in tissue injury (Chuluyan et al. 1995, Boring et al. 1997, Springer, 1994). Phosphorylation of Pyk2 at Tyr402 is required for its full activation. Since thrombin stimulation causes calcium release and given the dependency of Pyk2 activation on intracellular calcium, Bijli et al. undertook studies to determine the possible role of activated Pyk2 in thrombin-induced NF-κB activation and VCAM-1 and MCP-1 expression in human pulmonary artery endothelial cells (HPAEC). Unlike c-Src and Syk, these studies revealed that Pyk2 inhibition directly impacted the classical pathway of NF-κB activation. Inhibition of Pyk2 impaired IKK activation, IκBα phosphorylation, RelA/p65 Ser536 phosphorylation, and RelA/p65 DNA binding, thereby inhibiting NF-κB activity and inflammatory gene expression (Bijli et al. 2013). Thus, all the above studies demonstrate the unique and critical roles played by different tyrosine kinases in enhancing the thrombin-induced transcriptional activity of NF-κB and inflammatory gene expression in endothelial cells.

Cytoskeletal Changes Facilitate Endothelial NF-κB Activation

As earlier described, full NF-κB transcriptional activity depends on two key steps: its translocation from the cytoplasm into the nucleus for DNA binding and its transcriptional activation via post-translational modifications. Although its nuclear translocation is secondary to IκBα degradation, the underlying mechanisms that facilitate its nuclear translocation have remained elusive. Studies have shown that cytoskeletal proteins that serve structural functions inside the cell may be involved in this event. Actin cytoskeleton is dynamic, and the rates of polymerization and depolymerization of actin are critical determinants of many cellular responses, including transcriptional regulation (Hofmann et al. 2004, Miralles et al. 2003, Posern et al. 2002, Rivas et al. 2004). In HUVEC, thrombin was found to alter the actin cytoskeleton, and interfering with these alterations, whether by stabilizing or destabilizing the actin filaments, prevented thrombin-induced NF-κB activation and consequently expression of its target gene, ICAM-1 (Fazal et al. 2007). This blockade of NF-κB activation occurred downstream of IκBα degradation and was associated with impaired RelA/p65 nuclear translocation. Thrombin stimulation induced an association of RelA/p65 with actin; however, this interaction was sensitive to drugs, cytochalasin B and Latrunculin B that prevent stress fiber formation (formation of filamentous actin [F-actin]) and to the drug, jasplakinolide that stabilizes stress fibers. On the contrary, in parallel studies, stabilizing or destabilizing the actin filaments failed to inhibit RelA/p65 nuclear accumulation and ICAM-1 expression induced by pro-inflammatory cytokine, TNF-α. Thus, these studies reveal the existence of actin cytoskeleton-dependent and independent pathways that may be engaged in a stimulus-specific manner to facilitate RelA/p65 nuclear import and thereby ICAM-1 expression in endothelial cells (Fazal et al. 2007).

The above observations with thrombin led to further investigations on the mechanism of thrombin-induced stress fiber formation which is required for NF-κB nuclear translocation. A key signal mediating RelA/p65 activation by thrombin involves stimulation of the small GTPase RhoA and its effector Rho-associated kinase (ROCK) (Volovyk et al. 2006, Anwar et al. 2004). Activated RhoA/ROCK leads to activation of IKKβ, which in turn mediates phosphorylation and degradation of IκBα and thereby release of RelA/p65 for its nuclear uptake and binding to the ICAM-1 promoter (Anwar et al. 2004). One of the RhoA/ROCK effectors that mediate reorganization of the actin cytoskeleton is the actin-depolymerizing factor, cofilin, a family of small (15–20 kDa) proteins that bind monomeric and filamentous actin (Bamburg and Wiggan 2002, Chen et al. 2000). Cofilin regulates actin dynamics by depolymerizing actin filaments at their pointed ends or by creating new filament barbed ends for F-actin assembly through their severing activity (Hotulainen et al. 2005, Theriot 1997). This ability of cofilin depends on the status of its phosphorylation at Ser3 (Bamburg et al. 1999). Phosphorylation of cofilin renders it inactive and prevents it from binding to actin, thus facilitating actin polymerization (Bamburg et al. 1999). This phosphorylation event is catalyzed by LIM kinases (LIMK), which in turn are phosphorylated and activated by ROCK (Lawler 1999, Maekawa et al. 1999, Sumi et al. 2001, Ohashi et al. 2000). Stimulation of HUVEC with thrombin resulted in Ser3 phosphorylation (inactivation) of cofilin and formation of actin stress fibers in a ROCK-dependent manner (Fazal et al. 2009). However, the genetic knockdown of cofilin-1 stabilized the actin filaments and inhibited thrombin or RhoA-induced (using a constitutively active form of RhoA) NF-κB activity in these cells. Similarly, a constitutively inactive mutant of cofilin-1 (Cof1-S3D), known to stabilize the actin cytoskeleton, also inhibited NF-κB activity by thrombin. On the other extreme, overexpression of wild-type cofilin-1 or constitutively active cofilin-1 mutant (Cof1-S3A), known to destabilize the actin cytoskeleton, also impaired thrombin-induced NF-κB activity. Additionally, depletion of cofilin-1 was associated with a marked reduction in ICAM-1 expression induced by thrombin IκBα degradation and was a result of impaired nuclear translocation and DNA binding to NF-κB without any effect on IκBα degradation (Fazal et al. 2009). All the above observations suggested that thrombin induces a certain pool of inactive cofilin required to maintain an appropriate level of actin dynamics that favors NF-κB activation and ICAM-1 expression and that stabilizing or destabilizing the actin dynamics inhibits thrombin-induced inflammatory response.

The above central role of cofilin in thrombin response was further supported through another set of studies that demonstrated a dynamic mechanism in which LIM kinase 1 (LIMK1), a cofilin kinase, slingshot-1Long (SSH-1L), and a cofilin phosphatase are engaged by thrombin to regulate the actin dynamics. The knockdown of LIMK1 destabilized, whereas the knockdown of SSH-1L stabilized the actin filaments through modulation of cofilin phosphorylation. In either case, however, thrombin-induced NF-κB activity and expression of its target genes (ICAM-1 and VCAM-1) were inhibited. Investigation of underlying mechanisms revealed that knockdown of LIMK1 or SSH-1L each attenuated nuclear translocation and thereby DNA binding of RelA/p65. In addition, LIMK1 or SSH-1 depletion inhibited thrombin-induced RelA/p65 phosphorylation at Ser536. However, similar to earlier observations using TNF-α, LIMK1 or SSH-1L depletion failed to inhibit TNF-α-induced RelA/p65 nuclear translocation and pro-inflammatory gene expression (Leonard et al. 2013). In summary, all the above studies demonstrated the importance of actin dynamics in the regulation of endothelial cell inflammation associated with intravascular coagulation (involving thrombin) and that the involvement of actin dynamics in the inflammatory response is dependent upon the type of inflammatory stimulus.

Another finding that implicated cytoskeletal proteins in thrombin-induced NF-κB activation was the identification of myosin light chain kinase (MLCK), a calcium-calmodulin-dependent kinase dedicated to myosin II regulatory light chain (MLC) (Kamm and Stull 2001). This protein is expressed as two isoforms; smooth muscle MLCK (108–130 kDa) and nonmuscle MLCK (nmMLCK: 210 kDa) (Kamm and Stull 2001, Kudryashov et al. 1999), which is also known as EC-MLCK because of its abundance in endothelial cells. Earlier studies implicated nmMLCK as a key determinant of endothelial barrier disruption through its ability to regulate actomyosin contractility in EC stimulated with edemagenic agonists such as thrombin (Dudek and Garcia 2001, Mehta and Malik 2006). Consistent with this, nmMLCK knockout (nmMLCK−/−) mice were protected from ventilation- and endotoxin-induced ALI and also showed much better survival (Wainwright et al. 2003, Mirzapoiazova et al. 2011, Xu et al. 2008). Thrombin engages MLCK to phosphorylate MLC and thus increase actin-myosin interaction (Dudek and Garcia 2001, Mehta and Malik 2006). Knockdown of nmMLCK in HUVEC and HPAEC prevented thrombin-induced NF-κB activity and ICAM-1 expression. The knockdown of nmMLCK was found to inhibit thrombin-induced nuclear translocation and RelA/p65 Ser536 phosphorylation (Fazal et al. 2013). In strong support of these observations, *in vivo* studies using nmMLCK knockout mice revealed a significant reduction in lung PMN infiltration in mice challenged intraperitoneally (i.p.) with thrombin as compared to wild-type mice that showed elevated PMN in the lungs upon thrombin challenge. These observations provided clues that nmMLCK may be regulating thrombin-induced NF-κB activation by controlling actin dynamics. However, whether nmMLCK regulates NF-κB activation by directly phosphorylating IκBα and IKK remains unknown. Nevertheless, these findings provided mechanistic insights into lung inflammatory response associated with intravascular coagulation and identified nmMLCK as a critical target for the modulation of lung inflammation (Fazal et al. 2013).

Role of Autophagy in Endothelial NF-κB Activation and Inflammation

Autophagy is an evolutionarily conserved cellular process characterized by the formation of a double-membrane vesicle, called the autophagosome, which ensures clearance of damaged intracellular components (organelles and proteins) by delivering them to lysosomes for degradation (Mazushima 2007, Xie and Klionsky 2007). Recent studies have implicated autophagy in several inflammatory diseases involving aberrant endothelial cell responses, such as ALI. However, the mechanistic basis for the role of autophagy in endothelial cell inflammation has recently started emerging. Autophagy is accomplished in several sequential stages, including initiation, nucleation, elongation, and maturation, and requires the participation of a large number (> 30) of autophagy-related proteins (*Atg* genes) (Mazushima 2007, Xie and Klionsky 2007). Beclin1 is an autophagy regulator and plays a central role in autophagosome formation and maturation (Kang et al. 2011) and mediates the localization of other autophagy proteins to pre-autophagosomal structures (Kihara et al. 2001). Studies in HPAEC recently demonstrated the important role of Beclin1 in thrombin-induced NF-κB activation and pro-inflammatory gene expression (Leonard et al. 2019). Knockdown of Belicn1 in these cells resulted in decreased expression of pro-inflammatory genes in response to thrombin which was found to be associated with inhibition of both NF-κB DNA binding as well as RelA/p65 Ser536 phosphorylation. Beclin1 knockdown, however, showed no effect on thrombin-induced IκBα degradation in the cytosol suggesting that the inhibitory effect was secondary to thrombin-induced IκBα degradation. Additionally, silencing of Beclin-1 also protected against thrombin-induced endothelial cell barrier disruption by preventing the loss of VE-cadherin at adherens junctions. Furthermore, Beclin1 knockdown reduced thrombin-induced phosphorylation (inactivation) of actin-depolymerizing protein, cofilin-1, and thereby actin stress fiber formation required for EC permeability suggestive of a possible role of Beclin1 in actin dynamics for regulating RelA/p65 nuclear translocation (Leonard et al. 2019).

In another very recent study, Shadab et al. identified the role of ATG7, an important autophagy regulator in thrombin-induced endothelial cell inflammation. Knockdown of ATG7 in HPAEC significantly attenuated thrombin-induced expression of pro-inflammatory molecules such as IL-6, MCP-1, ICAM-1, and VCAM-1. Investigation of underlying mechanisms revealed reduced NF-κB activity attributable to the inhibition of endothelial inflammation in ATG7-silenced cells. Moreover, the depletion of ATG7 markedly reduced the binding of RelA/p65 to DNA in the nucleus. Similar to observations with Beclin1 depletion (Leonard et al. 2019), thrombin-induced degradation of IκBα in the cytosol was not affected in ATG7-depleted cells, suggesting a defect in the translocation of released RelA/p65 to the nucleus in these cells. This was likely due to the suppression of thrombin-induced phosphorylation and thereby inactivation of Cofilin1, an actin-depolymerizing protein, in ATG7-depleted cells. These observations suggested that ATG7, similar to Beclin-1 promotes thrombin-induced stress fiber formation required for RelA/p65 nuclear translocation. Similar to Belcin1 silencing, ATG7 silencing also reduced thrombin-induced endothelial cell permeability by inhibiting the disassembly of VE-cadherin at adherens junctions (Shadab et al. 2020).

The role of autophagy as a critical component of endothelial barrier disruption in ALI was provided recently through *in vivo* studies with an aerosolized bacterial lipopolysaccharide (LPS) inhalation mouse model of ALI. Administration of the autophagy inhibitor 3-methyladenine (3-MA), either prophylactically or therapeutically, reduced LPS-induced lung vascular leakage and tissue edema (Slavin et al. 2019). A 3-MA was also effective in reducing the levels of pro-inflammatory mediators and lung neutrophil sequestration induced by LPS. In this study, the knockdown of ATG5, another essential regulator of autophagy, in endothelial cells, attenuated thrombin-induced endothelial barrier disruption, confirming the involvement of autophagy in the inflammatory response. Similarly, exposure of cells to 3-MA, either before or after thrombin, protected against endothelial barrier dysfunction by inhibiting the cleavage and loss of vascular endothelial cadherin at adherens junctions, as well as the formation of actin stress fibers. The 3-MA also reversed LPS-induced EC barrier disruption (Slavin et al. 2019).

Together, all the above *in vitro* and *in vivo* observations strongly support the important role of autophagy in the inflammatory response in endothelial cells and in lung vascular injury. In particular, autophagy is required for promoting actin cytoskeletal dynamics upon thrombin stimulation to facilitate NF-κB nuclear translocation and DNA-binding function, pro-inflammatory gene expression as well as vascular leak via endothelial barrier disruption.

Other Mediators of Endothelial NF-κB Activation

Transglutaminase 2 (TG2)

It is a multifunctional enzyme and the most ubiquitous among the transglutaminase family of proteins (Lorand and Graham 2003). Among its several functions include calcium-dependent cross-linking of proteins, GTP binding and hydrolysis, and protein scaffolding (Lorand and Graham 2003). Under normal physiological conditions, TG2 exists as a catalytically inactive protein due to low Ca^{2+} concentrations (Siegel et al. 2008). However, under stress, loss in Ca^{2+} homeostasis (increase in calcium concentration) can activate intracellular TG2 resulting in cross-linking of cellular proteins (Siegel et al. 2008). TG2 has been shown to play a role in the activation of NF-κB in cancer cells (Mann et al. 2006) and conversely, its expression is also induced by NF-κB in liver cells (Kuncio et al. 1998). It has been implicated in a number of pathological processes, including celiac disease, cancer, tissue fibrosis, myocardial hypertrophy, wound healing, and inflammation (Lorand and Graham 2003, Lismaa et al. 2009). In one study (Oh et al. 2011) epithelial TG2 was identified as an important mediator of bleomycin-induced lung inflammation and fibrosis in mice. Studies in HPAEC depleted of TG2 demonstrated inhibition of thrombin-induced NF-κB activation and its target genes, VCAM-1, MCP-1, and IL-6 (interleukin 6) and this was attributed to inhibition of thrombin-induced DNA binding as well as serine phosphorylation of RelA/p65, a crucial event that controls the transcriptional capacity of the DNA-bound RelA/p65 (Bijli et al. 2014). These in vitro observations were strongly supported by *in vivo* studies that demonstrated a reduction in NF-κB activation, adhesion molecule expression, and lung PMN sequestration in TG2 knockout mice (TG2 –/– mice) compared with wild-type mice exposed to LPS. The mechanism by which TG2 regulates NF-κB in endothelial cells appears to be different from that in other cell types. Studies have shown that TG2 regulates NF-κB in other cell types primarily at the level of IκBα but via a non-canonical pathway, by causing polymerization of IκBα, which in turn leads to depletion of free IκBα and thereby nuclear translocation and DNA binding of NF-κB (Mann et al. 2006, Lee et al. 2004, Kumar and Mehta 2012). By contrast, TG2 regulation of thrombin-induced NF-κB activity in endothelial cells relies on RelA/p65 phosphorylation in addition to its DNA-binding activity (Bijli et al. 2014). Furthermore, this mechanism of NF-κB regulation by TG2 in endothelial cells appears to be stimulus-specific as TNFα-induced phosphorylation of RelA/p65 was insensitive to TG2 knockdown. These observations underscore the importance of TG2 in endothelial cell inflammation associated with intravascular coagulation (Bijli et al. 2014).

Phosphoinositide-Specific Phospholipase C-ε (PLC-ε)

It is a newly described member of the PLC family that hydrolyzes phosphatidylinositol 4, 5-bisphosphate (PIP2) to generate the second messenger's inositol 1,4,5-triphosphate (IP3) and diacylglycerol (DAG) (Bunney and Katan 2006, Kelley et al. 2001). The IP3 and DAG in turn lead to the generation of Ca^{2+} and activation of protein kinase C (PKC), respectively (Bunney and Katan 2006, Kelley et al. 2001). PLC-ε has been implicated in the development and function of the heart as well as tumor promotion and skin inflammation (Ikuta et al. 2008, Li et al. 2009, Wang et al. 2005). The primary sites of its expression are the heart and lungs. Although the role of PLC-ε in cardiac function and pathology has been established (Wang et al. 2005, Zhang et al. 2011), its relevance in ALI has not been much clear until recently. Bijli et al. recently performed studies in PLC-ε knockout [PLC-ε(–/–)] mice to address the role of PLC-ε in regulating lung vascular inflammation and injury in an aerosolized bacterial LPS inhalation mouse model of ALI. PLC-ε(–/–) mice showed a marked decrease in LPS-induced pro-inflammatory mediators including ICAM-1, VCAM-1, TNF-α, IL-1β, IL-6, macrophage inflammatory protein 2, keratinocyte-derived cytokine, monocyte chemoattractant protein 1, GMCSF, lung neutrophil infiltration and microvascular leakage, and loss of VE-cadherin compared with wild-type [PLC-ε(+/+)] mice. These data identified PLC-ε as a critical determinant of the pro-inflammatory and leaky phenotype of the lung. The same report also revealed that PLC-ε activity in HPAEC contributes to inflammation and barrier disruption. *In vitro* observations revealed that knockdown of PLC-ε in HPAEC inhibited NF-κB activity in response to diverse pro-inflammatory stimuli including thrombin, LPS, TNF-α, and the non-receptor agonist, such as PMA in these cells. Depletion of PLC-ε also inhibited thrombin-induced expression of VCAM-1. Importantly, PLC-ε knockdown protected against thrombin-induced endothelial barrier disruption by inhibiting the loss of VE-cadherin at adherens junctions and the formation of actin stress fibers required for NF-κB nuclear translocation (Bijli et al. 2016). All above *in vivo* and *in vitro* observations identify PLC-ε as a novel regulator of endothelial cell inflammation and permeability and implicate its important role in the pathogenesis of ALI.

NF-κB Activation as a Therapeutic Target

Different pharmacological agents have been shown to block NF-κB activity by targeting different events in the NF-κB activation pathway (Yamamoto and Gaynor 2001). For example, nonsteroidal anti-inflammatory agents such as sodium salicylate, aspirin, and sulindac exert their inhibitory effects partly, by inhibiting IKKβ activity. Similarly, naturally occurring flavonoids such as resveratrol, quercetin, and myricetin are thought to mediate their various biological effects through inhibition of IKK activity in cancer chemoprevention, suppression of inflammation, and protection from vascular disease. The anti-inflammatory effects of glucocorticoids such as prednisone and dexamethasone involve the expression of IκBα to increase cytosolic retention of NF-κB, thereby disturbing the interaction of RelA/p65 with the basal transcription machinery (Yamamoto and Gaynor 2001). Compounds such as peptide aldehyde MG132, lactacystin, and the immunosuppressive drug cyclosporine A (CsA) prevent NF-κB activation by inhibiting the protease activity of the proteasome that degrades IκBα, thus retaining NF-κB in the cytoplasm. Tacrolimus (FK506), another immunosuppressive drug, used to prevent rejection of organ transplants, inhibits NF-κB activation by preventing translocation of c-Rel from cytoplasm to the nucleus. In addition to the inhibition of key components of the canonical NF-κB pathway, an alternative choice has been to block its downstream targets or upstream stimulators. For example, since TNF-α is the activator and effector of the NF-κB pathway, the anti-TNF-α antibody has been applied in phase I and II clinical trials for treating cancer (Madhusudan et al. 2004, Madhusudan et al. 2005, Harrison et al. 2007), and the current FDA-approved anti-TNF-α antibodies include infliximab, adalimumab and golimumab (Mercogliano et al. 2020). Infliximab is proven to be well tolerated without dose-limiting toxic effects in advanced cancer by clinical studies (Brown et al. 2008).

One major concern associated with targeting the NF-κB signaling pathway is the specificity of drugs and the potential risk of toxicity since prolonged NF-κB blockade may interfere with host immune responses and result in liver apoptosis. In view of these challenges, an effective strategy for therapeutic interventions of diseases associated with chronic or dysregulated NF-κB activation would depend on achieving a delicate balance between suppressing NF-κB activity and interfering with normal cellular functions. Conditional targeting of specific NF-κB subunits, IκB proteins, or IKKs in a cell-specific manner can be a useful strategy to achieve this goal. For example, using an E-selectin promoter, it will be possible to direct the expression of super repressor IκBα, a dominant negative mutant of IKKs or short hairpin RNA (shRNA) targeting specific NF-κB subunits exclusively in endothelial cells and inflammation-specific manner, thereby providing control over the strength and duration of NF-κB activation, ensuring therapeutic efficacy and minimizing systemic toxicity. Such a strategy has been used to induce conditional and endothelial-specific expression of neutrophil inhibitory factor (NIF), a β_2-integrin antagonist, which in turn prevents lung PMN infiltration and vascular injury in a mouse model of gram-negative sepsis (Xu et al. 2002).

NF-κB in the Context of SARS COVID-19 Pandemic

The coronavirus disease 2019 (COVID-19) pandemic has affected healthcare systems in many parts of the world. Severe pneumonia and ARDS have been associated with COVID-19 infection in which post-viral activation of inflammation led to the release of cytokine/chemokines causing a "cytokine storm" resulting in tissue destruction mainly lungs. COVID-19 activates NF-κB in various cells such as macrophages present in the lung, liver, kidney, central nervous system, gastrointestinal system, and cardiovascular system, resulting in the production of IL-1, IL-2, IL-6, IL-12, TNF-α, LT-α, LT-β, GM-CSF, and various chemokines (Su et al. 2021). The sensitized NF-κB activation in the elderly population and patients with metabolic syndrome makes them highly susceptible to COVID-19 with the worst complications leading to high mortality (Kircheis et al. 2020).

Hyperactivation of the NF-κB pathway has been implicated in the pathogenesis of the severe/critical COVID-19 phenotype (Hirano and Murakami 2020). Studies during previous coronavirus outbreaks such as SARS-CoV and the Middle East Respiratory syndrome coronavirus (MERS-CoV) identified viral proteins such as nsp1, nsp3a, nsp7a, spike, and nucleocapsid protein that caused excessive NF-κB activation, possibly contributing to severe disease and high case-fatality rate (DeDiego et al. 2014, Oeckinghaus and Ghosh 2009, Liao et al. 2005). A study on SARS-CoV responsible for the outbreak in 2003 showed that the SARS-CoV nucleocapsid protein (N protein) activates NF-κB in Vero E6 cells in a dose-dependent manner (Liao et al. 2005). On the reverse side, SARS-CoV lacking the Envelope (E) gene (SARS-CoV-ΔE) showed reduced expression of pro-inflammatory cytokines, diminished neutrophil infiltration, reduced lung pathology, which resulted in increased survival of BALB (immunodeficient strain) mice (DeDiego et al. 2014, Day et al. 2009).

Many of the drugs that are currently effective in COVID disease have links to the NF-κB cascade of immune/inflammation regulation. For example, Remdesivir (GS-5734) is a nucleotide analog that blocks viral replication by inhibiting RNA-dependent RNA polymerase. Thus, by reducing dsRNA-related induction of the NF-κB pathway, it reduces the cytokine storm and severe disease. Administration of this drug showed quick recovery against placebo during the Adaptive COVID-19 Treatment Trial (ACTT-1) (Beigel et al. 2020). N-acetylcysteine is a potent NF-κB inhibitor by virtue of downregulating the phosphorylation of IκB, and also against TNF-α mediated activation of the NF-κB pathway (Oka et al. 2020). It has anti-oxidant properties (Wu et al. 2014) since it is a scavenger of ROS that is partly responsible for tissue damage during lung inflammation. It was reported to have a significant clinical improvement in critically ill COVID-19 patients (Assimakopoulos and Marangos 2020, ClinicalTrials.gov. 2020b).

Immunomodulation at the level of NF-κB activation and IκB degradation along with TNF-α inhibition bears the potential to the reduction of the cytokine storm and alleviation the severity of COVID-19 infection. Previous reports suggest that cytokine inhibitor therapy against TNF, IL-6, IL-17, IL-23, and IL-4 reduces the undesirable inflammatory response (Schett et al. 2020). Such approaches that mitigate the exaggerated immune response (by TNF and IL-6) and without impacting SARS-nCOV-2 clearance (by Interferon type I, IL-15, and IFN-γ) may exert beneficial effects against COVID-19 infection. Severe COVID-19 pneumonia also shares pathological similarities with severe bacterial pneumonia and sepsis by disrupting the hemostatic balance resulting in a pro-coagulant state (increased thrombin concentration and components of coagulation cascade) locally in the lungs and systemically, ultimately leading to the formation of microthrombi, disseminated intravascular coagulation and multi-organ failure. The deleterious effects of exaggerated inflammatory responses and activation of the coagulation cascade can lead to bystander tissue injury and are negatively associated with survival. In the past two decades, evidence from preclinical studies has led to the emergence of potential anticoagulant therapeutic strategies for the treatment of patients with pneumonia, sepsis, and ARDS, and some of these anticoagulant approaches have been put for clinical trials (Jose et al. 2020). Thus, anti-inflammatory together with anti-thrombin therapies could hold great potential in the management of disease severity associated with COVID-19 infections and other respiratory diseases that result in ALI and ARDS.

Concluding Remarks

The current status of research in the field of ARDS and ALI has vastly improved our understanding of the pathophysiological and biochemical mechanisms associated with lung disease and inflammation. Although newly emerging technologies in molecular biology, proteomics, genomics, and imaging have significantly reduced our efforts in our ability to understand the complexities associated with this disease condition, it is important to note that basic principles of protein biochemistry, immunological methods including Western blotting, enzyme-labeled immunosorbent assays (ELISA), as well as cell culture and basic molecular biology methods have greatly contributed to our fundamental understanding of biochemical mechanisms and associated pathology of ARDS/ALI over last several decades. With continued progress in our scientific understanding, it is anticipated that better management approaches will evolve shortly, that in turn will greatly help reduce mortality associated with this pathological condition and/or underlying physiology associated with both infectious or non-infectious diseases of the respiratory system.

Acknowledgments

In this book chapter, the author intended to provide a comprehensive, yet simplistic overview of the pathophysiology and molecular mechanisms of ALI. The author has tried to incorporate critical details from biochemical, immunological, and molecular-based research published by different experts in this field over the past several decades and has tried to explain critical findings on the crucial role of vascular cells (endothelial cells) in the mechanism of ALI. The author's main objective is to make this book chapter more clarifying and readable for a general scientific audience. While fully recognizing the countless invaluable contributions made, the author sincerely apologizes for not including research published by many other experts in this field.

References

Aarbiou, J., G. S. Tjabringa, R. M. Verhoosel, D. K. Ninaber, S. R. White, L. T. C. Peltenburg et al. (2006). Mechanisms of cell death induced by the neutrophil antimicrobial peptides alpha-defensins and LL-37. Inflamm. Res. 55: 119–127.

Abbassi, O., C. L. Lane, S. Krater, T. K. Kishimoto, D. C. Anderson, L. V. McIntire et al. (1991). Canine neutrophil margination mediated by lectin adhesion molecule-1 *in vitro*. J. Immunol. 147: 2107–2115.

Actor, J. K., S. A. Hwang, M. Olsen, M. Zimecki, R. L, Hunter Jr. and M. L. Kruzel. (2002). Lactoferrin immunomodulation of DTH response in mice. Int. Immunopharmacol. 2: 475–86.

Acute Respiratory Distress Syndrome Network., R. G Brower, M. A. Matthay, A. Morris, D. Schoenfeld, B. T. Thompson et al. (2000). Ventilation with lower tidal volumes as compared with traditional tidal volumes for acute lung injury and the acute respiratory distress syndrome. N. Engl. J. Med. 342: 1301–1308.

Agrawal, A., M. A. Matthay, K. N. Kangelaris, J. Stein, J. C. Chu, B. M. Imp et al. (2013). Plasma angiopoietin-2 predicts the onset of acute lung injury in critically ill patients. Am. J. Respir. Crit. Care Med. 187: 736–742.

Albelda, S. M., C. W. Smith and P. A. Ward. (1994). Adhesion molecules and inflammatory injury. FASEB J. 8: 504–512.

Anwar, K. N., F. Fazal, A. B. Malik and A. Rahman. (2004). RhoA/Rho-associated kinase pathway selectively regulates thrombin-induced intercellular adhesion molecule-1 expression in endothelial cells via activation of I kappa B kinase beta and phosphorylation of RelA/p65 J. Immunol. 173: 6965–6972.

Ashitani, J. I., H. Mukae, Y. Arimura, A. Sano, M. Tokojima and M. Nakazato. (2004). High concentrations of alpha-defensins in plasma and bronchoalveolar lavage fluid of patients with acute respiratory distress syndrome. Life Sci. 75: 1123–1134.

Assimakopoulos, S. F. and M. Marangos. (2020). N-acetyl-cysteine may prevent COVID-19-associated cytokine storm and acute respiratory distress syndrome. Med. Hypotheses. 140: 109778.

Auten, R. L. Jr., S. N. Mason, D. T. Tanaka, K. Welty-Wolf and M. H. Whorton. (2001). Anti-neutrophil chemokine preserves alveolar development in hyperoxia-exposed newborn rats. Am. J. Physiol. Lung Cell Mol. Physiol. 281: L336–344.

Auten, R. L., M. H. Whorton and S. Nicholas Mason. (2002). Blocking neutrophil influx reduces DNA damage in hyperoxia-exposed newborn rat lung. Am. J. Respir. Cell. Mol. Biol. 26: 391–397.

Avraham, H., S. Y. Park, K. Schinkmann and S. Avraham. (2000). RAFTK/Pyk2–mediated cellular signalling. Cell Signal. 12: 123–133.

Bachofen, M. and E. R. Weibel. (1982). Structural alterations of lung parenchyma in the adult respiratory distress syndrome. Clin. Chest. Med. 3: 35–56.

Bakaletz, L. O. (2017). Viral-bacterial co-infections in the respiratory tract. Curr. Opin. Microbiol. 35: 30–35.

Bamburg, J. A. and O'Neil P. Wiggan. (2002). ADF/cofilin and actin dynamics in disease. Trends Cell Biol. 12: 598–605.

Bamburg, J. R., A. McGough and S. Ono. (1999). Putting a new twist on actin: ADF/cofilins modulate actin dynamics. Trends Cell Biol. 9: 364–370.

Baraldo, S., G. Turato and M. Saetta. (2012). Pathophysiology of small airways in chronic obstructive pulmonary disease. Respiration 84: 89–97.

Barber, C. and D. Fishwick. (2016). Pneumoconiosis. Medicine 44: 355–358.

Barlow, P. G., L. Yuexin, T. S. Wilkinson, D. M. E Bowdish, Y. E. Lau, C. Cosseau et al. (2006). The human cationic host defense peptide LL-37 mediates contrasting effects on apoptotic pathways in different primary cells of the innate immune system. J. Leukoc. Biol. 80: 509–520.

Beigel, J. H., K. M. Tomashek, L. E. Dodd, A. K. Mehta, B. S. Zingman, A. C. Kalil et al. (2020). Remdesivir for the treatment of COVID-19—preliminary report.

Bijli, K. M., M. Minhajuddin, F. Fazal, M. A. O'Reilly, L. C. Platanias and A. Rahman. (2007). c-Src interacts with and phosphorylates RelA/p65 to promote thrombin-induced ICAM-1 expression in endothelial cells. Am. J. Physiol. Lung Cell Mol. Physiol. 292: L396–L404.

Bijli, K. M., F. Fazal, M. Minhajuddin and A. Rahman. (2008). Activation of Syk by protein kinase C-delta regulates thrombin-induced intercellular adhesion molecule-1 expression in endothelial cells via tyrosine phosphorylation of RelA/p65. J. Biol. Chem. 283: 14674–14684.

Bonizzi, G. and M. Karin. (2004). The two NF-κB activation pathways and their role in innate and adaptive immunity. Trends Immunol. 25: 280–288.

Boring, L., J. Gosling, S. W. Chensue, S. L. Kunkel, R. V. Farese Jr., H. E. Broxmeyer et al. 1997. Impaired monocyte migration and reduced type 1 (Th1) cytokine responses in C-C chemokine receptor 2 knockout mice. J. Clin. Invest. 100: 2552–2561.

Borregaard, N. and J. B. Cowland. (1997). Granules of the human neutrophilic polymorphonuclear leukocyte. Blood 89: 3503–21.

Bouwmwester, T., A. Bauch, H. Ruffner, P. O. Angrand, G. Bergamini, K. Croughton et al. (2004). A physical and functional map of the human TNFα/NF-κB signal transduction pathway. Nat. Cell. Biol. 6: 97–105.

Brizendine, K. D., J. W. Baddley and P. G. Pappas. (2011). Pulmonary cryptococcosis. Semin. Respir. Crit. Care Med. 32: 727–734.

Broermann, A., M. Winderlich, H. Block, M. Frye, J. Rossaint, A. Zarbock et al. (2011). Dissociation of VE-PTP from VE-cadherin is required for leukocyte extravasation and for VEGF-induced vascular permeability *in vivo*. J. Exp. Med. 208: 2393–2401.

Brown, E. R., K. A. Charles, S. A. Hoare, R. L. Rye, D. I. Jodrell, R. E. Aird et al. (2008). A clinical study assessing the tolerability and biological effects of infliximab, a TNF-alpha inhibitor, in patients with advanced cancer. Ann. Oncol. 19: 1340–1346.

Buc, M., M. Dzurilla, M. Vrlik and M. Bucova. (2009). Immunopathogenesis of Bronchial Asthma. Arch. Immunol. Ther. Exp. (Warsz.) 57: 331–44.

Bunney, T. D. and M. Katan. 2006. Phospholipase C epsilon: Linking second messengers and small GTPases. Trends Cell Biol. 16: 640–648.

Burns, A. R., D. C. Walker, E. S. Brown, L. T. Thurmon, R. A. Bowden, C. R. Keese et al. (1997). Neutrophil transendothelial migration is independent of tight junctions and occurs preferentially at tricellular corners. J. Immunol. 159: 2893.

Burns, L. J., J. C. Pooley, D. J. Walsh, G. M. Vercellotti, M. L. Weber and A. Kovacs. (1999). Intercellular adhesion molecule-1 expression in endothelial cells is activated by cytomegalovirus immediate early proteins. Transplantation 67: 137–144.

Calfee, C. S., L. B. Ware, D. V. Glidden, M. D. Eisner, P. E. Parsons, B. T. Thompson et al. (2011). Use of risk reclassification with multiple biomarkers improves mortality prediction in acute lung injury. Crit. Care Med. 39: 711–717.

Carden, D., F. Xiao, C. Moak, B. H. Willis, S. Robinson-Jackson and S. Alexander. (1998). Neutrophil elastase promotes lung microvascular injury and proteolysis of endothelial cadherins. Am. J. Physiol. 275: H385–392.

Carnesecchi, S., C. Deffert, A. Pagano, S. Garrido-Urbani, I. Métrailler-Ruchonnet, M. Schäppi et al. (2009). NADPH oxidase-1 plays a crucial role in hyperoxia-induced acute lung injury in mice. Am. J. Respir. Crit. Care Med. 180: 972–981.

Cernuda-Morollon, E. and A. J. Ridley. (2006). Rho GTPases and leukocyte adhesion receptor expression and function in endothelial cells. Circ. Res. 98: 757–767.

Chen, H., B. W. Bernstein and J. R. Bamburg. (2000). Regulating actin-filament dynamics *in vivo*. Trends Biochem. Sci. 25: 19–23.

Chen, L. F. and W. C. Greene. (2004). Shaping the nuclear activation of NF-κB. Nat. Mol. Cell Biol. 5: 392–401.

Cheng, J. J., Y. J. Chao and D. L. Wang. (2002). Cyclic strain activates redox sensitive proline-rich tyrosine kinase 2 (Pyk2) in endothelial cells. J. Biol. Chem. 277: 48152–48157.

Chiarugi, P., G. Pani, E. Giannoni, L. Taddei, R. Colavitti, G. Raugei et al. (2003). Reactive oxygen species as essential mediators of cell adhesion: The oxidative inhibition of a FAK tyrosine phosphatase is required for cell adhesion. J. Cell Biol. 161: 933–44.

Chuluyan, H. E., L. Osborn, R. Lobb and A. C. Issekutz. (1995). Domains 1 and 4 of vascular cell adhesion molecule-1 (CD106) both support very late activation antigen-4 (CD49d/CD29)–dependent monocyte transendothelial migration. J. Immunol. 155: 3135–3144.

Clunes, M. T. and R. C. Boucher. (2007). Cystic Fibrosis: The mechanisms of pathogenesis of an inherited lung disorder. Drug Discov. Today Dis. Mech. 4: 63–72.

Cochrane, C. G., R. G. Spragg, S. D. Revak, A. B. Cohen and V. W. McGuire. (1983). The presence of neutrophil elastase and evidence of oxidation activity in bronchoalveolar lavage fluid of patients with adult respiratory distress syndrome. Am. Rev. Respir. Dis. 127: S25–27.

Collins, T., M. A. Read, A. S. Neish, M. Z. Whitley, D. Thanos and T. Maniatis. (1995). Transcriptional regulation of endothelial cell adhesion molecules: NF-kappa B and cytokine-inducible enhancers. FASEB J. 9: 899–909.

Corada, M., M. Mariotti, G. Thurston, K. Smith, R. Kunkel, M. Brockhaus et al. (1999). Vascular endothelial–cadherin is an important determinant of microvascular integrity *in vivo*. Proc. Nat. Acad. Sci. 96: 9815–20.

Daniel, P. B., W. H. Walker and J. F. Habener. (1998). Cyclic AMP signaling and gene regulation. Annu. Rev. Nutr. 18: 353–383.

Day, C. W., R. Baric, S. X. Cai, M. Frieman, Y. Kumaki, J. D. Morrey et al. (2009). A new mouse-adapted strain of SARS-CoV as a lethal model for evaluating antiviral agents *in vitro* and *in vivo*. Virology 395: 210–222.

De la Rosa. G., D. Yang, P. Tewary, A. Varadhachary and J. J. Oppenheim. (2008). Lactoferrin acts as an alarmin to promote the recruitment and activation of APCs and antigen-specific immune responses. J. Immunol. 180: 6868–76.

DeDiego, M. L., J. L. Nieto-Torres, J. A. Regla-Nava, J. M. Jimenez-Guardeño, R. Fernandez-Delgado, C. Fett et al. (2014). Inhibition of NF-κB-mediated inflammation in severe acute respiratory syndrome coronavirus-infected mice increases survival. J. Virol. 15: 913–924.

Degitz, K., L. J. Li and S. W. Caughman. (1991). Cloning and characterization of the 5'-transcriptional regulatory region of the human intercellular adhesion molecule 1 gene. J. Biol. Chem. 266: 14024–14030.

Delacourt, C., S. Hérigault, C. Delclaux, A. Poncin, M. Levame, A. Harf et al. (2002). Protection against acute lung injury by intravenous or intratracheal pretreatment with EPI-HNE-4, a new potent neutrophil elastase inhibitor. Am. J. Respir. Cell Mol. Biol. 26: 290–297.

Delclaux, C., M. P. d'Ortho, C. Delacourt, F. Lebargy, C. Brun-Buisson, L. Brochard et al. (1997). Gelatinases in epithelial lining fluid of patients with adult respiratory distress syndrome. Am. J. Physiol. 272: L442–451.

Diacovo, T. G., S. J. Roth, J. M. Buccola, D. F. Bainton and T. A. Springer. (1996). Neutrophil rolling, arrest, and transmigration across activated, surface-adherent platelets via sequential action of P-selectin and the beta 2-integrin CD11b/CD18. Blood 88: 146–157.

Diamond, M. S., D. E. Staunton, A. R. de Fougerolles, S. A. Stacker, J. Garcia–Aguilar et al. (1990). ICAM-1 (CD54): A counter-receptor for Mac-1 (CD11b/CD18). J. Cell Biol. 111: 3129–3139.

Dolinay, T., Y. S. Kim, J. Howrylak, G. M. Hunninghake, C. H. An, L. Fredenburgh et al. (2012). Inflammasome-regulated cytokines are critical mediators of acute lung injury. Am. J. Respir. Crit. Care Med. 185: 1225–1234.

Donnelly, S. C., I. MacGregor, A. Zamani, M. W. Gordon, C. E. Robertson, D. J. Steedman et al. (1995). Plasma elastase levels and the development of the adult respiratory distress syndrome. Am. J. Respir. Crit. Care Med. 151: 1428–1433.

Doss, M., M. R. White, T. Tecle and K. L. Hartshorn. (2010). Human defensins and LL-37 in mucosal immunity. J. Leukoc. Biol. 87: 79–92.

Doyle, I. R., A. D. Bersten and T. E. Nicholas. (1997). Surfactant proteins-a and -B are elevated in plasma of patients with acute respiratory failure. Am. J. Respir. Crit. Care Med. 156: 1217–1229.

Dudek, S. M. and J. G. Garcia. (2001). Cytoskeletal regulation of pulmonary vascular permeability. J. Appl. Physiol. 91: 1487–1500.

Dustin, M. L. and T. A. Springer. (1988). Lymphocyte function-associated antigen-1 (LFA-1) interaction with intercellular adhesion molecule-1 (ICAM-1) is one of at least three mechanisms for lymphocyte adhesion to cultured endothelial cells. J. Cell Biol. 107: 321–331.

Eisner, M. D., P. Parsons, M. A. Matthay, L. Ware and K. Greene. (2003). Plasma surfactant protein levels and clinical outcomes in patients with acute lung injury. Thorax. 58: 983–988.

Fahy, R. J. and M. D. Wewers. (2005). Pulmonary defense and the human cathelicidin hCAP-18/ LL-37. Immunol. Res. 31: 75–89.

Fan, C., Q. Li, D. Ross and J. F. Engelhardt. (2003). Tyrosine phosphorylation of IκBα activates NF-κB through a redox-regulated and c-Src-dependent mechanism following hypoxia/reoxygenation. J. Biol. Chem. 278: 2072–2080.

Faurschou, M. and N. Borregaard. (2003). Neutrophil granules and secretory vesicles in inflammation. Microbes Infect. 5: 1317–1327.

Fein, A., R. F. Grossman, J. G. Jones, E. Overland, L. Pitts, J. F. Murray et al. (1979). The value of edema fluid protein measurement in patients with pulmonary edema. Am. J. Med. 67: 32–38.

Fligiel, S. E. G., T. Standiford, H. M. Fligiel, D. Tashkin, R. M. Strieter, R. L. Warner et al. (2006). Matrix metalloproteinases and matrix metalloproteinase inhibitors in acute lung injury. Hum. Pathol. 37: 422–430.

Fremont, R. D., T. Koyama, C. S. Calfee, W. Wu, L. A. Dossett, F. R. Bossert et al. (2010). Acute lung injury in patients with traumatic injuries: utility of a panel of biomarkers for diagnosis and pathogenesis. J. Trauma. 68: 1121–1127.

Fujimura, J. (2000). Pathology and pathophysiology of pneumoconiosis. Curr. Opin. Pulm. Med. 6: 140–144.

Gabe, L. M., J. Malo and K. S. Knox. (2017). Diagnosis and management of Coccidioidomycosis. Clin. Chest. Med. 38: 417–433.

Gajic, O., O. Dabbagh, P. K. Park, A. Adesanya, S. Y. Chang, P. Hou et al. (2011). Early identification of patients at risk of acute lung injury: Evaluation of lung injury prediction score in a multicenter cohort study. Am. J. Respir. Crit. Care Med. 183: 462–470.

Gautam, N., A. M. Olofsson, H. Herwald, L. F. Iversen, E. Lundgren-Akerlund, P. Hedqvist et al. (2001). Heparin-binding protein (HBP/CAP37): A missing link in neutrophilevoked alteration of vascular permeability. Nat. Med. 7: 1123–1127.

Gershman, E., R. Guthrie, K. Swiatek and S. Shojaee. (2019). Management of hemoptysis in patients with lung cancer. Ann. Transl. Med. 15: 358.

Ghosh, S. and M. Karin. (2002). Missing pieces in the NF-κB puzzle. Cell 109: S81–86.

Gilmore, T. D. (2006). Introduction to NF-kappaB: Players, pathways, perspectives. Oncogene 25: 6680–6684.

Ginzberg, H. H., P. T. Shannon, T. Suzuki, O. Hong, E. Vachon, T. Moraes et al. (2004). Leukocyte elastase induces epithelial apoptosis: Role of mitochondial permeability changes and Akt. Am. J. Physiol. Gastrointest. Liver Physiol. 287: G286–298.

Ginzberg, H. H., V. Cherapanov, Q. Dong, A. Cantin, C. A. McCulloch, P. T. Shannon et al. (2001). Neutrophil-mediated epithelial injury during transmigration: Role of elastase. Am. J. Physiol. Gastrointest. Liver Physiol. 281: G705–717.

Gopalan, P. K., A. R. Burns, S. I. Simon, S. Sparks, L. V. McIntire and C. W. Smith. (2000). Preferential sites for stationary adhesion of neutrophils to cytokine-stimulated HUVEC under flow conditions. J. Leukoc. Biol. 68: 47–57.

Greene, K. E., J. R. Wright, K. P. Steinberg, J. T. Ruzinski, E. Caldwell, W. B. Wong et al. (1999). Serial changes in surfactant-associated proteins in lung and serum before and after onset of ARDS. Am. J. Respir. Crit. Care Med. 160: 1843–1850.

Hagio, T., K. Kishikawa, K. Kawabata, S. Tasaka, S. Hashimoto, N. Hasegawa et al. (2008). Inhibition of neutrophil elastase reduces lung injury and bacterial count in hamsters. Pulm. Pharmacol. Ther. 21: 884–91.

Han, J., P. Thompson and B. Beutler. (1990). Dexamethasone and pentoxifylline inhibit endotoxin-induced cachectin/tumor necrosis factor synthesis at separate points in the signaling pathway. J. Exp. Med. 172: 391–394.

Harcourt, B. H., P. A. Rota, K. B. Hummel, W. J. Bellini and M. K. Offermann. (1999). Induction of intercellular adhesion molecule 1 gene expression by measles virus in human umbilical vein endothelial cells. J. Med. Virol. 57: 9–16.

Harrison, M. L., E. Obermueller, N. R. Maisey, S. Hoare, K. Edmonds, N. F. Li et al. (2007). Tumor necrosis factor alpha as a new target for renal cell carcinoma: Two sequential phase II trials of infliximab at standard and high dose. J. Clin. Oncol. 25: 4542–4549.

Hayden, M. S. and S. Ghosh. (2004). Signaling to NF-κB. Genes Dev. 18: 2195–2224.

Hendrickson, C. M. and M. A. Matthay. (2018). Endothelial biomarkers in human sepsis: Pathogenesis and prognosis for ARDS. Pulm. Circ. 8: 2045894018769876.

Herwald, H., H. Cramer, M. Mörgelin, W. Russell, U. Sollenberg, A. Norrby-Teglund et al. (2004). M protein, a classical bacterial virulence determinant, forms complexes with fibrinogen that induce vascular leakage. Cell 116: 367–379.

Heusch, M., L. Lin, R. Geleziunas and W. C. Greene. (1999). The generation of nfkb2 p52: Mechanism and efficiency. Oncogene 18: 6201–6208.

Hirano, T. and M. Murakami. (2020). COVID-19: A new virus, but a familiar receptor and cytokine release syndrome. Immunity 52: 731–733.

Hirozane, T., A. Matsumori, Y. Furukawa, S. Matsui, Y. Sato, Y. Matoba et al. (1995). Beneficial effect of amrinone on murine cardiac allograft survival. Clin. Exp. Immunol. 102: 186–191.

Hofmann, W. A., L. Stojiljkovic, B. Fuchsova, G. M. Vargas, E. Mavrommatis, V. Philimonenko et al. (2004). Actin is part of pre-initiation complexes and is necessary for transcription by RNA polymerase II. Nat. Cell Biol. 6: 1094–1101.

Hotulainen, P., E. Paunola, M. K. Vartiainen and P. Lappalainen. (2005). Actin-depolymerizing factor and cofilin-1 play overlapping roles in promoting rapid F-actin depolymerization in mammalian nonmuscle cells. Mol. Biol. Cell. 16: 649–664.

Huang, W. C., J. J. Chen, H. Inoue and C. C. Chen. (2003). Tyrosine phosphorylation of IKKα/β by protein kinase C-dependent c-Src activation is involved in TNF-α-induced cyclooxygenase-2 expression. **J. Immunol.** 170: 4767–4775.

Huxford, T., D. B. Huang, S. Malek and G. Ghosh. (1998). The crystal structure of IκBα/NF-κB complex reveals mechanisms of NF-κB inactivation. Cell 95: 759–70.

Iismaa, S. E., B. M. Mearns, L. Lorand and R. M. Graham. (2009). Transglutaminases and disease: Lessons from genetically engineered mouse models and inherited disorders. Physiol. Rev. 89: 991–1023.

Ikuta, S., H. Edamatsu, M. Li, L. Hu and T. Kataoka. (2008). Crucial role of phospholipase C epsilon in skin inflammation induced by tumor-promoting phorbol ester. Cancer Res. 68: 64–72.

Imai, Y., K. Kuba, G. G. Neely, R. Yaghubian-Malhami, T. Perkmann, G. V. Loo et al. (2008). Identification of oxidative stress and Toll-like receptor 4 signaling as a key pathway of acute lung injury. Cell 133: 235–249.

Imbert, V., R. A. Rupec, A. Livolsi, H. L. Pahl, E. B. Traenckner, C. Mueller-Dieckmann et al. (1996). Tyrosine phosphorylation of IκBα activates NF-κB without proteolytic degradation of IκBα. **Cell** 86: 787–798.

Jabaudon, M., R. Blondonnet, L. Roszyk, D. Bouvier, J. Audard, G. Clairefond et al. (2015). Soluble receptor for advanced glycation end-products predicts impaired alveolar fluid clearance in acute respiratory distress syndrome. Am. J. Respir. Crit. Care Med. 192: 191–199.

Jalkanen, V., R. Yang, R. Linko, H. Huhtala, M. Okkonen, T. Varpula et al. (2013). SuPAR and PAI-1 in critically ill, mechanically ventilated patients. Intensive Care Med. 39: 489–496.

Janusz, M. J. and M. Hare. (1994). Inhibition of human neutrophil elastase and cathepsin G by a biphenyl disulfonic acid copolymer. Int. J. Immunopharmacol. 16: 623–632.

Javaid, K., A. Rahman, K. N. Anwar, R. S. Frey, R. D. Minshall and A. B. Malik. (2003). Tumor necrosis factor-alpha induces early-onset endothelial adhesivity by protein kinase C zeta-dependent activation of intercellular adhesion molecule-1. Circ. Res. 92: 1089–1097.

Johnson, K. J., J. C. Fantone, J. Kaplan and P. A. Ward. (1981). *In vivo* damage of rat lungs by oxygen metabolites. J. Clin. Invest. 67: 983–93.

Jones, D. A., O. Abbassi, L. V. McIntire, R. P. McEver and C. W. Smith. (1993). P-selectin mediates neutrophil rolling on histamine-stimulated endothelial cells. Biophys. J. 65: 1560.

José, R. J., A. Williams, A. Manuel, J. S. Brown and C. Rachel. (2020). Targeting coagulation activation in severe COVID-19 pneumonia: Lessons from bacterial pneumonia and sepsis. Chambers European Respiratory Review 29: 200240.

Kai-Larsen, Y. and B. Agerberth. (2008). The role of the multifunctional peptide LL-37 in host defense. Front. Biosci. 13: 3760–3767.

Kamm, K. E. and J. T. Stull. (2001). Dedicated myosin light chain kinases with diverse cellular functions. J. Biol. Chem. 276: 4527–4530.

Kang, R., H. J. Zeh, M. T. Lotze and D. Tang. (2011). The Beclin 1 network regulates autophagy and apoptosis. Cell Death Differ. 18: 571–580.

Kansas, G. S. (1996). Selectins and their ligands: Current concepts and controversies. Blood 88: 3259–3287.

Kato, Jr, T., M. Delhase, A. Hoffmann and M. Karin. (2003). CK2 is a c-terminal IKK responsible for NF-κB activation during the UV response. Mol. Cell 12: 829–839.

Kawabata, K., T. Hagio, S. Matsumoto, S. Nakao, S. Orita, Y. Aze et al. (2000). Delayed neutrophil elastase inhibition prevents subsequent progression of acute lung injury induced by endotoxin inhalation in hamsters. Am. J. Respir. Crit. Care Med. 161: 2013–2018.

Kelley, G. G., S. E. Reks, J. M. Ondrako and A. V. Smrcka. (2001). Phospholipase C(epsilon): A novel Ras effector. EMBO J. 20: 743–754.

Keogh, R. J., R. A. Houliston and C. P. Wheeler-Jones. (2002). Human endothelial Pyk2 is expressed in two isoforms and associates with paxillin and p130Cas. Biochem. Biophys. Res. Commun. 290: 1470–1477.

Kettritz, R., M. Choi, S. Rolle, M. Wellner and F. C. Luft. (2004). Integrins and cytokines activate nuclear transcription factor-kappaB in human neutrophils. J. Biol. Chem. 279: 2657–2665.

Kihara, A., Y. Kabeya, Y. Ohsumi and T. Yoshimori. (2001). Beclin-phosphatidylinositol 3-kinase complex functions at the trans-Golgi network. EMBO Rep. 2: 330–335.

Kim, G. -L., S. -H. Seon and D. -K. Rhee. (2017). Pneumonia and *Streptococcus pneumoniae* vaccine. Arch. Pharm. Res. 40: 885–893.

Kim, I., S. O. Moon, S. H. Kim, H. J. Kim, Y. S. Koh, G. Y. Koh et al. (2001). Vascular endothelial growth factor expression of intercellular adhesion molecule 1 (ICAM-1), vascular cell adhesion molecule 1 (VCAM-1), and E-selectin through nuclear factor-kappa B activation in endothelial cells. J. Biol. Chem. 276: 7614–7620.

Kimes, K. E., S. N. Kasule and J. E. Blair. (2020). Pulmonary Coccidioidomycosis. Semin. Respir. Crit. Care Med. 41: 42–52.

Kinkade, S. and N. A. Long. (2016). Acute Bronchitis. Am. Fam. Physician. 94: 560–565.

Kircheis, R., E. Haasbach, D. Lueftenegger, W. T. Heyken, M. Ocker and O. Planz. (2020). NF-κB pathway as a potential target for treatment of critical stage COVID-19 patients. Front. Immunol. 11: 598444.

Koh, H., S. Tasaka, N. Hasegawa, K. Asano, T. Kotani, H. Morisaki et al. (2008). Vascular endothelial growth factor in epithelial lining fluid of patients with acute respiratory distress syndrome. Respirology 13: 281–284.

Konrad, J., E. Eber and V. Stadlbauer. (2020). Changing paradigms in the treatment of gastrointestinal complications of cystic fibrosis in the era of cystic fibrosis transmembrane conductance regulator modulators. Pediatr. Respir. Rev. 24: S1526–0542.

Kristof, A. S., P. Goldberg, V. Laubach and S. N. Hussain. (1998). Role of inducible nitric oxide synthase in endotoxin-induced acute lung injury. Am. J. Respir. Crit. Care Med. 158: 1883–1889.

Kudryashov, D. S., M. V. Chibalina, K. G. Birukov, T. J. Lukas, J. R. Sellers, L. J. Van Eldik et al. (1999). Unique sequence of a high molecular weight myosin light chain kinase is involved in interaction with actin cytoskeleton. FEBS Lett. 463: 67–71.

Kumar, S. and K. Mehta. (2012). Tissue transglutaminase constitutively activates hif-1α promoter and nuclear factor-κb via a non-canonical pathway. PLoS One 7: e49321.

Kuncio, G. S., M. Tsyganskaya, J. Zhu, S. L. Liu, L. Nagy, V. Thomazy et al. (1998). Tnf-alpha modulates expression of the tissue transglutaminase gene in liver cells. Am. J. Physiol. 274: G240–245.

Lane, T. A., G. E. Lamkin, E. V. Wancewicz. (1990). Protein kinase C inhibitors block the enhanced expression of intercellular adhesion molecule-1 on endothelial cells activated by interleukin-1, lipopolysaccharide and tumor necrosis factor. Biochem. Biophys. Res. Commun. 172: 1273–1281.

Lawler, S. (1999). Regulation of actin dynamics: The LIM kinase connection. Curr. Biol. 9: R800–R802.

Lawrence, M. B. and T. A. Springer. (1993). Neutrophils roll on E-selectin. J. Immunol. 151: 6338.

Ledebur, H. C. and T. P. Parks. (1995). Transcriptional regulation of the intercellular adhesion molecule-1 gene by inflammatory cytokines in human endothelial cells. Essential roles of a variant NF-kappa B site and p65 homodimers. J. Biol. Chem. 270: 933–943.

Lee, C. T., A. M. Fein, M. Lippmann, H. Holtzman, P. Kimbel and G. Weinbaum. (1981). Elastolytic activity in pulmonary lavage fluid from patients with adult respiratory-distress syndrome. N. Engl. J. Med. 304: 192–196.

Lee, J., Y. S. Kim, D. H. Choi, M. S. Bang, T. R. Han, T. H. Joh et al. (2004). Transglutaminase 2 induces nuclear factor-kappab activation via a novel pathway in bv-2 microglia. J. Biol. Chem. 279: 53725–53735.

Lev, S., H. Moreno, R. Martinez, P. Canoll, E. Peles, J. M. Musacchio et al. (1995). Protein tyrosine kinase PYK2 involved in Ca(2+)-induced regulation of ion channel and MAP kinase functions. Nature 376: 727–729.

Levay, P. F. and M. Viljoen. (1995). Lactoferrin: A general review. Haematologica. 80: 252–267.

Li, K. J., M. C. Lu, S. C. Hsieh, C. H. Wu, H. S. Yu, C. Y. Tsai et al. (2006). Release of surface-expressed lactoferrin from polymorphonuclear neutrophils after contact with CD4+ T cells and its modulation on Th1/Th2 cytokine production. J. Leukoc. Biol. 80: 350–358.

Li, M., H. Edamatsu, R. Kitazawa, S. Kitazawa and T. Kataoka. (2009). Phospholipase Cepsilon promotes intestinal tumorigenesis of Apc(Min/+) mice through augmentation of inflammation and angiogenesis. Carcinogenesis 30: 1424–1432.

Li, Q., D. Van Antwerp, F. Mercurio, K. F. Lee and I. M. Verma. (1999). Severe liver degeneration in mice lacking the IKK2 gene. Science 284: 321–325.

Liao, Q. J., L. B. Ye, K. A. Timani, Y. C. Zeng, Y. L. She, L. Ye. et al. (2005). Activation of NF-kB by the full-length nucleocapsid protein of the SARS coronavirus. Acta Biochim. Biophys. 37: 607–612.

Ling, L., Z. Cao and D. V. Goeddel. (1998). NF-kappaB-inducing kinase activates IKK-alpha by phosphorylation of Ser-176. Proc. Natl. Acad. Sci. USA 95: 3792–3797.

Lorand, L. and R. M. Graham. (2003). Transglutaminases: Crosslinking enzymes with pleiotropic functions. Nat. Rev. Mol. Cell Biol. 4: 140–156.

Lugo, R. A and M. C. Nahata. (1993). Pathogenesis and treatment of bronchiolitis. Clin. Pharm. 12: 95–116.

Maddox, L. and D. A. Schwartz. (2002). The pathophysiology of Asthma. Ann. Rev. Med. 53: 477–498.

Madhusudan, S., M. Foster, S. R. Muthuramalingam, J. P. Braybrooke, S. Wilner, K. Kaur et al. (2004). A phase II study of etanercept (Enbrel), a tumor necrosis factor alpha inhibitor in patients with metastatic breast cancer. Clin. Cancer Res.10: 6528–6534.

Madhusudan, S., S. R. Muthuramalingam, J. P. Braybrooke, S. Wilner, K. Kaur, C. Han et al. (2005). Study of etanercept, a tumor necrosis factor-alpha inhibitor, in recurrent ovarian cancer. J. Clin. Oncol. 23: 5950–5959.

Maekawa, M., T. Ishizaki, S. Boku, N. Watanabe, A. Fujita, A. Iwamatsu. et al. (1999). Signaling from Rho to the actin cytoskeleton through protein kinases ROCK and LIM-kinase. Science 285: 895–898.

Mahabeleshwar, G. H. and G. C. Kundu. (2003). Tyrosine kinase p56lck regulates cell motility and NF-κB-mediated secretion of urokinase type plasminogen activator through tyrosine phosphorylation of IκBα following hypoxia/reoxygenation. **J. Biol. Chem.** 278: 52598–52612.

Malik, A. B and S. K. Lo. (1996). Vascular endothelial adhesion molecules and tissue inflammation. Pharmacol. Rev. 48: 213–229.

Mann, A. P., A. Verma, G. Sethi, B. Manavathi, H. Wang, J. Y. Fok et al. (2006). Overexpression of tissue transglutaminase leads to constitutive activation of nuclear factor-kappab in cancer cells: Delineation of a novel pathway. Cancer Res. 66: 8788–8795.

Matthay, M. A. (2014). Resolution of pulmonary edema. Thirty years of progress. Am. J. Respir. Crit. Care Med. 189: 1301–1308.

Matthay, M. A., L. B. Ware and G. A. Zimmerman. (2012). The acute respiratory distress syndrome. J. Clin. Invest. 122: 2731–2740.

Matthay, M. A., H. G. Folkesson and C. Clerici. (2002). Lung epithelial fluid transport and the resolution of pulmonary edema. Physiol. Rev. 82: 569–600.

Matthay, M. A., R. L. Zemans, G. A. Zimmerman, Y. M. Arabi, J. R. Beitler, A. Mercat et al. (2019). Acute respiratory distress syndrome. Nat. Rev. Dis. Primers. 5: 18.

Mehta, D. and A. B. Malik. (2006). Signaling mechanisms regulating endothelial permeability. Physiol. Rev. 86: 279–367.

Mercogliano, M. F., S. Bruni, P. V. Elizalde and R. Schillaci. (2020). Tumor necrosis factor α blockade: An opportunity to tackle breast cancer. Front. Oncol. 10: 584.

Miles, J. S. and S. Islam. (2019). Point of care ultrasound in thoracic malignancy. Ann. Transl. Med. 7: 350.

Minami, T. and W. C. Aird. (2005). Endothelial cell gene regulation. Trends Cardiovasc. Med. 15: 174–184.

Miralles, F., G. Posern, A. I. Zaromytidou and R. Treisman. (2003). Actin dynamics control SRF activity by regulation of its coactivator MAL. Cell 113: 329–342.

Mirzapoiazova, T., J. Moitra, L. Moreno-Vinasco, S. Sammani, J. R. Turner, E. T. Chiang et al. (2011). Non-muscle myosin light chain kinase isoform is a viable molecular target in acute inflammatory lung injury. Am. J. Respir. Cell Mol. Biol. 44: 40–52.

Mizushima, N. (2007). Autophagy: Process and function. Genes Dev. 21: 2861–2873.

Moalli, R., J. M. Doyle, H. R. Tahhan, F. M. Hasan, S. S. Braman and T. Saldeen. (1989). Fibrinolysis in critically ill patients. Am. Rev. Respir. Dis. 140: 287–293.

Moule, M. G. and J. D. Cirillo. (2020). Mycobacterium tuberculosis dissemination plays a critical role in pathogenesis. Front. Cell Infect. Microbiol. 10: 65–76.

Murray, J. F. (2011). Pulmonary edema: Pathophysiology and diagnosis. Int. J. Tuberc. Lung Dis. 15: 155–160.

Nagaoka, I., H. Tamura and M. Hirata. (2006). An antimicrobial cathelicidin peptide, human CAP18/LL-37, suppresses neutrophil apoptosis via the activation of formyl-peptide receptorlike 1 and P2X7. J. Immunol. 176: 3044–3052.

Nygaard, S. D., T. Ganz and M. W. Peterson. (1993). Defensins reduce the barrier integrity of a cultured epithelial monolayer without cytotoxicity. Am. J. Respir. Cell Mol. Biol. 8: 193–200.

Oeckinghaus, A. and S. Ghosh. (2009). The NF-kappaB family of transcription factors and its regulation. Cold Spring Harb. Perspect. Biol. 1: a000034.

Oh, K., H. B. Park, O. J. Byoun, D. M. Shin, E. M. Jeong, Y. W. Kim et al. (2011). Epithelial transglutaminase 2 is needed for t cell interleukin-17 production and subsequent pulmonary inflammation and fibrosis in bleomycin-treated mice. J. Exp. Med. 208: 1707–1719.

Ohashi, K., K. Nagata, M. Maekawa, T. Ishizaki, S. Narumiya, K. Mizuno et al. (2000). Rho-associated kinase ROCK activates LIM-kinase 1 by phosphorylation at threonine 508 within the activation loop J. Biol. Chem. 275: 3577–3582.

Oka, S., H. Kamata, K. Kamata, H. Yagisawa and H. Hirata. (2000). N-acetylcysteine suppresses TNF-induced NF-kappaB activation through inhibition of IkappaB kinases. FEBS Lett. 472: 196–202.

Okigaki, M., C. Davis, M. Falasca, S. Harroch, D. P. Felsenfeld, M. P. Sheetz et al. (2003). Pyk2 regulates multiple signaling events crucial for macrophagy morphology and migration. Proc. Natl. Acad. Sci. USA 100: 10740–10745.

Oliva, J. and O. Terrier. (2021). Viral and bacterial co-infections in the lungs: Dangerous liaisons. Viruses 13: 1725.

Ollivier, V., G. C. Parry, R. R. Cobb, D. de Prost and N. Mackman. (1996). Elevated cyclic AMP inhibits NF-κB-mediated transcription in human monocytic cells and endothelial cells. J. Biol. Chem. 271: 20828–20835.

Phua, J., J. R. Badia, N. K. J. Adhikari, J. O. Friedrich, R. A. Fowler, J. M. Singh et al. (2009). Has mortality from acute respiratory distress syndrome decreased over time?: A systematic review. Am. J. Respir. Crit. Care Med. 179: 220–227.

Posern, G., A. Sotiropoulos and R. Treisman. (2002). Mutant actins demonstrate a role for unpolymerized actin in control of transcription by serum response factor. Mol. Biol. Cell. 13: 4167–4178.

Prabhakaran, P., L. B. Ware, K. E. White, M. T. Cross, M. A. Matthay and M. A. Olman. (2003). Elevated levels of plasminogen activator inhibitor-1 in pulmonary edema fluid are associated with mortality in acute lung injury. Am. J. Physiol. Lung Cell. Mol. Physiol. 285: L20–L28.

Pugin, J., G. Verghese, M. C. Widmer and M. A. Matthay. (1999). The alveolar space is the site of intense inflammatory and profibrotic reactions in the early phase of acute respiratory distress syndrome. Crit. Care Med. 27: 304–312.

Qing, G., Z. Qu and G. Xiao. (2005). Stabilization of basally translated NF-kappaB-inducing kinase (NIK) protein functions as a molecular switch of processing of NF-kappaB2 p100. J. Biol. Chem. 280: 40578–40582.

Quagliaro, L., L. Piconi, R. Assaloni, R. Da Ros, A. Maier, G. Zuodar et al. (2005). Intermittent high glucose enhances ICAM-1, VCAM-1 and E-selectin expression in human umbilical vein endothelial cells in culture: The distinct role of protein kinase C and mitochondrial superoxide production. Atherosclerosis 183: 259–267.

Rabe, K. F. and H. Watz. (2017). Chronic obstructive pulmonary disease. Lancet 389: 1931–1940.

Rahman, A., K. N. Anwar, A. L. True and A. B. Malik. (1999a). Thrombin-induced p65 homodimer binding to downstream NF-kappa B site of the promoter mediates endothelial ICAM-1 expression and neutrophil adhesion. J. Immunol. 162: 5466–5476.

Rahman, A., K. N. Anwar, M. Minhajuddin, K. M. Bijli, K. Javaid, A. L. True et al. (2004). cAMP targeting of p38 MAP kinase inhibits thrombin-induced NF-kappaB activation and ICAM-1 expression in endothelial cells. Am. J. Physiol. Lung Cell Mol. Physiol. 287: L1017–1024.

Rahman, A., M. Bando, J. Kefer, K. N. Anwar and A. B. Malik. (1999b). Protein kinase C-activated oxidant generation in endothelial cells signals intercellular adhesion molecule-1 gene transcription. Mol. Pharmacol. 55: 575–583.

Regnier, C. H., H. Y. Song, X. Gao, D. V. Goeddel, Z. Cao and M. Rothe. (1997). Identification and characterization of an IκB kinase. Cell 90: 357–383.

Ricou, B., L. Nicod, S. Lacraz, H. G. Welgus, P. M. Suter and J. M. Dayer. (1996). Matrix metalloproteinases and TIMP in acute respiratory distress syndrome. Am. J. Respir. Crit. Care Med. 154: 346–352.

Rivas, F. V., J. P. O'Keefe, M. L. Alegre and T. F. Gajewski. (2004). Actin cytoskeleton regulates calcium dynamics and NFAT nuclear duration. Mol. Cell Biol. 24: 1628–1639.

Roebuck, K. A. and A. Finnegan. (1999). Regulation of intercellular adhesion molecule-1 (CD54) gene expression. J. Leukoc. Biol. 66: 876–888.

Roper, J. M., D. J. Mazzatti, R. H. Watkins, W. M. Maniscalco, P. C. Keng and M. A. O'Reilly. (2004). *In vivo* exposure to hyperoxia induces DNA damage in a population of alveolar type II epithelial cells. Am. J. Physiol. Lung Cell Mol. Physiol. 286: L1045–1054.

Ruthman, C. A. and E. Festic. (2015). Emerging therapies for the prevention of acute respiratory distress syndrome. Ther. Adv. Respir. Dis. 9: 173–187.

Ryndak, M. B. and S. Laal. (2019). Mycobacterium tuberculosis primary infection and dissemination: A critical role for alveolar epithelial cells. Front. Cell Infect. Microbiol. 9: 299–314.

Sakamoto, N., H. Mukae, T. Fujii, H. Ishii, S. Yoshioka, T. Kakugawa et al. (2005). Differential effects of {alpha}- and {beta}-defensin on cytokine production by cultured human bronchial epithelial cells. Am. J. Physiol. Lung Cell Mol. Physiol. 288: L508–513.

Sato, H., M. E. J. Callister, S. Mumby, G. J. Quinlan, K. I. Welsh, R. M. DuBois et al. (2004). KL-6 levels are elevated in plasma from patients with acute respiratory distress syndrome. Eur. Respir. J. 23: 142–145.

Schulte, D., V. Küppers, N. Dartsch, A. Broermann, H. Li, A. Zarbock et al. (2011). Stabilizing the VE-cadherin–catenin complex blocks leukocyte extravasation and vascular permeability. The EMBO Journal 30: 4157–4170.

Scott, M. G., D. J. Davidson, M. R. Gold, D. Bowdish and R. E. W. Hancock. (2002). The human antimicrobial peptide LL-37 is a multifunctional modulator of innate immune responses. J. Immunol. 169: 3883–3891.

Sen, R. and D. Baltimore. (1986). Multiple nuclear factors interact with the immunoglobulin enhancer sequences. Cell 46: 705–716.

Senftleben, U., Y. Cao, G. Xiao, F. R. Greten, G. Krähn, G. Bonizzi et al. (2001). Activation of IKKα of a second, evolutionary conserved, NF-κB signaling pathway. Science 293: 1495–99.

Serkkola, E. and M. Hurme. (1993). Activation of NF-κB by cAMP in human myeloid cells. FEBS Lett. 334: 327–330.

Setianingrum, F., R. R. Richardson and D. W. Denning. (2019). Pulmonary cryptococcosis: A review of pathobiology and clinical aspects. Med. Mycol. 57: 133–150.

Shim, J. Y. (2020). Current perspectives on atypical pneumonia in children. Clin. Exp. Pediatr. 63: 469–476.

Shirasawa, M., N. Fujiwara, S. Hirabayashi, H. Ohno, J. Lida, K. Makita et al. 2004. Receptor for advanced glycation end-products is a marker of type I lung alveolar cells. Genes Cells. 9: 165–174.

Siegel, M., P. Strnad, R. E. Watts, K. Choi, B. Jabri, M. B. Omary et al. (2008). Extracellular transglutaminase 2 is catalytically inactive, but is transiently activated upon tissue injury. PLoS One 3(3): e1861.

Sigel, K., R. Pitts and K. Crothers. (2016). Lung Malignancies in HIV Infection. Semin. Respir. Crit. Care Med. 37: 267–276.

Simon, S. I. and C. E. Green. (2005). Molecular mechanics and dynamics of leukocyte recruitment during inflammation. Annu. Rev. Biomed. Eng. 7: 151–185.

Simon, S. I. and H. L. Goldsmith. (2002). Leukocyte adhesion dynamics in shear flow. Ann. Biomed. Eng. 30: 315–332.

Smith, C. W., S. D. Marlin, R. Rothlein, C. Toman and D. C. Anderson. (1989). Cooperative interactions of LFA-1 and Mac-1 with intercellular adhesion molecule-1 in facilitating adherence and transendothelial migration of human neutrophils *in vitro*. J. Clin. Invest. 83: 2008–2017.

Soehnlein, O. and L. Lindbom. (2009). Neutrophilderived azurocidin alarms the immune system. J. Leukoc. Biol. 85: 344–351.

Soehnlein, O. and L. Lindbom. (2010). Phagocyte partnership during the onset and resolution of inflammation. Nat. Rev. Immunol. 10: 427–439.

Soehnlein, O., X. Xie, H. Ulbrich, E. Kenne, P. Rotzius, H. Flodgaard et al. (2005). Neutrophil-derived heparin-binding protein (HBP/CAP37) deposited on endothelium enhances monocyte arrest under flow conditions 164. J. Immunol. 174: 6399–6405.

Soehnlein, O., S. Oehmcke, X. Ma, A. G. Rothfuchs, R. Frithiof, N. van Rooijen et al. (2008a). Neutrophil degranulation mediates severe lung damage triggered by streptococcal M1 protein 172. Eur. Respir. J. 32: 405–412.

Soehnlein, O., Y. K. Larsen, R. Frithiof, O. E. Sorensen, E. Kenne, K. Scharffetter-Kochanek et al. (2008b). Neutrophil primary granule proteins HBP and HNP1–3 boost bacterial phagocytosis by human and murine macrophages 168. J. Clin. Invest. 118: 3491–3502.

Sommer, N., P. A. Loschmann, G. H. Northoff, M. Weller, A. Steinbrecher, J. P. Steinbach et al. (1995). The antidepressant rolipram suppresses cytokine production and prevents autoimmune encephalomyelitis. Nat. Med. 1: 1244–1248.

Soong, L. B., T. Ganz, A. Ellison and G. H. Caughey. (1997). Purification and characterization of defensins from cystic fibrosis sputum. Inflamm. Res. 46: 98–102.

Springer, T. A. (1990). Adhesion receptors of the immune system. Nature 346: 425–434.

Springer, T. A. (1994). Traffic signals for lymphocyte recirculation and leukocyte emigration: The multistep paradigm. Cell 76: 301–314.

Staunton, D. E., S. D. Marlin, C. Stratowa, M. L. Dustin and T. A. Springer. (1988). Primary structure of ICAM-1 demonstrates interaction between members of the immunoglobulin and integrin supergene families. Cell 52: 925–933.

Staunton, D. E., V. J. Merluzzi, R. Rothlein, R. Barton, S. D. Marlin and T. A. Springer. (1989). A cell adhesion molecule, ICAM-1, is the major surface receptor for rhinoviruses. Cell 56: 849–853.

Steinberg, J., G. Fink, A. Picone, B. Searles, H. Schiller, H. M. Lee et al. (2001). Evidence of increased matrix metalloproteinase-9 concentration in patients following cardiopulmonary bypass. J. Extra Corpor. Technol. 33: 218–222.

Su, C. M., L. Wang and D. Yoo. (2021). Activation of NF-κB and induction of proinflammatory cytokine expressions mediated by ORF7a protein of SARS-CoV-2. Sci. Rep. 11: 13464.

Sumi, T., K. Matsumoto and T. Nakamura. (2001). Specific activation of LIM kinase 2 via phosphorylation of threonine 505 by ROCK, a Rho-dependent protein kinase. J. Biol. Chem. 276: 670–676.

Sun, S. C. (2012). The noncanonical NF-κB pathway. Immunol. Rev. 246: 125–140.

Takada, Y. and B. B. Aggarwal. (2004). TNF activates Syk protein tyrosine kinase leading to TNF-induced MAPK activation, NF-kappaB activation, and apoptosis. J. Immunol. 173: 1066–1077.

Takada, Y., A. Mukhopadhyay, G. C. Kundu, G. H. Mahabeleshwar, S. Singh and B. B. Aggarwal. (2003). Hydrogen peroxide activates NF-kappa B through tyrosine phosphorylation of I kappa B alpha and serine phosphorylation of p65: Evidence for the involvement of I kappa B alpha kinase and Syk protein-tyrosine kinase. J. Biol. Chem. 278: 24233–24241.

Tanaka, M., M. E. Fuentes, K. Yamaguchi, M. H. Durnin, S. A. Dalrymple, K. L. Hardy et al. 1999. Embryonic lethality, liver degeneration, and impaired NF-κB activation in IKKβ-deficient mice. Immunity 10: 421–429.

Taylor, S. S., J. A. Buechler and W. Yonemoto. (1990). cAMP-dependent protein kinase: Framework for a diverse family of regulatory enzymes. Annu. Rev. Biochem. 59: 971–1005.

Tecle, T., S. Tripathi and K. L. Hartshorn. (2010). Review: Defensins and cathelicidins in lung immunity. Innate Immun. 16: 151–159.

Terpstra, M. L., J. Aman, G. P. van Nieuw Amerongen and A. B. Groeneveld. (2014). Plasma biomarkers for acute respiratory distress syndrome: A systematic review and meta-analysis. Crit. Care Med. 42: 691–700.

Theriot, J. A. (1997). Accelerating on a treadmill: ADF/cofilin promotes rapid actin filament turnover in the dynamic cytoskeleton. J. Cell Biol. 136: 1165–1168.

Thompson, P. W., A. M. Randi and A. J. Ridley. (2002). Intercellular adhesion molecule (ICAM)-1, but not ICAM-2, activates RhoA and stimulates c-fos and rhoA transcription in endothelial cells. J. Immunol. 169: 1007–1013.

Tobón, A. M. and B. L. Gómez. (2021). Pulmonary histoplasmosis. Mycopathologia 186(5): 697–705.

Torii, K., K. Iida, Y. Miyazaki, S. Saga, Y. Kondoh, H. Taniguchi et al. (1997). Higher concentrations of matrix metalloproteinases in bronchoalveolar lavage fluid of patients with adult respiratory distress syndrome. Am. J. Respir. Crit. Care Med. 155: 43–46.

Tremblay, G. M., E. Vachon, C. Larouche and Y. Bourbonnais. (2002). Inhibition of human neutrophil elastase-induced acute lung injury in hamsters by recombinant human pre-elafin (trappin-2). Chest. 121: 582–588.

Ulanova, M., L. Pattagunta, M. Marcet-Palacios, M. Duszyk, U. Steinhoff, F. Duta et al. (2005). Syk tyrosine kinase participates in beta1-integrin signaling and inflammatory responses in airway epithelial cells. Am. J. Physiol. 288: L497–L507.

Van der Does, A. M., H. Beekhuizen, B. Ravensbergen, T. Vos, T. H. M. Ottenhoff, J. T. van Dissel et al. (2010). LL-37 Directs macrophage differentiation toward macrophages with a pro-inflammatory signature. J. Immunol. 185: 1442–1449.

Van, W. S., S. P. Mannesse-Lazeroms, J. H. Dijkman and P. S. Hiemstra. (1997). Effect of neutrophil serine proteinases and defensins on lung epithelial cells: Modulation of cytotoxicity and IL-8 production. J. Leukoc. Biol. 62: 217–226.

Viatour, P., M. P. Merville, V. Bours and A. Chariot. (2005). Phosphorylation of NF-κB and IκB proteins: Implications in cancer and inflammation. Trends Biochem. Sci. 30: 43–52.

Vielma, S. A., G. Krings and M. F. Lopes–Virella. (2003). Chlamydophila pneumoniae induces ICAM-1 expression in human aortic endothelial cells via protein kinase C-dependent activation of nuclear factor-kappaB. Circ. Res. 92: 1130–1137.

Volovyk, Z. M., M. J. Wolf, S. V. Prasad and H. A. Rockman. (2006). Agonist-stimulated beta-adrenergic receptor internalization requires dynamic cytoskeletal actin turnover. J. Biol. Chem. 281: 9773–9780.

Voraberger, G., R. Schafer and C. Stratowa. (1991). Cloning of the human gene for intercellular adhesion molecule 1 and analysis of its 5'-regulatory region. Induction by cytokines and phorbol ester. J. Immunol. 147: 2777–2786.

Wada, T., S. Jesmin, S. Gando, Y. Yanagida, A. Mizugaki, S. N. Sultana et al. (2013). The role of angiogenic factors and their soluble receptors in acute lung injury (ALI)/acute respiratory distress syndrome (ARDS) associated with critical illness. J. Inflamm. (London England) 10: 6–6.

Wainwright, M. S., J. Rossi, J. Schavocky, S. Crawford, D. Steinhorn, A. V. Velentza et al. (2003). Protein kinase involved in lung injury susceptibility: evidence from enzyme isoform genetic knockout and *in vivo* inhibitor treatment. Proc. Natl. Acad. Sci. U S A 100: 6233–6238.

Wang, H., E. A. Oestreich, N. Maekawa, T. A. Bullard, K. L. Vikstrom, R. T. Dirksen et al. 2005. Phospholipase C epsilon modulates beta-adrenergic receptor-dependent cardiac contraction and inhibits cardiac hypertrophy. Circ. Res 97: 1305–1313.

Wang, W., Y. Suzuki, T. Tanigaki, D. R. Rank and T. A. Raffin. (1994). Effect of the NADPH oxidase inhibitor apocynin on septic lung injury in guinea pigs. Am. J. Respir. Crit. Care Med. 150: 1449–1452.

Ware, L. B. and C. S. Calfee. (2016). Biomarkers of ARDS: What's new? Intensive Care Med. 42: 797–799.

Ware, L. B., T. Koyama, D. D. Billheimer, W. Wu, G. R. Bernard, B. T. Thompson et al. (2010). Prognostic and pathogenetic value of combining clinical and biochemical indices in patients with acute lung injury. Chest 137: 288–296.

Waris, G., A. Livolsi, V. Imbert, J. F. Peyron and A. Siddiqui. (2003). Hepatitis C virus NS5A and subgenomic replicon activate NF-κB via tyrosine phosphorylation of IκBα and its degradation by calpain protease. J. Biol. Chem. 278: 40778–40787.

Wawryk, S. O., P. N. Cockerill, I. P. Wicks and A. W. Boyd. (1991). Isolation and characterization of the promoter region of the human intercellular adhesion molecule-1 gene. Int. Immunol. 3: 83–93.

Weyant, R. B., D. Kabbani, K. Doucette, C. Lau and C. Cervera. 2021. *Pneumocystis jirovecii*: A review with a focus on prevention and treatment. Expert. Opin. Pharmacother. 12: 1579–1592.

Wilson, R. and C. F. Rayner. (1995). Bronchitis. Curr. Opin. Pulm. Med. 1: 177–182.

Wojciak–Stothard, B., L. Williams and A. J. Ridley. (1999). Monocyte adhesion and spreading on human endothelial cells is dependent on Rho-regulated receptor clustering. J. Cell Biol. 145: 1293–1307.

Wu, S. Q. and W. C. Aird. (2005). Thrombin, TNF-alpha, and LPS exert overlapping but nonidentical effects on gene expression in endothelial cells and vascular smooth muscle cells. Am. J. Physiol. Heart Circ. Physiol. 289: H873–H885.

Wu, X., A. Luo, Y. Zhou and J. Ren. (2014). N-acetylcysteine reduces oxidative stress, nuclear factor-κB activity and cardiomyocyte apoptosis in heart failure. Mol. Med. Rep. 10: 615–624.

Xiao, G., A. Fong and S. C. Sun. (2004). Induction of p100 processing by NIK involves docking IKKα to p100 and IKKα-mediated phosphorylation. J. Biol. Chem. 279: 30099–30105.

Xie, Z. and D. J. Klionsky. (2007). Autophagosome formation: Core machinery and adaptations. Nat. Cell Biol. 9: 1102–1109.

Xing, K., S. Murthy, W. C. Liles and J. M. Singh. (2012). Clinical utility of biomarkers of endothelial activation in sepsis—A systematic review. Crit. Care 16: R7.

Xu, J., X. P. Gao, R. Ramchandran, Y. Y. Zhao, S. M. Vogel and A. B. Malik. (2008). Nonmuscle myosin light-chain kinase mediates neutrophil transmigration in sepsis-induced lung inflammation by activating beta2 integrins. Nat. Immunol. 9: 880–886.

Xu, N., X. P. Gao, R. D. Minshall, A. Rahman and A. B. Malik. (2002). Time-dependent reversal of sepsis-induced PMN uptake and lung vascular injury by expression of CD18 antagonist. Am. J. Physiol. Lung Cell Mol. Physiol. 282: L796–802.

Yamamoto, Y. and R. B. Gaynor. (2001). Therapeutic potential of inhibition of the NF-κB pathway in the treatment of inflammation and cancer. J. Clin. Invest. 107: 135–42.

Zemans, R. L., S. P. Colgan and G. P. Downey. (2009). Transepithelial migration of neutrophils: Mechanisms and implications for acute lung injury. Am. J. Respir. Cell Mol. Biol. 40: 519–535.

Zhang, L., S. Malik, G. G. Kelley, M. S. Kapiloff and A. V. Smrcka. (2011). Phospholipase C epsilon scaffolds to muscle-specific A kinase anchoring protein (mAKAPbeta) and integrates multiple hypertrophic stimuli in cardiac myocytes. J. Biol. Chem. 286: 23012–23021.

Zhang, Q., M. J. Lenardo, D. Baltimore. (2017). 30 Years of NF-κB: A blossoming of relevance to human pathobiology. Cell 168: 37–57.

Zhao, Z., N. Wickersham, K. N. Kangelaris, A. K. May, G. R. Bernard, M. A. Matthay et al. (2017). External validation of a biomarker and clinical prediction model for hospital mortality in acute respiratory distress syndrome. Intensive Care Med. 43: 1123–1131.

Chapter 6

MALDI-TOF MS Fingerprinting for the Diagnosis of Infectious Diseases

Hercules Moura,[1,*] *Glauber Wagner,*[2] *Renato Simões,*[2]
Yulanda Williamson[1] *and John R. Barr*[1]

Introduction

Mass Spectrometry (MS) is an analytical technique that measures the mass-to-charge ratio (*m/z*) of different positive or negative ions. It is used as a reliable analytical tool with several diverse applications. Mass spectrometers evolved over 100 years from devices that separated ionized particles, into complex instruments that can detect, identify, and quantify small and large molecules, such as entire proteins (Siuzdak 2006) with high resolution and high mass accuracy. The basic components of a mass spectrometer are an ion source that generates ions, a mass analyzer that separates the ions, and an ion detector. Among the soft ionization methods, matrix-assisted laser-desorption ionization (MALDI) is used for different biological applications such as protein and peptide sequencing, image analysis, and microbial identification.

MALDI-time-of-flight (TOF) MS is changing the workflow for microbial identification in microbiology laboratories. For early diagnosis, clinical microbiology laboratories continue to use more arduous and time-consuming classical methods, such as staining and microscopy; culture, biochemical, and antigenic techniques; and antimicrobial susceptibility tests. However, because of its high resolving power and analytical sensitivity, MALDI-TOF MS decreases cultured organism labor and time to the final result by markedly reducing the need for biochemical and antigenic techniques (Korstrzewa 2018). Cost per specimen is another reason to use MALDI-

---
[1] Clinical Chemistry Branch, Division of Laboratory Sciences, National Center for Environmental Health, Centers for Disease Control and Prevention, Chamblee Campus, 4770 Buford Hwy NE, Atlanta, GA 30341-3724, USA.
[2] Universidade Federal de Santa Catarina, Brazil.
* Corresponding author: Hercul.Moura@gmail.com

TOF MS in the clinical microbiology laboratory (Tran et al. 2015). The initial cost of a dedicated MS instrument is relatively high, but anecdotal observation shows that with robust use, the cost of such instruments is offset over time (Doern et al. 2016). Commercial and customized research databases are imperative for accurate microbial identification of the wide range of organisms potentially encountered in clinical samples. Using these databases has allowed one to identify microorganisms at the genus, species, and sometimes strain level (Hou et al. 2019, Tsuchida et al. 2020). Moreover, when the biochemical analysis is not sufficient, the specificity of these databases has aided in the identification of several difficult-to-identify bacteria, such as non-fermenting Gram-negative bacteria and anaerobes (Kostrzewa et al. 2019). Lastly, beyond the clinical setting, MALDI-TOF MS has applications for veterinary and food microbiology and environmental analysis (Yaemsiri and Sykes 2018, Akimowicz and Bucka-Kolendo 2020, Yan et al. 2020). Here, we review the literature on MALDI-TOF MS applications in microbiology and summarize our work spanning over 15 years of successfully applying MS classification workflows for microbial identification.

The MALDI-TOF MS Instrument

MALDI-TOF MS are analytical instruments used for different chemical and biological applications. Such instruments work well for microorganism identification because MALDI is tolerant to sample impurity, and TOFs have a virtually unlimited mass range (Siuzdak 2006, Liyanage 2006). The MALDI source generates ions through a soft ionization mechanism when a metal target plate containing a dried solid deposit of co-crystallized analyte and a matrix consisting of low-mass organic compound is irradiated by a UV laser beam (337 nm or 355 nm Nd:YAG) or infrared lasers (Figure 1). Current MALDI-TOF MS instruments typically have neodymium-doped yttrium aluminum garnet (Nd:YAG) lasers (355 nm). MALDI matrixes, crystalline solids with strong absorbance at laser wavelengths, include among others alpha-cyano-4-hydroxycinnamic acid (CHCA), 3,5-dimethoxy-4-hydroxycinnamic (SA), and 2,5-dihydroxybenzoic acid (DHB) that are used for peptide and protein analysis. Ion formation occurs by pulsed laser desorption of the analyte/matrix from the solid phase into the gas phase to generate a plume. High voltage accelerates the ions in the plume area, which then enter the TOF mass analyzer. The ion packets are separated according to their mass-to-charge (*m/z*) ratios. Linear TOF is the most used analyzer for microbial identification. It is simple and can easily separate small concentrations of ions with virtually infinite high masses. Once the mass analyzer separates the ions, they reach the electron multiplier detector, which generates a current signal further reported as spectra (Liyanage 2006, Siuzdak 2006).

MS Applications to Identify Microorganisms

Whole-cell fingerprinting of Gram-positive and Gram-negative microorganisms started earlier than the first introduction in 1987 of MS soft ionization methods such as MALDI (Fenselau and Demirev 2001, Siuzdak 2006). The first method

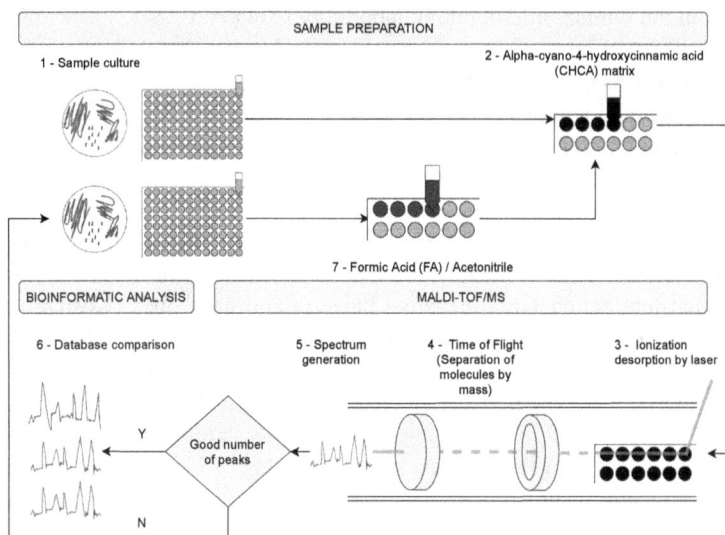

Figure 1. Overview of MALDI-TOF MS sample preparation and analysis for microbial identification. (1) Direct method is plating a small amount of biomass from a fresh individual colony on a MALDI target plate (2) and overlaying it with alpha-cyano-4-hydroxycinnamic acid (CHCA) matrix. (3) After drying, the plate is introduced to the mass spectrometer and irradiated by a UV laser beam. Ion formation occurs by pulsed laser desorption of the analyte/matrix from the solid phase into the gas phase to generate a plume. (4) High voltage accelerates the ions in the plume area, which then enter the TOF mass analyzer. The ion packets are separated according to their mass-to-charge (m/z) ratios. Linear TOF is the most used analyzer for microbial identification. It is simple and can easily separate small concentrations of ions with virtually infinite high masses. (5) Once the mass analyzer separates the ions, they reach the electron multiplier detector which generates a current signal further reported as spectra. (6) If quality spectra with a good number of peaks are not obtained, an alternative method should be used. (7) An alternative method consists of introducing an extra step to induce cell lysis by adding a small drop of FA after colony plating and before adding the matrix.

proposed and demonstrated for microbial identification was pyrolysis-MS in 1975 (Anhalt and Fenselau 1975, Fenselau and Demirev 2001). Subsequent attempts at MS applications for microorganism characterization included different desorption/ ionization techniques such as plasma desorption, laser desorption, and fast atom bombardment (FAB) (Fenselau and Demirev 2001). However, it was MALDI-TOF that delivered the most sensitive and specific results (Liyanage 2006, Clark et al. 2013, Shah 2016). Early attempts for bacterial identification using MALDI-TOF MS considered different aspects of sample collection and preparation, instrumentation, and data analysis algorithms. Comprehensive studies explored such issues, from determining the best culture conditions for MS analysis to sample preparation methods, including techniques to plate intact cells or extract biomarkers (Saenz et al. 1999). Additionally, such studies determined which MALDI matrixes should be employed as well. In early studies determining the effect of culture conditions on MALDI analysis, the main problem found was the lack of spectral reproducibility. In addition to optimal database construction, these findings underscored the importance of analyzing biological replicates (at least three separate multi-day cultures) and technical replicates (MALDI spectra of the same culture on several days) to document expected spectral variability. However, the high spectral variability generated increased uncertainty because at that point there was no consensus about the nature of the peaks detected by MS (Fenselau and Demirev 2001). Only after the demonstration that the majority of MS peaks consisted of basic peptides and small proteins, mostly very conserved ribosomal proteins, were the reservations about which culture media to use prior to MS analysis considered of less importance. These studies emphasized that the main requirement is that culture conditions should be as robust and reproducible as possible, suitable for the target organisms, and compatible with achieving good MALDI signals. Importantly, one should use biological and technical replicates when generating spectra for database construction.

Sample Preparation for MALDI-TOF MS Analysis

From the very beginning it was clear that because of microbial diversity, sample preparation should be specific. For instance, cells of most Gram-negative organisms could be easily disrupted, while cells of Gram-positive organisms were more difficult to break. In addition, other forms such as bacterial spores, mycobacteria, and fungi would need special disruption procedures prior to analysis. Several studies attempted to determine the best conditions yielding specific and consistent spectra. In contrast, because the final goal was the use of MALDI-TOF MS for the timely and accurate identification of cultured microorganisms in clinical laboratories, there was a need for a simple, universal method to be used for different groups of organisms. After several studies, a consensus method was devised: plating a small amount of biomass from a fresh individual colony on a MALDI target plate and overlaying it with alpha-cyano-4-hydroxycinnamic acid (CHCA) matrix (Clark et al. 2013, Korstrzewa 2018, Wolk and Clark 2018). After drying, the plate is introduced into a MALDI-TOF MS instrument for spectra acquisition. If quality spectra with a good number of peaks are not obtained, an alternative method should be used. An initial tentative method consisted of introducing an extra step to induce cell lysis by adding a small drop of formic acid (FA) after colony plating and before adding the matrix. Another variation of sample preparation of difficult-to-break bacteria included the use of FA and acetonitrile for extracting proteins in a tube and plating the resulting extract. In addition, special procedures were designed for spores, fungi, and mycobacteria identification and consisted of chemical inactivation followed by mechanical extraction (Figure 1). In summary, when using MALDI-TOF MS for research purposes, one can choose among different culture methods, sample preparation, MALDI matrixes, and data acquisition methods to be tried to improve the study of a particular microorganism. However, MALDI-TOF MS systems dedicated to clinical uses are required to comply with strict adherence to Standard Operation Procedures (SOPs) for complete sample work-up to report a result.

Optimization of spectra acquisition, spectral processing, and fingerprinting techniques were all very important for fast and accurate microbial identification. The spectral acquisition was easily standardized through instrument software, with special attention to collecting a few MALDI spectra required for the desired algorithm. The most difficult part was determining a standard way for data processing.

Fingerprinting algorithms used for further database construction need to come from standardized data processing. Furthermore, those reporting microbial identification results from clinical laboratories are required to follow regulatory agency-approved standard operating procedures. These steps have been fulfilled by the two current benchtop systems available in the market, each with European and North American regulatory approval for use in clinical microbiology laboratories.

The strict application of safety precautions, as appropriate for each organism, is very important when using MALDI-TOF MS for microbial identification. Although most vegetative forms of organisms are lysed by matrix and solvents used for MALDI analysis, especially after FA extraction, potentially contaminated samples should still be processed in a Class II biological safety cabinet (BSL-2). Special attention should be paid to bacilli and other spore-forming bacteria because their preparations are different. If the laboratorian suspects that the material potentially contains spores of highly infectious organisms, they can gamma-irradiate the material to render the organisms non-infectious without any effect on MALDI identification, as happens after autoclavation (Shaw et al. 2004, Moura et al. 2008, Woolfitt et al. 2011, Tracz et al. 2013). For instance, such safety measures were strictly followed in two of our early MALDI-TOF MS studies using select agents cultured organisms to differentiate *Coxiella* forms and bacilli species. All culture preparations were done in a BSL-3 laboratory; the cultures were then gamma-irradiated. The material was processed for MALDI analysis only after 21 days when viability tests were confirmed negative. Figure 2 depicts Gram-stained acid *Bacillus anthracis* vegetative cells and spores after gamma-irradiation or autoclavation (Woolfitt et al. 2011).

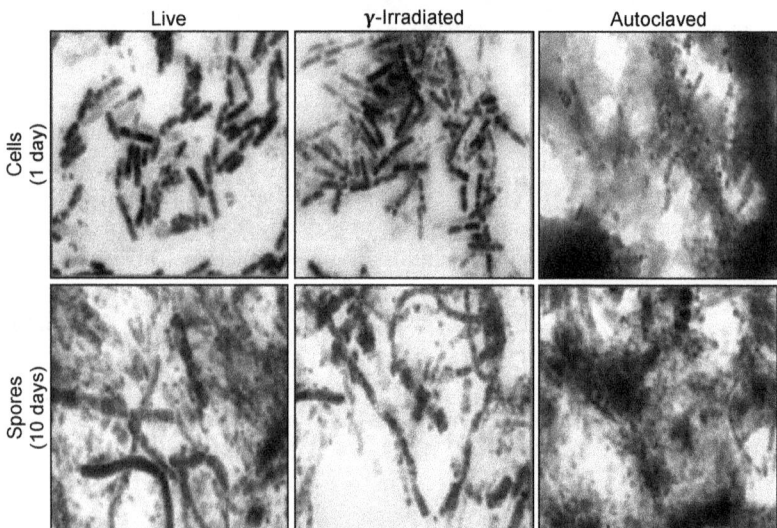

Figure 2. Gram-stained acid *Bacillus anthracis* vegetative cells and spores after gamma-irradiation or autoclavation. Gamma-irradiation renders the organisms non-infectious without any effect on MALDI identification. Instance of spores and vegetative cells of *Bacillus anthracis* highly infectious organism. Note that autoclavation destroys the morphology of the organisms which will not generate good spectra for identification.

Peak Detection and Extraction for Database Identification

In the early days of microbial identification in research laboratories using research instruments, peak detection, and extraction for fingerprinting definition, comparison, and microbial identification was done by eye or by manually comparing a list of peaks, which is not recommended (Figure 3). The term "MALDI protein fingerprinting" was used to define a MALDI spectrum obtained from whole cells; they consisted typically of peptides and small proteins in the range of 2–14 kDa that did not require determination of their function or identity (Figure 4). The benefit of advanced statistical methods for analysis made them the preferred way for microbial identification after pioneer work by different authors (Saenz et al. 1999, Jarman et al. 1999, Jarman et al. 2000). Several methods were tested, most with successful results, such as principal component analysis (PCA), partial least squares-discriminant analysis (PLS-DA), neural networks, dendrograms and clustering, and the random forest algorithm. Furthermore, matching spectra with biologically relevant protein databases was applied to microbial identification with relative success (Demirev et al. 1999, Pineda et al. 2000). In particular, Random forest has been increasingly used for the characterization of spectra generated by MALDI-TOF MS instruments (Satten et al. 2004, Moura et al. 2008, Woolfitt et al. 2011). Software that allowed computer-based analysis for fast microbial identification to the genus and species level was developed and optimized over time; our group, among others, developed powerful research toolboxes with several workflows to accomplish microbial

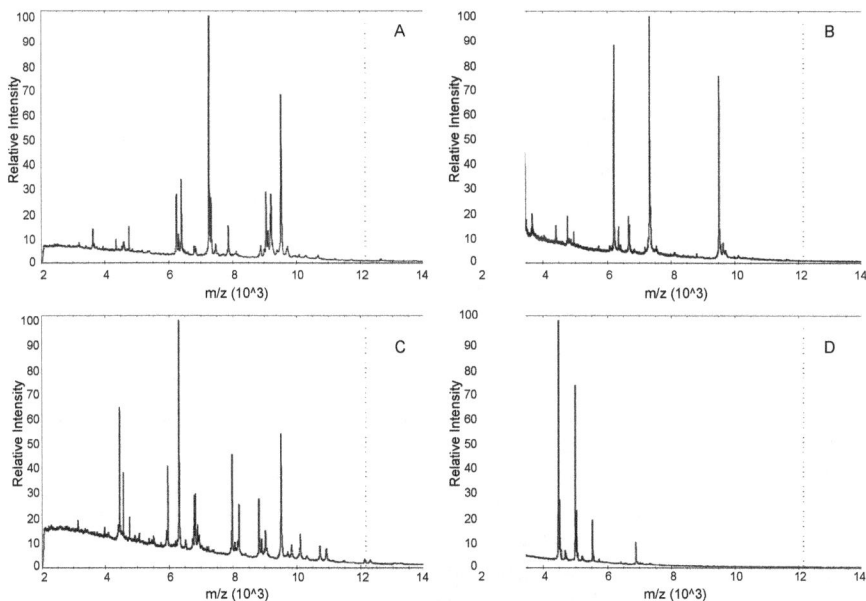

Figure 3. This is an example of raw spectra for MALDI fingerprinting. Visual analysis of four species depicting a clear difference among each other. Peak detection and extraction for fingerprinting definition, comparison, and microbial identification were done by eye or by manually comparing a list of peaks. (A) *Escherichia coli*; (B) *Enterococcus faecalis*; (C) *Streptococcus pyogenes*; and (D) *Staphylococcus aureus*.

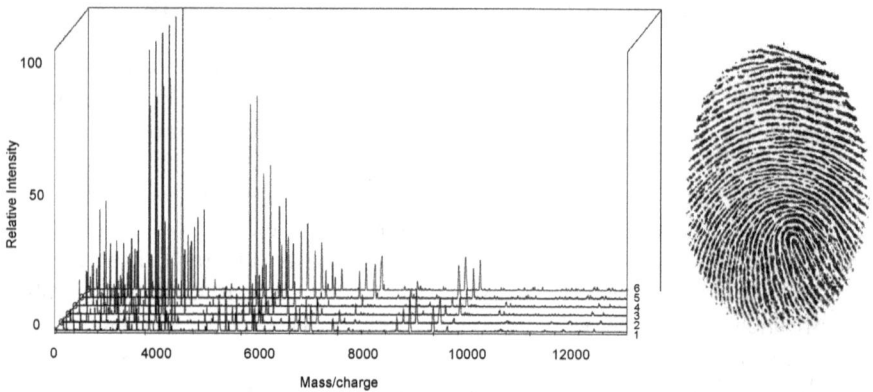

Figure 4. MALDI protein fingerprinting. MALDI spectra obtained from whole cells consist typically of peptides and small proteins in the range of 2–14 kDa that did not require determination of their function or identity.

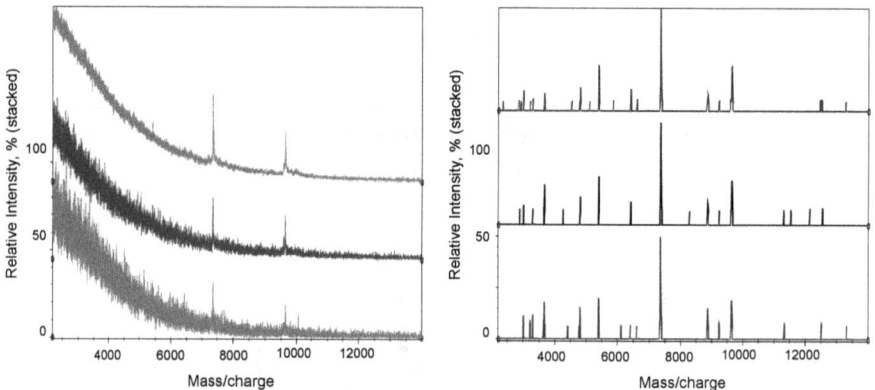

Figure 5. Instances of preprocessing for MALDI fingerprinting. (A) Replicate raw spectra near minimum quality. (B) The same spectra were de-noised after processing.

identification, with special attention to peak picking and peak detection. Currently, MALDI fingerprinting research has several preprocessing options. Scientists should (1) obtain a continuum (profile) spectra from different instrument formats, (2) trim to good *m/z* range, (3) normalize intensities in all spectra, (4) interpolate, so all spectra have identical *m/z* points, (5) sum replicate spectra, (6) should be smooth, (7) background-subtract, (8) de-noise, (9) reformat for classification algorithms, and finally (10) choose an algorithm, i.e., PLS-DA, hierarchical clustering, or random forest. While our toolbox uses VB.Net modules, some alternative programming environments include C#, MATLAB®/Octave, R, and Python. Instances of preprocessing for MALDI fingerprinting are depicted in Figure 5 along with a way to visualize the reproducibility of multiple spectra collected for library development using an in-house developed program (Gel view). Interestingly, the two systems that are dedicated to clinical diagnosis use different proprietary bioinformatic approaches applying a similar concept that will be detailed later.

The Journey in Microbiology Laboratories

Studies of microorganism identification were reported by a small number of research groups in the early 2000s. They developed initial MALDI-TOF MS algorithms for bacterial identification using the research instruments available in mass spectrometry laboratories. Most initial studies collected mass spectra in the range of 2,000 to 20,000 *m/z*. The development of such exploratory proof-of-concept projects using research instruments had the advantage of extra freedom to investigate and discover better methods for sample preparation, MS acquisition, and further spectra analysis. Most projects aimed at microorganism identification at the genus and species level (Lay 2000). Nevertheless, the main goal for most authors was the identification beyond species, with the potential to discriminate to the level of strains and subtypes. Initially, as a proof of concept, organisms such as *Staphylococcus* spp., *Streptococcus* spp., and *Escherichia coli* were studied. Other organisms, including fungi and protozoans, were studied as well. Among the latter, *Cryptosporidium* spp. and microsporidia, in the mid-1980 were major causes of diarrhea in immunocompromised people (Magnuson et al. 2000, Moura et al. 2004). Interestingly, MALDI-TOF MS studies on cultivated microsporidia, then classified as protozoans and further reclassified and now studied among the fungi, allowed the differentiation of four species infecting humans (Moura et al. 2004). Furthermore, such early studies were seminal to improve innovative data analysis methods using fingerprint libraries, statistical methods, and bioinformatics that were later essential for microorganism identification. For instance, BioNumerics (Applied Maths, Ghent, Belgium) is an attractive resource for MALDI-TOF MS data analysis. The software has been applied on different occasions to process data generated using research MS instruments to successfully differentiate the pathogenic protozoan *Naegleria fowleri* from other non-pathogenic species (Moura et al. 2015). Even more, BioNumerics has been used recently to process MALDI Biotyper data, e.g., for *S. pneumoniae* serotype differentiation (Pinto et al. 2017) or as additional elements for validation of *Vagococcus bubulae* and *Vagococcus vulneris* and two new species of the catalase-negative, Gram-stain positive genus *Vagococcus* (Shewmaker et al. 2019).

Quality control procedures for verification and validation of MALDI-TOF MS performance are convenient and can be accomplished using a positive control (e.g., *E. coli*) for instrument calibration. While not common, because $\sim 10^4$–10^5 colony-forming units are needed to generate a good MS signal, one option would be the use of a negative control to check for plate contamination. The number of publications over time using MALDI-TOF MS for microbial identification provides a good idea of the acceptance of the method by microbiologists. The few papers published prior to the early 2000s were proof of concept showing that the methods were effective in identifying microorganisms. From 2005 to 2010, the number of papers published each year slowly increased. After that was a flurry of MALDI-TOF MS applications using Gram-positive and Gram-negative bacterial species, yeasts, molds, and protozoans (Figure 6). Interestingly, the increase in publications coincided with the introduction of new instrumentation in the market. Indeed, MS applications for bacterial identification became better known after the availability

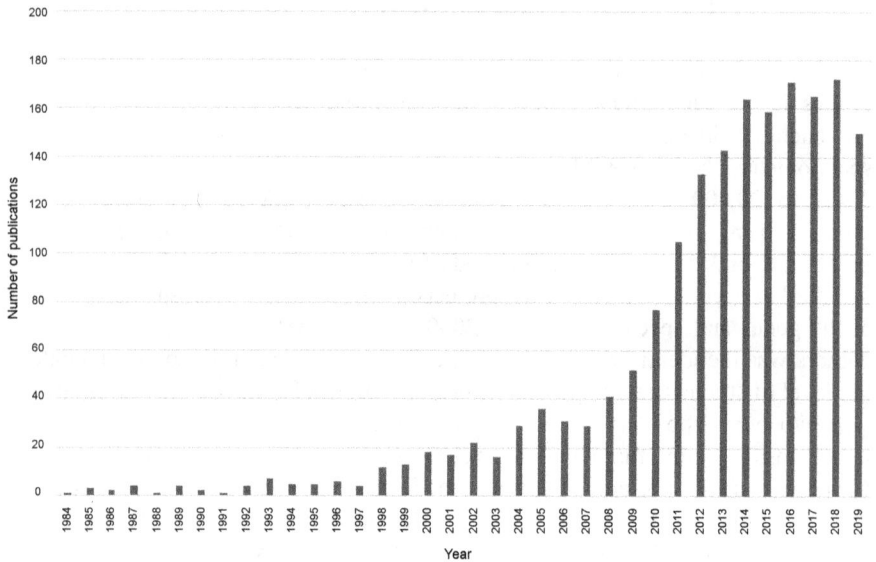

Figure 6. Publications about rapid identification of microorganisms by mass spectrometry. The few papers published prior to the early 2000s were proof of concept showing that the methods were effective in identifying microorganisms. From 2005 to 2010, the number of papers published each year slowly increased. After that was a flurry of MALDI-TOF MS applications using Gram-positive and Gram-negative bacterial species, yeasts, molds, and protozoans. The increase in publications coincided with the introduction of new instrumentation in the market. Indeed, MS applications for bacterial identification became better known after the availability of two dedicated clinical systems by two different manufacturers.

of two dedicated clinical systems by two different manufacturers: Vitek-MS (BioMerieux, France) and MALDI Biotyper (Bruker Daltonics GmbH, Germany.) The instruments are designed for high-performance microorganism identification and have now European and North American regulatory approval for use in clinical microbiology laboratories. Both systems are currently available in different countries and have been in use in microbiology laboratories for a few years with reported good results. Both systems can be used in two versions, with databases validated for use in *in vitro* diagnosis (IVD) for reporting identification results or a Research Use Only (RUO) version. As defined by the manufacturers following regulatory agencies, the user in clinical labs must follow standard operating procedures for complete IVD work-up, with fixed data processing using sealed databases with regulatory compliance and approval. In addition, databases are approved from time to time for genus and species determination.

The database used for microbial identification on the Vitek-MS platform is the SARAMIS database (AnagnosTec GmbH). The Vitek-MS system uses two different algorithms in the IVD and RUO modes (Clark et al. 2013, Kostrzewa et al. 2019). The IVD is based on supervised machine learning that divides acquired spectra into 1,300 segments used for species identification (Kostrzewa et al. 2019). The RUO mode uses SuperSpectra, which comprises processed spectra acquired from 15 different isolates from the same species submitted to different culture media and conditions. Spectra from unknown isolates are processed into a list of peaks and intensities queried against the database for final identification. A perfect match has a value of 99.9%, while values between > 60% to 99.8% are considered a good match (Clark et al. 2013, Kostrzewa et al. 2019).

The BioTyper bioinformatic approach is the same for both IVD and RUO analyses. The software package uses a pattern approach of mass spectra acquired with the Microflex LT MALDI-TOF mass spectrometer (Bruker) and a database containing individual references, each named Main Spectral Profiles (MSP). The analysis is done using spectrum peak frequency, position, and intensity. An MSP database of several bacteria and yeasts, provided with the software, is used to compare data from unknown specimens for identification. Results of the spectral database are provided as a log (score) value and correlated with genus and species. Scores ranging from 2.3 to 3.0 indicate a "high confidence identification" (Clark et al. 2013, Kostrzewa et al. 2019).

Because of the recurrent use of MALDI-TOF MS instruments for bacterial identification, the Centers for Disease Control & Prevention (CDC) included the search by protein profile as part of MicrobeNet (https://www.cdc.gov/microbenet/index.html), a free online resource and database publicly available upon request on the CDC's website, that provides detailed information on rare and emerging bacteria and fungi. CDC's subject matter experts curate the RUO database. The user can submit the spectra acquired using a Biotyper instrument to obtain identification.

Besides clinical laboratory IVD use, several authors have been using such dedicated instruments in RUO mode to study different organisms and characterization below the species level. Following a sensible plating method and applying a comprehensive database, scientists can easily differentiate almost all organisms at least to the genus level and frequently to the species level. The amount of work done so far indicates that nowadays, the most probable cause of misidentification of an organism by MALDI-TOF MS is the absence of spectra for the organism in the database. Another useful application of the MALDI-TOF MS system is that it can be rapidly adapted to the identification of emerging pathogens and new species. This can be accomplished by extending databases in the RUO mode as described for *Elizabethkingia* species (Cheng et al. 2019). Again, when used for clinical diagnosis, MALDI-TOF MS systems should follow guidelines from the Clinical and Laboratory Standards Institute and the College of American Pathologists.

A comprehensive review of MALDI-TOF MS applications in clinical microbiology was published by (Clark et al. 2013) with convincing early evidence of its usefulness. Further studies confirmed the value of MALDI-TOF MS reproducibility, accuracy, and robustness for the identification of organisms. Identification of microorganisms using MALDI-TOF MS is a dynamic subject with the application easily repurposed and amplified; in fact, new applications are continuously being described using the instrumentation currently available in the market. Almost every bacterial group has been tested using commercial MALDI-TOF MS (Table 1). We summarize below the key points for each group.

Table 1. Sample list of selected publications improving MALDI-TOF MS identification of bacterial species.

Genus	Study Type	Reference	PubMed*
Achromobacter	DB** review	(Garrigos et al. 2021)	32283265
Acinetobacter	CSF detection	(Brunetti et al. 2018)	29112767
Bacillus	Isolate id***	(Shu and Yang 2017)	29138467
Bacteroides	DB Accuracy	(Sárvár et al. 2017)	28889758
Bordetella	Rare species id	(Kukla et al. 2020)	32189223
Borrelia	Isolate id	(Neumann-Cip et al. 2020)	32373099
Brachyspira	Rare species id	(Warneke et al. 2014)	25012082
Brucella	DB review	(Christoforidou et al. 2020)	32068074
Burkholderia	DB Accuracy	(Wong et al. 2020)	32597748
Campylobacter	DB Accuracy	(Hsieh et al. 2018)	28899453
Clostridium	DB Accuracy	(Sulaiman et al. 2021)	33982069
Corynebacterium	Rare species id	(Bernard et al. 2019)	31755876
Escherichia	Isolate id	(Kubo et al. 2021)	33745812
Enterococcus	Isolate id	(Christ et al. 2017)	28318563
Francisella	DB review	(Regoui et al. 2020)	32731606
Haemophilus	Isolate id	(Månsson et al. 2015)	25926500
Helicobacter	Isolate id	(Berlamont et al. 2021)	33803832
Klebsiella	Isolate id	(Huang et al. 2020)	32027671
Lactobacillus	Isolate id	(Huang and Huang 2018)	29153517
Legionella	DB review	(Pascale et al. 2020)	33384668
Leptospira	DB review	(Girault et al. 2020)	32632856
Listeria	Isolate id	(Jadhav 2021)	32975763
Mycobacteria	Rare species id	(Oliva et al. 2021)	33664176
Mycoplasma	DB review	(Baudler et al. 2019)	31184287
Neisseria	DB review	(Hong et al. 2019)	30287414
Nocardia	Rare species id	(Yaemsiri and Sykes 2018)	29105868
Porphyromonas	DB review	(Zamora-Cintas et al. 2018)	30541687
Prevotella	DB review	(Toprak et al. 2019)	31813262
Salmonella	Isolate id	(Fukuyama et al. 2019)	31697871
Staphylococcus	Isolate id	(Liu et al. 2021)	33053243
Streptococcus	DB review	(Ikryannikova et al. 2013)	23331578

*https://pubmed.ncbi.nlm.nih.gov/.
**DB = database.
***id = identification.

Gram-Positive Cocci

Gram-positive cocci such as streptococci and staphylococci have been investigated. Within the commonly disease-associated staphylococci group, *Staphylococcus aureus* is routinely identified with high accuracy in clinical laboratories using regular phenotypic protocols. MALDI-TOF MS can identify genus and species as well, but identification below species requires the application of subtyping methods (Liu et al. 2021). In addition, the main requirement for *S. aureus* after identification is the determination of their antimicrobial resistance. The latter and bacterial subtyping will be discussed below, along with the emerging applications of MALDI-TOF MS. Other non-*S. aureus*, coagulase-positive staphylococci in the *Staphylococcus intermedius* group, and the opportunistic coagulase-negative species can be accurately identified by MALDI-TOF MS as well. The method can potentially provide epidemiological data for methicillin-resistant *S. aureus* (MRSA) isolates. Until now, Micrococci have been identified only at the genus level because of limited entries in the MALDI-TOF databases.

Several species and serogroups comprising the genus *Streptococcus* (e.g., *Streptococcus pyogenes*, *Streptococcus agalactiae*) can be differentiated by MALDI-TOF MS and identification can be accomplished below species (Moura et al. 2008). For some time, a commonly reported problem was that *Streptococcus pneumoniae* isolates were difficult to identify by MALDI-TOF MS using current instrument databases. The problem was solved with better bioinformatic processes and updated databases on both commercial systems (Doern et al. 2016). Previous studies using research MALDI-TOF MS instruments demonstrated the differentiation of non-typeable, non-encapsulated *S. pneumoniae* conjunctivitis outbreak strains (Williamson et al. 2008). Furthermore, in a recent report, 492 isolates of capsulated *S. pneumoniae* were discriminated and typed using spectra obtained using a MALDI Biotyper instrument and further analysis by BioNumerics. A combination of MALDI-TOF and BioNumerics analysis strongly correlated with current methods of serological typing (Pinto et al. 2017). Another study reported the differentiation of *S. pneumoniae* and other *S. mitis* group streptococci using an improved MALDI Biotyper database and a novel result interpretation algorithm (Harju et al. 2017). Furthermore, Viridans group streptococci could be identified at the species level. Within non-Enterococcus group D streptococci, the *S. bovis-S.equinis* complex can be reliably identified at the species level. Few studies have addressed the nutritionally variant streptococci and related genera. Enterococci can be generally characterized by MALDI-TOF MS. *Lactococcus* spp. can be differentiated by MALDI-TOF MS and identification can be accomplished below species.

Gram-Positive Bacilli

The ubiquitous genus *Bacillus* comprises over 200 species that are differentiated using 16S rRNA gene-based taxonomy. A comprehensive study using MALDI-TOF MS to differentiate among close species of members of the *Bacillus subtilis* group and *Bacillus cereus* group indicated the importance of the control of culture conditions for successful differentiation (Shu and Yang 2017). However, MALDI-TOF MS analysis of some species within the Gram-positive bacilli such as *Bacillus* spp. is not as frequently described as it is for other organisms. For instance, *Bacillus anthracis* is a Category A bioterrorism agent which requires select agent laboratories to work with those organisms. Early studies in our laboratory using an Applied Biosystems (AB) 4700 Proteomics Analyzer research MALDI-TOF instrument provided data that permitted the unambiguous differentiation of spores and vegetative stages of six species within the genus *Bacillus*, including the very closely related *B. cereus* and *B. anthracis* (Woolfitt et al. 2011). For the first time, a combination of spectra preprocessing steps was used. The steps consisted in applying normalization, summing, background subtraction and smoothing, and standardizing and denoising to generate only statistically significant peaks to be submitted to a range of statistical algorithms. Even more, such analyses allowed the separation of seven *B. anthracis* strains belonging to different genotypes (Woolfitt et al. 2011).

Gram-Negative Bacteria

Gram-negative organisms can be identified by MALDI-TOF MS. The three main groups, Enterobacteriaceae (lactose fermenting), the non-fermenting, and the fastidious Gram-negative bacteria are ubiquitous members of the human microbiota and can be involved in a wide range of infections. Most Enterobacteriaceae can be easily grouped, and the MALDI-TOF MS method is very promising for serovar identification of *Salmonella* species. However, MALDI-TOF MS cannot differentiate between pathogenic and non-pathogenic *E. coli* isolates, including *E. coli* and *Shigella* spp. Although closely related to Enterobacteriaceae, Cronobacter species can be differentiated from the group; several foodborne pathogens have been identified by MALDI-TOF MS which has been accepted to confirm and identify species of *Cronobacter*, *Salmonella*, and *Campylobacter* (Bastin et al. 2019). Among the non-fermenting Gram-negative bacteria, species of *Pseudomonas*, *Achromobacter*, and *Burkholderia* have been analyzed and confirmed MALDI-TOF identification at least to the species level (Garrigos et al. 2021, Wong et al. 2020). Improved results have been reported for the fastidious Gram-negative bacteria (Christoforidou et al. 2020, Hsieh et al. 2018, Månsson et al. 2015, Berlamont et al. 2021, Pascale et al. 2020).

Anaerobes

The use of MALDI-TOF MS to identify anaerobes works as efficiently as for aerobic bacteria and is dependent on the presence of their specific mass spectra on reliable databases. A recent report detailed the validation and expansion of a MALDI-TOF MS Biotyper database of clinical anaerobe isolates which improved confidence in anaerobe identification (Veloo et al. 2018). Overall, the two commercial systems can identify Gram-negative genera and species of *Bacteroides*, *Porphyromonas*, and *Prevotella*. Even species difficult to differentiate can be unequivocally identified by MALDI-TOF MS (Kostrzewa et al. 2019). *Clostridioides difficile* is an important Gram-positive anaerobe organism causing healthcare-associated infections. Toxigenic *C. difficile* isolates can secrete two major toxins: TcdA (an enterotoxin) and TcdB, which is a potent cytotoxin and can cause outbreaks. Epidemic and hypervirulent strains generate substantial mortality, morbidity, and economic burden.

Both toxigenic and non-toxigenic isolates belong to many types that are differentiated using specialized and time-consuming methods. Thus, the determination of *C. difficile* ribotypes using simpler and faster methods is important for epidemiological purposes. Early studies provided promising data for *C. difficile* ribotyping (Reil et al. 2011, Rizzardi and Åkerlund 2015, Emele et al. 2019, Carneiro et al. 2021).

Emerging Applications and Limitations of MALDI-TOF MS

Emerging applications of MALDI-TOF MS that are useful in clinical labs are culture-independent microbial identification directly from patient specimens, such as urine, secretions, cerebral spinal fluid, and faster identification of blood cultures with improving attempts for extraction before analysis (Ponderand et al. 2020). Although several studies have been published, these valuable applications are still under development. Organisms causing mixed infections are still difficult to identify using MALDI-TOF MS because of their low performance. Fast antibiotic susceptibility tests (AST) are another ambition in clinical microbiology. Promising studies have been published including organisms that are resistant to penicillin, carbapenem, methicillin, or vancomycin (Rees and Barr 2017, Wolk and Clark 2018). Strain typing, although difficult to standardize, is another promising application of MALDI-TOF MS that attracts attention, with great potential to provide epidemiological data. In addition, other MALDI-TOF MS applications for microbial identification and determination of antibiotic-resistant organisms have been proposed, such as a quick lipid extraction followed by lipid analysis (Sorensen et al. 2020).

Limitations of the MALDI-TOF MS method exist and should be considered when used as a method for bacterial identification, the most relevant being the absence of the organism in the database used for the identification (Doern et al. 2016). Trying to remediate this issue, several recent publications describe database review and improvement (Table 1), while clinical laboratories using the two systems frequently update their databases, and CDC's Microbenet provides free identification for rare organisms. Again, when used for clinical diagnosis of MALDI-TOF MS, systems should follow guidelines from the Clinical and Laboratory Standards Institute and the College of American Pathologists.

In summary, MALDI-TOF MS instruments can be used for rapid whole-organism fingerprinting and could discriminate to the level of strains and subtypes. Clinical MALDI-TOF MS systems became increasingly accepted as powerful tools for rapid and reliable microorganism identification because of strengths such as cost-effectiveness with low consumable costs, rapid turnaround time, high throughput, automation, reproducibility, single colony requirement, and broad applicability. Additional uses for the MALDI-TOF MS systems are under development, such as antibiotic susceptibility testing and rapid blood culture analysis.

Acknowledgments

The content is solely the responsibility of the authors and does not necessarily represent the official position of the Centers for Disease Control and Prevention.

Use of trade names is for identification only and does not imply endorsement by the Centers for Disease Control and Prevention, the Public Health Service, or the U.S. Department of Health and Human Services.

References

Akimowicz, Monika and Joanna Bucka-Kolendo. (2020). MALDI-TOF MS - application in food microbiology. Acta Biochim. Pol. 67: 327–332.

Anhalt, John P. and Catherine Fenselau. (1975). Identification of bacteria using mass spectrometry. Analytical Chemistry 47: 219–235.

Bastin, B., P. Bird, M. J. Benzinger, J. Agin, D. Goins, M. Timke et al. (2019). Confirmations and identification of Salmonella spp., Cronobacter spp., and other gram-negavitive organisms by the bruker MALDI biotyper method: Collaborative study method extension to include campylobacter species, Revised First Action 2017.09. J. AOAC Int. 102: 1595–1616.

Baudler, Liane, Sandra Scheufen, Luisa Ziegler, Franca Möller Palau-Ribes, Christa Ewers and Michael Lierz. (2019). Identification and differentiation of avian Mycoplasma species using MALDI-TOF MS. J. Vet. Diagn. Invest. 31: 620–624. https://pubmed.ncbi.nlm.nih.gov/31184287/.

Berlamont, Helena, Chloë De Witte, Sofie De Bruyckere, James G. Fox, Steffen Backert, Annemieke Smet et al. (2021). Differentiation of gastric helicobacter species using MALDI-TOF mass spectrometry. Pathogens 10: 366. https://pubmed.ncbi.nlm.nih.gov/33803832/.

Bernard, K. A., A. L. Pacheco, T. Burdz and D. Wiebe. (2019). Increase in detection of Corynebacterium diphtheriae in Canada: 2006–2019. Can. Commun. Dis. Rep. 45: 296–301.

Brunetti, Grazia, Giancarlo Ceccarelli, Alessandra Giordano, Anna S. Navazio, Pietro Vittozzi, Mario Venditti et al. (2018). Fast and reliable diagnosis of XDR Acinetobacter baumannii meningitis by matrix-assisted laser desorption/ionization time-of-flight mass spectrometry. New Microbiol. 41: 77–79.

Carneiro, L. G., T. C. A. Pinto, H. Moura, J. Barr, R. M. C. P. Domingues and E. O. Ferreira. (2021). MALDI-TOF MS: An alternative approach for ribotyping Clostridioides difficile isolates in Brazil. Anaerobe 69: 102351. https://pubmed.ncbi.nlm.nih.gov/33621659/.

CDC, Microbenet. https://www.cdc.gov/microbenet/index.html.

Cheng, Y. H., C. L. Perng, M. J. Jian, S. Y. Lee, J. R. Sun and H. S. Shang. (2019). Multicentre study evaluating matrix-assisted laser desorption ionization time of flight mass spectrometry for identification of clinically isolated Elizabethkingia species and analysis of antimicrobial susceptibility. Clinical Microbiology and Infection 25: 340–345. https://pubmed.ncbi.nlm.nih.gov/29689427/.

Christ, Ana Paula Guarnieri, Solange Rodrigues Ramos, Rodrigo Cayô, Ana Cristina Gales, Elayse Maria Hachich and Maria Inês Zanoli Sato. (2017). Characterization of Enterococcus species isolated from marine recreational waters by MALDI-TOF MS and Rapid ID API® 20 Strep system. Mar. Pollut. Bull. 118: 376–381. https://pubmed.ncbi.nlm.nih.gov/28318563/.

Christoforidou, Sofia, Maria Kyritsi, Evridiki Boukouvala, Loukia Ekateriniadou, Antonios Zdragas, Georgios Samouris et al. (2020). Identification of Brucella spp. isolates and discrimination from the vaccine strain Rev. 1 by MALDI-TOF mass spectrometry. Mol. Cell Probes 51: 101533. https://pubmed.ncbi.nlm.nih.gov/32068074/.

Clark, Andrew E., Erin J. Kaleta, Amit Arora and Donna M. Wolk. (2013). Matrix-assisted laser desorption ionization-time of flight mass spectrometry: A fundamental shift in the routine practice of clinical microbiology. Clinical Microbiology Reviews 26: 547–603.

Demirev, P. A., Y. P. Ho, V. Rhyzhov and C. Fenselau. (1999). Microorganism identification by mass spectrometry and protein database searches. Anal. Chem. 71: 2732–8.

Doern, Christopher D., Robert C. Jerris and Mark D. Gonzalez. (2016). Matrix assisted laser desorption ionization time-of-flight mass spectrometry for the clinical labortaory. In MALDI-TOF Mass Spectrometry in Microbiology, by Markus Kostrzewa and Soren Schubert, 9–31. Norfolk, UK: Caister Academic Press.

Emele, M. F., F. M. Joppe, T. Riedel, J. Overmann, M. Rupnik, P Cooper et al. (2019). Proteotyping of clostridioides difficile as alternate typing method to ribotyping is able to distinguish the ribotypes RT027 and RT176 from other ribotypes. Front. Microbiol. 10: 2087. doi:doi: 10.3389/fmicb.2019.02087.

Fenselau, Catherine and Plamen A. Demirev. (2001). Characterization of intact microorganisms by MALDI mass spectrometry. Edited by 20. Mass Spectrometry Reviews, 157–171.

Fukuyama, Yuko, Teruyo Ojima-Kato, Satomi Nagai, Keisuke Shima, Shinji Funatsu, Yoshihiro Yamada et al. (2019). Improved MALDI-MS method for the highly sensitive and reproducible detection of biomarker peaks for the proteotyping of Salmonella serotypes. J. Mass Spectrom. 54: 966–975. https://pubmed.ncbi.nlm.nih.gov/31697871/.

Garrigos, T., C. Neuwirth, A. Chapuis, J. Bador, L. Amoureux and Collaborators. (2021). Development of a database for the rapid and accurate routine identification of Achromobacter species by matrix-assisted laser desorption/ionization-time-of-flight mass spectrometry (MALDI-TOF MS). Clin. Microbiol. Infect. 126e1–126e5.

Girault, Dominique, Malia Kainiu, Emilie Barsac, Roman Thibeaux and Cyrille Goarant. (2020). Use of MALDI-ToF mass spectrometry for identification of leptospira. Methods Mol. Biol., 23–29. https://pubmed.ncbi.nlm.nih.gov/32632856/.

Harju, Inka, Christoph Lange, Markus Kostrzewa, Thomas Maier, Kaisu Hantakokko-Jalava and Marjo Haanpera. (2017). Improvged differentiation of *Streptococcus pneumoniae* and other *S. mitis* group Streptococci by MALDI biotyper using an improved MADI biotyper database contant and a novel result interpretation algorithm. Journal of Clinical Microbiology 55: 914–922.

Hong, E., Y. Y. Bakhalek and M. -K. Taha. (2019). Identification of Neisseria meningitidis by MALDI-TOF MS may not be reliable. Clin. Microbiol. Infect. 25: 717–722. https://pubmed.ncbi.nlm.nih.gov/30287414/.

Hou, T. Y., Chiang-Ni Chuan and SHih-Hua Teng. (2019). Current status of MALDI-TOF mass spectrometry in clinical microbiology. Jounal Food Drug Analysis 27: 404–414.

Hsieh, Ying-Hsin, Yun F. Wang, Hercules Moura, Nancy Miranda, Steven Simpson, Ramnath Gowrishankar et al. (2018). Application of MALDI-TOF MS systems in the rapid identification of Campylobacter spp. of public health importance. J. AOAC Int. 101: 761–768.

Huang, Chien-Hsun and Lina Huang. (2018). Rapid species- and subspecies-specific level classification and identification of Lactobacillus casei group members using MALDI Biotyper combined with ClinProTools. J. Dairy Sci. 979–991. https://pubmed.ncbi.nlm.nih.gov/29153517/.

Huang, Tsi-Shu, Susan Shin-Jung Lee, Chia-Chien Lee and Fu-Chuen Chang. (2020). Detection of carbapenem-resistant Klebsiella pneumoniae on the basis of matrix-assisted laser desorption ionization time-of-flight mass spectrometry by using supervised machine learning approach. PLoS One e0228459. https://pubmed.ncbi.nlm.nih.gov/32027671/.

Ikryannikova, L. N., L. N. Filimonova, M. V. Malakhova, T. Savinova, O. Filimonova, E. N. Ilina et al. (2013). Discrimination between *Streptococcus pneumoniae* and *Streptococcus mitis* based on sorting of their MALDI mass spectra. Clin. Microbiol. Infect. 19: 1066–71. https://pubmed.ncbi.nlm.nih.gov/23331578/.

Jadhav, Snehal R., Rohan M. Shah and Enzo A. Palombo. (2021). MALDI-ToF MS: A rapid methodology for identifying and subtyping Listeria monocytogenes. Methods Mol. Biol. 17–29. https://pubmed.ncbi.nlm.nih.gov/32975763/.

Jarman, Kristin H., Don S. Daly, Catherine E. Petersen, Adam J. Saenz, Nancy B. Valentine et al. (1999). Extracting and visualizing matrix-assisted laser desorption/ionization time-of-flight mass spectral fingerprints. Rapid Communications in Mass Spectrometry 13: 1586–1594.

Jarman, Kristin H., Sharon T. Cebula, Adam J. Saenz, Catherine E. Petersen, Nancy B. Valentine and Karen L. Wahl. (2000). An Algorithm for automated bacterial identification using matrix-assisted laser desorption/ionization mass spectrometry. Analytical Chemistry 72: 1217–1223.

Korstrzewa, M. (2018). Application of the MALDI Biotyper to clinical microbiology: Progress and potential. Expert. Rev. Proteomics 15: 191–202.

Kostrzewa, M., E. Nagy, P. Schrottner and A. B. Pranada. (2019). How MALDI-TOF mass spectrometry can aid the diagnosis of hard-to-identify pathogenic bacteria - the rare and the unknown. Expert. Review of Molecular Diagnostics 19: 667–682.

Kubo, Yumi, Osamu Ueda, Sawa Nagamitsu, Hachiro Yamanishi, Akihiro Nakamura and Masaru Komatsu. (2021). Novel strategy of rapid typing of Shiga toxin-producing Escherichia coli using MALDI Biotyper and ClinProTools analysis. J. Infect. Chemother. S1341–321.

Kukla, Rudolf, Michal Svarc, Radka Bolehovska, Lenka Ryskova, Pavla Paterova, Miroslav Fajfr et al. (2020). Isolation of Bordetella trematum from the respiratory tract of a patient with lung cancer: A case report. Folia Microbiol. (Praha) 65: 623–627.

Lay, J. O. (2000). MALDI-TOF mass spectrometry and bacterial taxonomy. Trends Anal. Chem. 19: 507–516.

Liu, Xin, Taojunfeng Su, Yen-Michael S. Hsu, Hua Yu, He Sarina Yang, Li Jiang et al. (2021). Rapid identification and discrimination of methicillin-resistant Staphylococcus aureus strains via matrix-assisted laser desorption/ionization time-of-flight mass spectrometry. Rapid Commun. Mass Spectrom. 35: e8972. https://pubmed.ncbi.nlm.nih.gov/33053243/.

Liyanage, R. and J. O. Lay. (2006). An introduction to MALDI-TOF MS. In Identification of Microorganisms by Mass Spectrometry, by C.L. & Lay, J.O. Wilkins, 39–69. Hoboken, New Jersey: John Wiley & Sons, Inc.

Magnuson, Matthew L., James H. Owens and Catherine A. Kelty. (2000). Characterization of cryptosporidium parvum by matrix-assisted laser desorption ionization-time of flight mass spectrometry. Appl. Environm. Microbiol. 66: 4720–4724.

Månsson, Viktor, Fredrik Resman, Markus Kostrzewa, Bo Nilson and Kristian Riesbeck. (2015). Identification of Haemophilus influenzae Type b isolates by use of matrix-assisted laser desorption ionization-time of flight mass spectrometry. J. Clin. Microbiol. 53: 2215–24. https://pubmed.ncbi.nlm.nih.gov/25926500/.

Moura, Hercules, Adrian R. Woolfitt, Maria G. Carvalho, Antonis Pavlopoulos, Lucia M. Teixeira, Glen A. Satten et al. (2008). MALDI-TOF mass spectrometry as a tool for differentiation of invasive and noninvasive Streptococcus pyogenes isolates. FEMS Immunology & Medical Microbiology 53: 333–342.

Moura, Hercules, Fernando Izquierdo, Adrian R. Woolfitt, Glauber Wagner, Tatiana Pinto, Carmen del Aguila et al. (2015). Detection of biomarkers of pathogenic naegleria fowleri through mass spectrometry and proteomics. The Journal of Eukariotic Microbiology 62: 12–20.

Moura, Hercules, M. Ospina, A. R. Woofitt, John R. Barr and Govinda S. Visvesvara. (2004). Analysis of four human microsporidian isolates by MALDI-TOF mass spectrometry. Journal Eukaryotic Microbiology 50: 156–163.

Neumann-Cip, Anna-Cathrine, Volker Fingerle, Gabriele Margos, Reinhard K. Straubinger, Evelyn Overzier, Sebastian Ulrich et al. (2020). A Novel Rapid Sample Preparation Method for MALDI-TOF MS permits Borrelia burgdorferi sensu lato species and isolate differentiation. Front. Microbiol. 11: 690.

Oliva, Ester, Marco Arosio, Ester Mazzola, Miriam Mascheroni, Annarosa Cerro, Marina Cuntró et al. (2021). Rapid identification of non-tuberculous mycobacteria with MALDI-TOF mass spectrometry. Infez. Med. 29: 79–84. https://pubmed.ncbi.nlm.nih.gov/33664176/.

Pascale, Maria Rosaria, Marta Mazzotta, Silvano Salaris, Luna Girolamini, Antonella Grottola, Maria Luisa Simone et al. (2020). Evaluation of MALDI-TOF mass spectrometry in diagnostic and environmental surveillance of Legionella species: A comparison with culture and mip-gene sequencing technique. Front. Microbiol. 589369. https://pubmed.ncbi.nlm.nih.gov/33384668/.

Pierce, Carrie L., John R. Barr, Adrian R. Woolfitt, H. Moura, Edward I. Shaw, Herbert A. Thompson et al. (2007). Strain and phase identification of the U.S. category B agent Coxiella burnetti by matrix assisted laser desrption/ionization time-of-flight mass spectrometry and multivariate pattern recognition. Analytica Chimica Acta 583: 23–31.

Pineda, F. J., J. S. Lin, C. Fenselau and P. A. Demirev. (2000). Testing the significance of microorganism identification by mass spectrometry and proteome database search. Anal. Chem. 72: 3739–44.

Pinto, Tatiana C. A., Natalia S. Costa, Luciana F. S. Castro, Rachel L. Ribeiro, Ana C. N. Botelho, Felipe P. G. Neves et al. (2017). Potential of MALDI-TOF MS as an alternative approach for capsular typing Streptococcus pneumoniae isolates. Scientific Reports 45572.

Ponderand, Lea, Patricia Pavese, Daniele Maubon, Emmanuelle Giraudon, Thomas Girard, Caroline Landelle et al. (2020). Evaluation of rapid sepsityper protocol and specific MBT-sepsityper module (Bruker Daltonics) fo rthe rapid diagnosis of bacteriemia and fungemia by MALDI-TOF MS. Ann. Clin. Microbiol. Antimicrob. 60: 403.

Rees, Jon C. and John R. Barr. (2017). Detection of methicillin-resistant *Staphylococcus* aureus using phage amplification combined with matrix-assisted laser desorption/ionization mass spectrometry. Analytical Bionalytical Chemistry 409: 1379–1386.

Regoui, Sofiane, Aurélie Hennebique, Thomas Girard, Sandrine Boisset, Yvan Caspar and Max Maurin. (2020). Optimized MALDI TOF mass spectrometry identification of Francisella tularensis Subsp. holarctica. Microorganisms 8: 1143. https://pubmed.ncbi.nlm.nih.gov/32731606/.

Reil, M., M. Erhard, E. J. Kuijper, M. Kist and H. Zaiss. (2011). Recognition of Clostridium difficile PCR-ribotypes 001, 027 and 126/078 using an extended MALDI-TOF MS system. Eur. J. Clin. Microbiol. Infect. Dis. 30: 1431–1436.

Rizzardi, Kristina and Thomas Åkerlund. (2015). High molecular weight typing with MALDI-TOF MS—A novel method for rapid typing of Clostridium difficile. PLoS One 10: e0122457. https:// pubmed.ncbi.nlm.nih.gov/25923527/.

Saenz, Adam J., Catherine E. Petersen, Valentine, Nancy B., Gantt, Stephanie L. et al. (1999). Reproducibility of matrix-assisted laser desorption/ionization time-of-flight mass spectrometry for replicate bacterial culture analysis. Rapid Communications in Mass Spectrometry 13: 1580–1585.

Sárvár, Károly Péter, József Sóki, Miklós Iván, Cecilia Miszti, Krisztina Latkóczy, Szilvia Zsóka Melegh et al. (2017). MALDI-TOF MS versus 16S rRNA sequencing: Minor discrepancy between tools in identification of Bacteroides isolates. Acta Microbiol. Immunol. Hung. 65: 173–181. https:// pubmed.ncbi.nlm.nih.gov/28889758.

Satten, Glen A., Somnath Datta, Hercules Moura, Adrian R. Woolfitt, Maria G. Carvalho, George M. Carlone et al. (2004). Standardization and denoising algorithms for mass spectra to classify whole organism bacterial species. Bioinformatics 20: 1–9.

Shah, Haroun N. (2016). Introduction—A personal Vision of the MALDI-TOF MS journey from obscurity to frontline diagnostics. In MALDI-TOF Mass Spectrometry in Microbiology, by Markus Kostrzewa and Soren Schubert, 1–7. Norfolk, UK: Caister Academic Press.

Shaw, Edward I., Hercules Moura, Adrian R. Woolfitt, M. Ospina, Herbert A. Thompson and John R. Barr. (2004). Identification of biomarkers of whole Coxiella burnetti Phase I by MALDI-TOF mass spectrometry. Analytical Chemistry 76: 4017–4022.

Shewmaker, Patricia L., Anne M. Whitney, Christopher A. Gulvik, Ben W. Humrighouse, Jarret Gartin, Hercules Moura et al. (2019). Vagococcus bubulae sp. nov., isolated from ground beef, and Vagococcus vulneris sp. nov., isolated from a human foot wound. International Journal of Systematic and Evolutionary Microbiology 69: 2268–2276.

Shu, Lin-Jie and Yu-Liang Yang. (2017). Bacillus classification based on matrix-assisted laser desorption ionization time-of-flight mass spectrometry-effects of culture conditions. Sci. Rep. 15546. https:// pubmed.ncbi.nlm.nih.gov/29138467/.

Siuzdak, Gary. (2006). The Expanding Role of Mass Spectrometry in Biotechnology. San Diego: MCC Press.

Sorensen, Matthew, Courtney E. Chandler, Francesca M. Gardner, Salma Ramadan, Prasanna D. Khot, Lisa M. Leung et al. (2020). Rapid microbial identification as colistin resistance detection via MALDI-TOF MS using a novel on-target extraction of membrane lipids. Scientific Reports 10: 21536.

Sulaiman, Irshad M., Nancy Miranda and Steven Simpson. (2021). MALDI-TOF Mass Spectrometry and 16S rRNA gene sequence analysis for the identification of foodborne Clostridium spp. J. AOAC Int. InPrint.

Toprak, Nurver Ulger, Alida C. M. Veloo, Edit Urban, Ingrid Wybo, Helene Jean-Pierre, Trefor Morris et al. (2019). Comparing identification of clinically relevant Prevotella species by VITEK-MS and MALDI biotyper. Acta Microbiol. Immunol. Hung. 67: 6–13. https://pubmed.ncbi.nlm.nih. gov/31813262/.

Tracz, Dobryan M., Stuart J. McCorrister, Garrett R. Westmacott and Cindi R. Corbet. (2013). Effect of gamma radiation on the identification of bacterial pathogensby MALDI-TOF MS. Journal of Microbiological Methods 92: 132–134. https://pubmed.ncbi.nlm.nih.gov/23201167/.

Tran, Anthony, Kevin Alby, Alan Kerr, Melissa Jones and Peter H. Gilligan. (2015). Cost savings realized by implementation of routine microbiological identification by Matrix-Assisted Laser Desorption Ionization-Time of Flight Mass Spectrometry. Journal of Clinical Microbiology 53: 2473–9.

Tsuchida, Sachio, Hiroshi Umemura and Tomohiro Nakayama. (2020). Current status of Matrix-Assisted Laser Desorption/Ionization Time-of-Flight mass spectrometry (MALDI-TOF MS) in clinical diagnostic microbiology. Molecules 25: 4775.

vanBelkum, Alex, Martin Welker, David Pincus, Jean-Philippe Charrier and Victoria Girard. (2017). Matrix-assisted laser desorption ionization time-of-flight mass spectrometry in clinical microbiology: What are the current issues? Annals of Laboratory Medicine 37: 475–483.

Veloo, A. C. M., H. Jean-Pierre, U. S. Justesen, T. Morris, E. Urban, I. Wybo et al. (2018). Validation of MALDI-TOF MS Biotyper database optimized for anaerobic bacteria: The ENRIA workgroup. Anarobe 54: 224–230.

Warneke, Hallie L., Joann M. Kinyon, Leslie P. Bower, Eric R. Burrough and Timothy S. Frana. (2014). Matrix-assisted laser desorption ionization time-of-flight mass spectrometry for rapid identification of Brachyspira species isolated from swine, including the newly described "Brachyspira hampsonii". J. Vet. Diagn. Invest. 26: 635–9.

Williamson, Yulanda M., Hercules Moura, Adrian R. Woolfitt, James L. Pirkle, John R. Barr, Maria G. Carvalho et al. (2008). Differentiation of Streptococcus pneumoniae congunctivitis outbreak isolates by matrix-assisted laser desorption ionization-time of flight mass spectrometry. Applied and Environmental Microbiology 74: 5891–5897.

Wolk, Donna M. and Andrew E. Clark. (2018). Matrix-assisted laser desorption time of flight mass spectrometry. Clinical Laboratory Medicine 38: 471–486.

Wong, Kendrew, S. K., Suk Dhaliwal, Jennifer Bilawka, Jocelyn A. Srigley, Sylvie Champagne, Marc G. Romney et al. (2020). Matrix-assisted laser desorption/ionization time-of-flight MS for the accurate identification of Burkholderia cepacia complex and Burkholderia gladioli in the clinical microbiology laboratory. J. Med. Microbiol. 69: 1105–1113. https://pubmed.ncbi.nlm.nih.gov/32597748/.

Woolfitt, Adrian R., Anne E. Boyer, Conrad P. Quinn, Alex R. Hoffmaster, Thomas R. Kozel, Barun K. De et al. (2011). Matrix assisted laser desorption ionization mass spectrometric analysis of Bacillus anthracis: From fingerprint analysis of the bacterium to quantification of its toxins in clinical samples. In Detection of Biological Agents for the Prevention of Bioterrorism, NATO Science for Peace and Security Series A: Chemistry and Biology, by Joseph Banoub, 83–97. Dordrecht, The Netherlands: Springer.

Yaemsiri, S. and J. E. Sykes. (2018). Successful treatment of dissemicated Nocardiosis caused by Nocardia veterana in a dog. J. Vet. Intern. Med. 32: 418–422.

Yan, W., Jing Qian, Y. Ge, C. Zhou and H. Zhang. (2020). Principal component analysis of MALDI-TOF MS of whole-cell foodborne pathogenic bacteria. Analytical Biochemistry 592: 113582.

Zamora-Cintas, Maribel, Marín Mercedes, Lidia Quiroga, Andrea Martínez, María Antonia Fernández-Chico, Emilio Bouza et al. (2018). Identification of Porphyromonas isolates from clinical origin using MALDI-TOF Mass Spectrometry. Anaerobe 54: 197–200. https://pubmed.ncbi.nlm.nih.gov/30541687/.

Chapter 7

Proteomics Fundamentals and Applications in Microbiology

Glauber Wagner,[1] Guilherme Augusto Maia,[1]
John Robert Barr[2] and Hercules Moura[2,]*

Introduction

Since the late 20th century, with the advent of DNA sequencing automated methods, the elucidation of parasite genomes and their hosts has grown rapidly. Innumerable inferences regarding these organisms have been made, and new questions have arisen. Although DNA technologies provide information about the genetic content of such organisms, more details were needed about the expression of their genes and, consequently, the proteins they express.

In the early 1980s, the identification of proteins in a protein extract became possible, thanks to the development of ionization methods of compounds, which were then analyzed using mass spectrometers and thus starting the golden age of proteomics.

In this chapter, we summarize the main aspects of proteomic analysis and how it can be applied in the clinical ground, especially to characterize organisms or identify diagnostic markers. Some topics may be further explored from supplementary references at the end of this chapter.

The term proteome was first used by Marc Wilkins in 1994 at a conference in Siena, Italy, and further described afterward (Wilkins et al. 1996). Wilkins adapted the already established concept of the genome (global study of an organism's genes) to proteome referring to the global study of an organism's proteins. Furthermore, it can

[1] Department of Microbiology, Immunology and Parasitology, Federal University of Santa Catarina, Florianópolis, SC, 88040-900, Brazil.
[2] Division of Laboratory Sciences, National Center for Environmental Health, Centers for Disease Control and Prevention, Atlanta, Georgia, 30341, USA.
* Corresponding author: Hercul.Moura@gmail.com

be inferred that there is a proteome for the entire genome. In addition, the dynamics of gene expression change over time; some genes may be expressed constitutively, while others are only expressed at certain moments of the cell life cycle, in different tissues, or even in different cell compartments. In a sense, the proteome is nothing more than a snapshot of a moment in the life of an organism, tissue, or cell.

In general, proteomic analysis requires four steps: (1) protein preparation and extraction, (2) protein/peptide separation, (3) measurement of the mass/charge (m/z) ratio of proteins/peptides, and (4) protein identification. In the first step, different methods of protein extraction can be used. The method of choice will depend on the desired cell fraction, type of tissue, and proteomic approach to be performed. The second stage can be performed using sodium dodecyl sulfate-polyacrylamide gel electrophoresis (SDS-PAGE), high-performance liquid chromatography (HPLC), or methods of obtaining proteins by affinity. In the third stage, the mass/charge ratio of the protein/peptide is gauged using a mass spectrometer. For this, the proteins/peptides are charged during the ionization process, producing ions. These ions are separated in a mass analyzer, to be further identified in a detector (details will be described later). In the last stage, the detected ions are processed and used to identify the amino acids that make up a given peptide and later to identify the protein itself through different search algorithms in databases.

Proteomic Study Strategies

Two strategies are used for proteomic studies: top-down, in which the intact protein is analyzed; and bottom-up in which the peptides resulting from the proteolytic digestion of a protein are identified (Figure 1) (Lovric 2011, Price 2011).

In the top-down strategy, proteins are subjected to analysis using mass spectrometers without any previous proteolytic treatment. The m/z ratio of the intact protein is measured. In some cases, the protein interaction with sugars, lipids, metals, or other compounds can be identified. This approach also can be used to identify and classify organisms based on the standard protein mass profile or protein mass fingerprinting (PMF), which will be described later.

In the bottom-up strategy, the protein is digested before mass spectrometry (MS) analysis and then identified based on the measurement of the m/z ratio of peptides, resulting from controlled proteolytic digestion.

These strategies have been used for qualitative analysis of microorganisms to characterize proteins (Parodi-Talice et al. 2004, Cuervo et al. 2007, Zarean et al. 2015, Goos et al. 2017) and identify post-translational modifications (Nakayasu et al. 2009, Meevissen et al. 2011, Zilberstein 2015). Proteomics also can be used to characterize the response of microorganisms to drugs (Andrade et al. 2008, Singh and Sundar 2017, Wang et al. 2019c, Iftikhar et al. 2020, Wang et al. 2020d) and to identify candidate vaccine antigens (Ndao et al. 2010, Yeng et al. 2010, Huang et al. 2012, Kamali et al. 2012, Nakayasu et al. 2012, Singh 2012, da Costa et al. 2013, Eyford et al. 2013, Thézénas et al. 2013, Wagner et al. 2013, Moura et al. 2015, Kardoush et al. 2017, Yadav et al. 2017, Chang et al. 2020, Wareth et al. 2020).

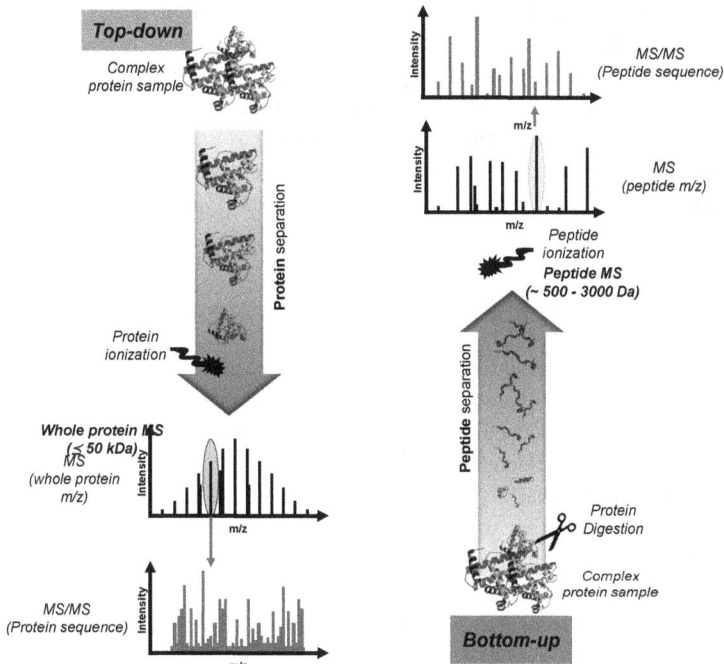

Figure 1. Strategies used in top-down and bottom-up proteomics. In the top-down strategy, intact proteins are separated and ionized for measuring their *m/z* ratios using mass spectrometers, which later can be fragmented within the instrument for better characterization of the protein. In the bottom-up strategy, proteins are digested, and the resulting peptides are separated and ionized to measure their *m/z* ratios. Selected peptides are then fragmented and analyzed by mass spectrometry. The peptide amino acid sequence can be determined, and protein identification is achieved by analyzing these fragments.

Quantitative analysis is also used to measure the expression levels of a particular protein (Pollo-Oliveira et al. 2013, Singh et al. 2015) to evaluate the differential expression of proteins between the life stages of a parasite (Hong et al. 2013, Zhou et al. 2016, Jesus et al. 2017), or even track the alteration of the proteins expressed in infected tissues (Campos et al. 2017, Elhosseiny et al. 2019).

Relative quantification of proteins is carried out to compare amounts of proteins between two samples, whereas absolute quantification is applied for the precise determination of a specific protein or peptide in a sample (Bantscheff et al. 2012). Relative quantification can be performed by incorporating labels into proteins or peptides (label-based method) or without these labels (label-free method). In the label-based method, labels can be generated by incorporating amino acids with stable isotopes into the proteins of a cell in culture (stable isotope labeling with amino acids in cell culture; SILAC) (Ong et al. 2003, Ong and Mann 2007) or by adding a tagged isobaric N-terminal region of the peptides (isobaric tag for relative and absolute quantitation; iTRAQ) (Wiese et al. 2007, Zhou et al. 2016). In the label-free method, proteins are quantified by comparing the spectral number of a peptide obtained in different samples (spectral counting) (Lundgren et al. 2010, Zhu et al. 2010, Nahnsen et al. 2013).

Absolute quantification of proteins can be performed using iTRAQ or an approach known as selected reaction monitoring (SRM). SRM is used to quantify a specific protein in a sample. For this purpose, a peptide derived from the protein of interest is chemically synthesized with heavy isotopes such as 13C or 15N, which increases the mass of these peptides. After spiking a known concentration of the heavy peptide in the digest, the final protein concentration can be determined by comparing the amounts of heavy and light peptides (Gerber et al. 2003, Duncan et al. 2009).

Sample Preparation for Proteomics+

Sample preparation is essential for comprehensive protein identification. Protein extraction methods vary according to the biological question, the strategy, or the proteomic approach to be used. For example, a proteomic map of soluble proteins of a microorganism by 2D electrophoresis can be followed by protein identification by MS. This can be performed by starting from an extract of soluble proteins obtained through a simple extraction of protein in buffer (e.g., Tris-HCl 40 mM/1% Triton X-100) subjected to strong homogenization using vortex equipment. On the other hand, a better understanding of proteins on cell surfaces is possible after enrichment for hydrophobic proteins using a nonionic detergent, e.g., Triton X-114 (Cordero et al. 2009, Wagner et al. 2013). Furthermore, if the interest is to analyze secreted proteins or those in exosomes, specific commercial kits or ultracentrifugation can be used to obtain such protein fractions (Théry et al. 2006, Nten et al. 2010, Marcilla et al. 2012, Ujang et al. 2016, Li et al. 2017). Note that contaminants, such as detergents, lipids, salts, and other chemical compounds, must be removed after detergent extraction. The use of several commercial kits available or even precipitation of the extracted proteins can be performed using 20% trifluoroacetic acid (TCA) in acetone (Görg et al. 2004, Hao et al. 2015).

After extraction, samples can still be enriched with proteins of specific interest, using chromatographic methods (automated or not) with columns or resins that show affinity to specific ligands in some proteins. Examples include resins or particles containing metals that bind to phosphorylated proteins (Machida et al. 2007, Nakayasu et al. 2009, Rainer and Bonn 2015) or those containing lectins that bind to glycosylated proteins (Wuhrer et al. 2011, Ongay et al. 2012). Size exclusion columns also can be used to analyze proteins in a specific molecular weight range (Ayub et al. 2009). Proteins that bind to certain antibodies (Pillay et al. 2013) or even to a set of antibodies also can be identified, as in the case of the antibodies in patient serum that has been exposed to a specific infection (Nakayasu et al. 2012, Kamali et al. 2012, Wagner et al. 2013, Singh and Sundar 2017).

For gel-based analysis, regardless of the protein extract applied, the extracted proteins must be denatured for better migration in the gel. Denatured proteins also better expose cleavage sites for the proteolytic digestion process. This step can be performed after the extraction process or during protein solubilization. Different compounds can be used to improve digestion, such as buffers containing sodium dodecyl sulfate, and another chemical, such as β-mercaptoethanol, used as reducing agents (for use in 1D gels). Another option is the use of buffers containing urea, followed by treatment with a reducing agent (dithiothreitol; DTT) and an alkylating agent (iodoacetamide) (for use in 2D gels and digestion in solution) (Walker 2002). Recently, surfactants such as Rapigest are applied for the digestion of proteins in solution (Yu et al. 2003).

Protein Digestion

Protein digestion and the consequent generation of peptides is the basic principle of the bottom-up proteomic strategy, which is used for most studies in proteomics. In this process, endopeptidases are used to cleave the peptide bonds of proteins, generating small pieces (peptides), which in turn will be subjected to MS analysis (Switzar et al. 2013).

Currently, several endopeptidases can be used in proteomic studies, each with specific protein cleavage sites. Table 1 lists a few endopeptidases and their respective protein cleavage sites. Trypsin is the most used endopeptidase in proteomic studies. It has remarkable characteristics that make it an excellent choice, especially when the amino acid composition of the proteins to be analyzed is unknown. Such characteristics include the following:

- High specificity at the cleavage site (after arginine or lysine, if not followed by proline).
- Few cleavage failures (missed cleavages) when compared with other enzymes.
- Many peptides are generated with an ideal size for analysis of MS (approximately 8–12 amino acids long) because of the abundance of the amino acids arginine and lysine that compose the protein cleavage sites.
- Easily produced and purified in heterologous expression systems, making it less costly than other enzymes.
- Can be used to cleave proteins in a solution, gel, or even on surfaces.

In addition, the last residue of the peptide is arginine or lysine, which are basic amino acids and thus possess a proton (H^+) in the amino group. After cleavage, a positive ion will be generated, which is essential for analysis using mass spectrometers that operate in a positive mode (Eidhammer et al. 2007, Lovric 2011).

Table 1. Examples of endopeptidases used in proteomics and their respective cleavage sites.

Enzyme	Cleavage Site	Description
Trypsin	(R|K).[^P]	Cleaves the C-terminal region of an arginine (R) or lysine (K) if these are not followed by a proline (P)
Chymotrypsin	(W|Y|F).[^P]	Cleaves the C-terminal region of tryptophan (W), tyrosine (Y), or phenylalanine (F) if these are not followed by a proline (P)
Glu C	(E|D).[^P]	Cleaves the C-terminal region of a glutamic acid (E) or cysteine (D) if these are not followed by a proline (P)
Lys C	(K).	Cleaves the C-terminal region of a lysine (K)
Aps N	.(D)	Cleaves the N-terminal region of an aspartic acid (D)

The choice of which enzyme to use will depend on the composition of the protein of interest and the ability to generate peptides compatible with analysis by MS. For instance, highly basic proteins will be composed of a large amount of arginine (R) or lysine (K), whereas proteins with an acidic characteristic will have a predominance of aspartic acid (D) and glutamic acid (E) residues. Thus, using trypsin to cleave a basic protein will generate many peptides with ideal sizes for MS. This does not occur with acidic proteins, which would be better cleaved by enzymes such as Glu-C or Asp-C (Eidhammer et al. 2007, Lovric 2011).

In some cases, especially for improving the coverage of the identified protein (percentage of protein with peptides determined by MS), a combination of endopeptidases can be used, such as trypsin and Glu-C, to digest a protein. In such cases, to correctly identify the studied protein, be aware that these enzymes might generate peptides with distinct C-terminal regions during the bioinformatics analysis.

Proteomic Approaches with or without Gel

After protein solubilization, two basic approaches can be applied to the study of cells, tissue, or organism proteomes (Figure 2). The first classic approach, known as gel-based proteomics, uses gel electrophoresis systems to separate proteins from a complex sample. After separation, gel bands or spots are excised, and proteins are digested and analyzed by MS. A second approach, known as gel-free proteomics or proteomics does not use gel electrophoresis to separate proteins. In gel-free

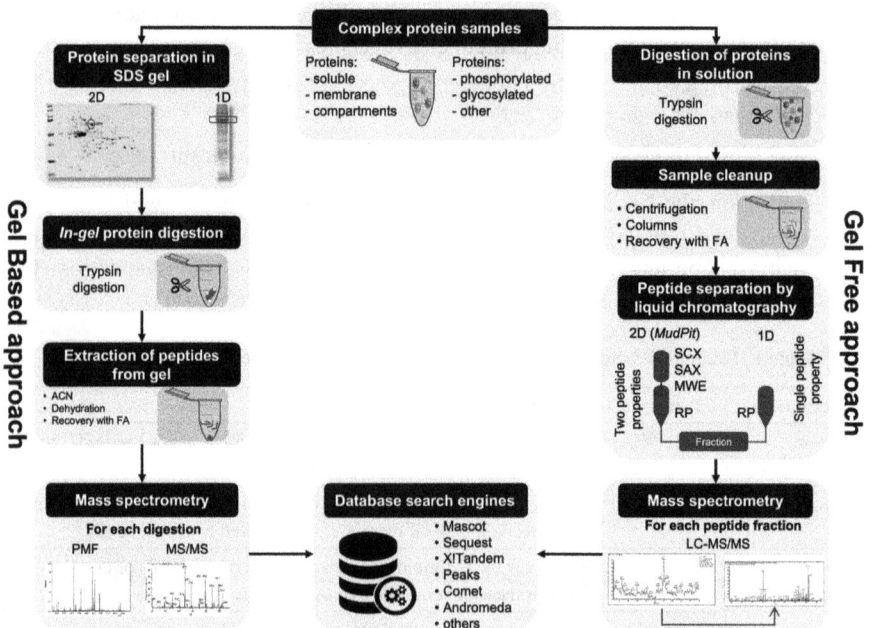

Figure 2. Schematic flowchart of two approaches applied in proteomics, with the use of gel (gel-based) and without the use of gel (gel-free), starting from the same biological sample.

proteomics, the separation of proteins can occur using chromatography or other systems. In addition, peptides resulting from in-solution protein digestion can be separated using chromatography systems, and liquid chromatography separation systems may be coupled directly to mass spectrometers.

Gel-based Proteomics

In gel-based proteomics, electrophoretic profiles are generated in one (1D) or two dimensions (2D), followed by protein digestion in the gel fragments and characterization of the peptides by MS. This approach has been widely used, with good results in identifying proteins isolated from microorganisms (Paba et al. 2004, Parodi-Talice et al. 2004, Wu and Craig 2006, Andrade et al. 2008, Sodré et al. 2009, Alcolea et al. 2011, Esquivel-Velázquez et al. 2011, Hong et al. 2013, Zhou et al. 2014, Brunoro et al. 2016).

In unidimensional electrophoresis (1D), as described by Laemmli (Laemmli 1970), the proteins in a mixture are separated according to a single characteristic of the protein, its molecular mass. The molecular mass of a protein is determined by the sum of the molecular masses of the atoms that constitute an amino acid. Thus, the molecular mass of a protein is expressed in unified atomic mass units or daltons (Da). Various books list the molecular mass of each atom (Eidhammer et al. 2007, Lovric 2011, Price 2011).

Two-dimensional electrophoresis (2D), on the other hand, separates proteins from a complex mixture using two intrinsic characteristics of proteins, their protein isoelectric point (pI) and molecular mass. The isoelectric point is the pH of a solution at which the net charge of a protein becomes electrically neutral, that is when the number of electron donor sites is equivalent to the number of receptor sites. Based on these properties, a protein extract is subjected to isoelectric focusing and subsequently to electrophoresis (SDS-PAGE). The proteins are separated by their pI and molecular mass, thus generating separation in two dimensions of these proteins.

In the first dimension, isoelectric focusing, proteins are subjected to a pH gradient in a polymer. After applying an electric current, the proteins migrate in this polymer until they find a pH equivalent to their pI. Until 1982, this targeting was carried out in a non-immobilized or balanced pH gradient, so the reproducibility of the experiments was low. Recently, Bjellqvist and collaborators (Bjellqvist et al. 1982) developed a plastic strip containing a polymer with an immobilized pH gradient, improving the reproducibility of protein targeting and consequently the 2D profile. For the second dimension, these proteins resolved based on their respective pI are separated according to their molecular mass through SDS-PAGE electrophoresis (Laemmli 1970).

Thousands of proteins can be separated using this methodology. However, even with recent advances, there are problems with profile reproducibility. This emphasizes the importance of including sample replicates in the experiment, which is essential to ensure the reproducibility of the 2D profiles. Two types of replicates can be used: technical and biological. Technical replicates can point out possible experimental errors through repetitions of the same biological sample, by showing variations in the position of a specific protein on the gel. Biological replicates can disclose biological variations in the biological samples under study.

After a protein extract profile (1D or 2D) and gel slices are obtained, the proteins are subjected to proteolytic digestion, with subsequent analysis of the resulting peptides by MS, as described next.

Gel-free Proteomics

The gel-free approach is also known as shotgun proteomics. It was developed to overcome limitations of the gel-based approach in identifying low-expressed proteins, or proteins with a high degree of hydrophobicity that are difficult to solubilize and resolve using gel electrophoresis (Wu and Maccoss 2002).

In the gel-free approach, proteins are digested in solution (see next section), and the peptides resulting from the digestion are subjected to separation by liquid chromatography using HPLC or nano-HPLC (McMaster 2007). The latter improves sensitivity, thus allowing lower concentrations of proteins to be used. Low flow rates (e.g., below 300 nanoliters/min) favor the generation of smaller droplets and better ion formation, as detailed in the section on electrospray ionization.

Other authors have written extensively about chromatography for peptide characterization (McMaster 2007, Lovric 2011). Briefly, peptides are separated using liquid chromatography. The peptide mixture is dissolved in a solvent called the mobile phase and carried through a system containing a stationary phase. Different peptides have different affinities for the stationary phase, causing them to separate at a particular retention time, providing important information for peptide characterization (McMaster 2007).

Chromatography used for peptide separation in most proteomics studies is carried out with a reverse phase column. This column is composed of a hydrophobic stationary phase due to its aliphatic chains of methylene (CH_2) radicals, ranging from 2 (C2) to 18 (C18) with C8 and C18 columns being the most used in proteomics. The analytes (peptides) bind to these chains, in accordance with their hydrophobic composition, and are gradually released from the stationary phase as the hydrophobicity of the mobile phase changes. At the beginning of this process, most peptides bind to the stationary phase and contaminants such as salts are removed from the sample. As the solvent concentration of the mobile phase increases, the peptides are released, first the more hydrophilic (with less interaction with the stationary phase) and then the more hydrophobic (McMaster 2007, Lovric 2011).

An interesting method uses nano-HPLC with two different columns to separate peptides. In this method, the peptides are separated using one column, and the resulting fractions are collected and then undergo a second separation, which is done in line. That is, the eluate (fraction) from the first column is subjected to a second column in the same equipment. The latter approach has been described as a multidimensional protein identification technology or MudPIT (Washburn et al. 2001, Washburn et al. 2002). In this approach, at least two columns are used, for instance, one with strong cation exchange (SCX) followed by a reverse phase column. The SCX column is formed by negatively charged polymers, so the peptides bind to them when in a low pH environment, which is generated by the addition of formic acid to the solvent upon sample injection. After that, with a gradient of sodium chloride and potassium chloride, the peptides are eluted according to their ability to interact with the stationary phase. Less positively charged peptides are eluted more easily at low salt concentrations in the stationary stage. Peptides with a greater positive charge are eluted when the salt contraction increases. Each fraction obtained in the SCX chromatography is subjected to a reverse phase column and the separation of the analytes occurs as previously described, fraction by fraction, and the peptides are then subjected to analysis by MS.

Mass Spectrometry as a Tool for the Identification of Proteins in a Proteome

The study of proteomics aims to identify proteins present in a biological sample, and so we must apply methods that allow such identification. In this context, regardless of the origin of the proteins or peptides, MS is applied in a large number of basic and clinical studies.

MS is an analytical technique used with greater emphasis since the 1950s in the analysis of chemicals. It is essential for the identification of the components of a molecule based on the atomic or molecular mass of which it is composed (Gross 2006, Cole 2011). MS has evolved over more than a hundred years. Improvements in mass analyzers, and especially of ionization sources, have made it possible to use this technique to detect, quantify and characterize peptides and proteins in the study of proteomics.

Mass spectrometers have three essential components: (1) an ionization source, (2) a mass analyzer, and (3) a detector. In recent models, a computer controls all instrument parameters for data acquisition, analysis, and storage (Figure 3).

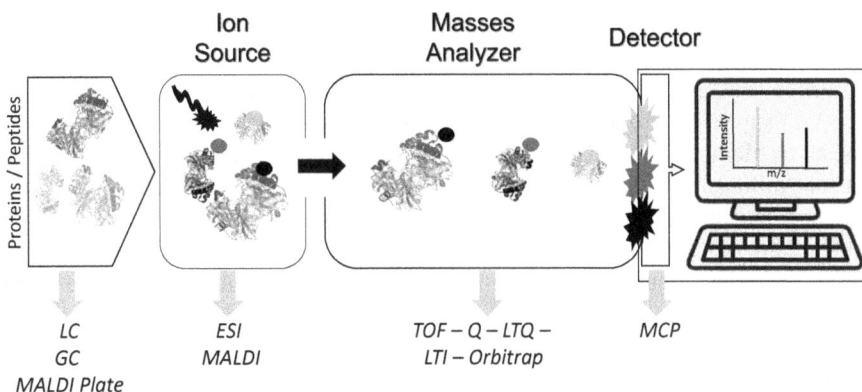

Figure 3. Schematic of mass spectrometer components: ion source (matrix-assisted laser desorption/ionization [MALDI] or electrospray ionization [ESI]), mass analyzer (time of flight [TOF], quadrupole [Q], linear ion trap [LIT or LTQ], or Orbitrap) and detector (microchannel plates [MCP]). Before MS, protein and peptides are separated and submitted to MS by means of liquid chromatography (LC), gas chromatography (GC), or using MALDI plates. The mass spectrometer is coupled to a computer that controls the equipment and analyzes the detected ions.

Conceptually, the molecules are ionized on the source (receive or lose protons), and then the ions are introduced into the mass spectrometer to be analyzed. In the mass analyzer, the ionized compounds are separated according to their mass-to-charge ratio (m/z). In the third stage, the ionized compounds are detected, and the results are presented as a mass spectrum, a plot of intensity as a function of the m/z ratio. This chapter only describes some of the components of the various ionization sources, mass analyzers, and detectors that are mostly used in proteomics studies.

Ionization Sources

Ionization is a key factor in measuring the nominal molecular mass of a protein or peptide. Before explaining the different sources of ionization, we need to review a few essential concepts for understanding the process:

- Amino acids, with very few exceptions, have specific nominal molecular masses (Eidhammer et al. 2007, Lovric 2011).
- To form a protein, amino acids are joined by peptide bonds, a type of covalent bond between the carboxyl group of one amino acid and the amino group of another amino acid.
- These bonds, when broken, either by the action of an enzyme or by the mechanical collision of atoms, generate binding sites for one or more ions.

In this way, a protein or a peptide can be ionized by receiving or losing one or more protons (H^+). Thus, what is measured by the mass spectrometer is the relationship between the nominal molecular mass of the protein or peptide (m), divided by the number of charges that this molecule received (z). The collection of those peaks is what is used to represent the mass spectrum (Figure 4A) (Cole 2011, Lovric 2011). For instance, suppose that a hypothetical small protein with a nominal molecular mass of 10,000 Da (10 kDa) has been subjected to ionization and this protein has received only one H^+, so the m/z ratio of this ion is 10,000. If this same protein is double charged (receives two H^+), its m/z ratio is 5,000, that is 10,000/2; if it is triply charged (receives three H^+), its m/z ratio is 3,333 (Figure 4B).

We can select from various ways to ionize a molecule. However, when it comes to biomolecules such as proteins, peptides, and nucleic acids, the method must be mild enough to ionize the molecule without fragmenting it, while also being efficient. In this context, two ionization techniques are widely used for soft peptide and protein ionization. One, electrospray ionization (ESI), produces gaseous ionized molecules from a liquid solution, creating a fine spray of highly charged droplets in the presence of a strong electric field (Yamashita and Fenn 1984a, Yamashita and Fenn 1984b, Siuzdak 2006). The other, matrix-assisted laser desorption/ionization (MALDI), uses a laser energy-absorbing matrix to create ions from molecules with minimal fragmentation (Karas et al. 1985, Hillenkamp et al. 1986).

In ESI, proteins or peptides are carried to the ionization source by the liquid flow of a solvent, for example, a mixture of water and acetonitrile. When the solvent reaches the tip of a capillary that is being subjected to high voltage and high temperature, it begins to form droplets. As the solvent evaporates, these droplets break down into

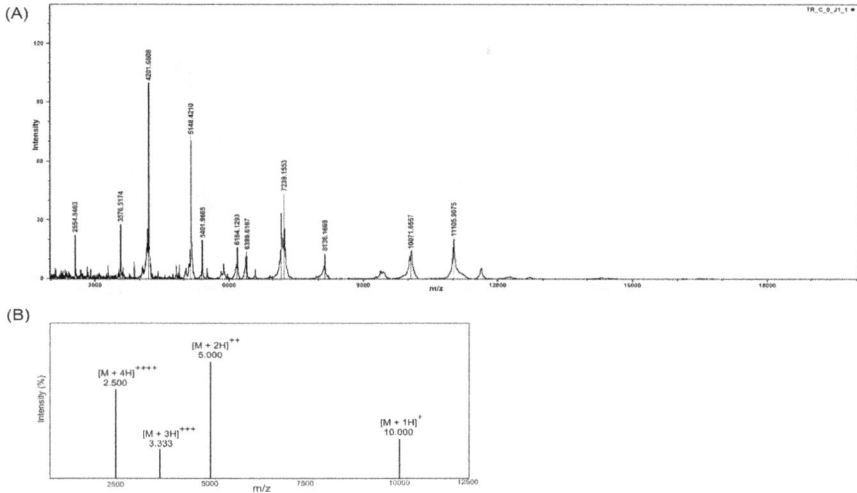

Figure 4. Example of the mass spectrum. (A) Mass spectrum from a matrix-assisted laser desorption/ionization-time of flight (MALDI-TOF) mass spectrometry equipment. (B) Representative schematic of a mass spectrum of a hypothetical 10 kDa (M) protein that received charges of 1, 2, 3, and 4 H+, and the peaks corresponding to the m/z ratio for each ion.

even smaller droplets, forming small, highly surface-charged droplets capable of producing ions in a gas phase. In the presence of a magnetic field, the proteins or peptides detach themselves from the surface of these droplets, already loaded with one or more protons (H$^+$) (Gross 2006, Venter et al. 2006, Cole 2011, Lovric 2011). In ESI, the same protein or peptide can be ionized with more than two ions, which will give different values of *m/z* for the same molecule.

In MALDI, these molecules remain in a solid phase formed by the crystallization of the sample, together with a matrix on a metal surface, but ionization also occurs in a gas phase. In MALDI, laser pulses are focused on the crystal matrix. The matrix absorbs the energy, undergoing a desorption process by sublimation, transitioning from a solid state to a gaseous state (Gross 2006, Cole 2011, Lovric 2011). In the gas phase, the ionized matrix transfers a portion of the ions (most commonly H$^+$) to the protein or peptide, thus forming the molecular ions that will be directed to the mass analyzer. In MALDI, unlike in ESI, ions generally receive only one or, in some cases, two or more protons (H$^+$). This entire event occurs under a vacuum, allowing the ions that are being produced during the desorption process to be introduced into the mass analyzer.

In MALDI, matrices have a fundamental role in generating ions and might play an important role in protecting proteins or peptides from breakage caused by laser energy. Different matrices are used in proteomic analysis, each differing in the way they transfer energy (ions) to the analytes, which reflects the ability to generate ions in different ranges of *m/z* ratios. The most used matrices in proteomics analysis are α-cyano-4-hydroxycinnamic acid (HCCA) and sinapinic acid (SA). HCCA favors the formation of ions with less than 10,000 Da, while SA is ideal for proteins heavier than 10,000 Da (Lovric 2011). The user determines the best matrix based on the expected size of the ions be analyzed, and after testing in the mass spectrometer.

Among the various ways to prepare samples for MALDI analysis, the most common is the dried droplet method, in which a drop (0.5–2 μL) of the sample is deposited on a specific place of the metal plate (known as a spot). After this drop dries, at room temperature, the same volume of the supersaturated matrix (10 mg/mL) is added over the sample. The same volumes of matrix and sample can be mixed before adding a drop of the mixture on the spot. Two matrices can be combined in a sandwich-like preparation, for instance, depositing 0.5 μL of SA, letting it dry, and depositing 0.5–1 μL of the sample, and finally the same volume of HCCA (Shah and Gharbia 2010, Lovric 2011). Regardless of the method or matrix is chosen, the sample must be free of salts and other impurities, such as those resulting from digestion or protein extraction buffers. Salts and impurities can interfere negatively with the desorption process and consequently interfere with matrix crystallization and ion production (Shah and Gharbia 2010, Lovric 2011).

Mass Spectrometers

Before we discuss the types of equipment used in proteomics, three important concepts must be understood:

- Sensitivity is the ability to detect and identify ions in low concentrations, such as picomoles, femtomoles, or even attomoles.
- Resolution or resolving power is defined as the ability to discriminate two ions with adjacent *m/z* peaks of similar intensity.
- Mass accuracy is the measure of agreement between the measured mass and the true mass expressed as a ratio in parts per million (ppm) (Price 2011).

Some devices have high resolution but low sensitivity, and different instruments might perform differently for the same protein sample. Thus, it is important to notice that the choice of equipment depends on the purpose of the analysis.

Another important concept is a monoisotopic mass of ions, which can be defined by the mass of an ion calculated from the empirical formula of the molecule, considering only the exact mass of the most abundant isotopes, such as carbon (C): 12.000000 Da, hydrogen (H): 1.007825 Da, and oxygen (O): 15.994915 Da (Price 2011). In high-resolution equipment, the monoisotopic mass can be used to determine the capacity of the mass spectrometer to distinguish the isotopes (Hoffman and Stroobant 2007).

The measurement of ions is performed by mass spectrometers, which are mass analyzer machines. After the proteins or peptides have been ionized, the highly charged droplets are electrostatically attracted to the mass spectrometer inlet. The ions are focused and transferred from the ionization source to the mass analyzer, which will discriminate the ions according to the *m/z* ratio and direct them to the detector.

Among the available mass analyzers, the most used in proteomics are time-of-flight (TOF), quadrupole (Q), ion-trap (quadrupole ion-trap (QIT), linear ion-trap (LIT or LTQ), and Fourier transform, or hybrids that combine different analyzers (Han et al. 2008). We do not explain all the technical details and the fundamentals of each different analyzer in this chapter but include an extensive bibliography of books on the topic (Gross 2006, Siuzdak 2006, Cole 2011, Lovric 2011). The basic principles of these analyzers are covered in those references.

TOF MS (Figure 5A) achieves mass analysis by accelerating ions through an electric field, followed by a field-free drift region under a high vacuum. All ions reach the same kinetic energy; therefore, high m/z ions travel slower than low m/z ions, which reach the detector earlier. The time taken to reach the detector can be converted into mass, according to the travel length. Longer drift tubes yield a higher mass resolution or a secondary electrostatic field at the end of the drift region can increase resolution as in the case of a reflectron. This corrects for energy spread in the velocity of ions at the time of formation. TOF MS is predominantly used with MALDI because it is a pulsed system (Gross 2006, Siuzdak 2006, Lovric 2011).

The linear quadrupole (Figure 5B) is composed of four metal rods (monopoles) in parallel, equally spaced apart, that form a circular or hyperbolic channel down the length of the quadrupole. Alternate pairs of rods are electrically connected. A radio frequency voltage ($V_o \cos wt$) and a direct current voltage are applied to provide an oscillating field in the quadrupole. The oscillating field can be set so that only selected m/z will pass through the quadrupole, and all other m/z ions will be filtered out, or the voltages can be ramped to allow all ions to be scanned through

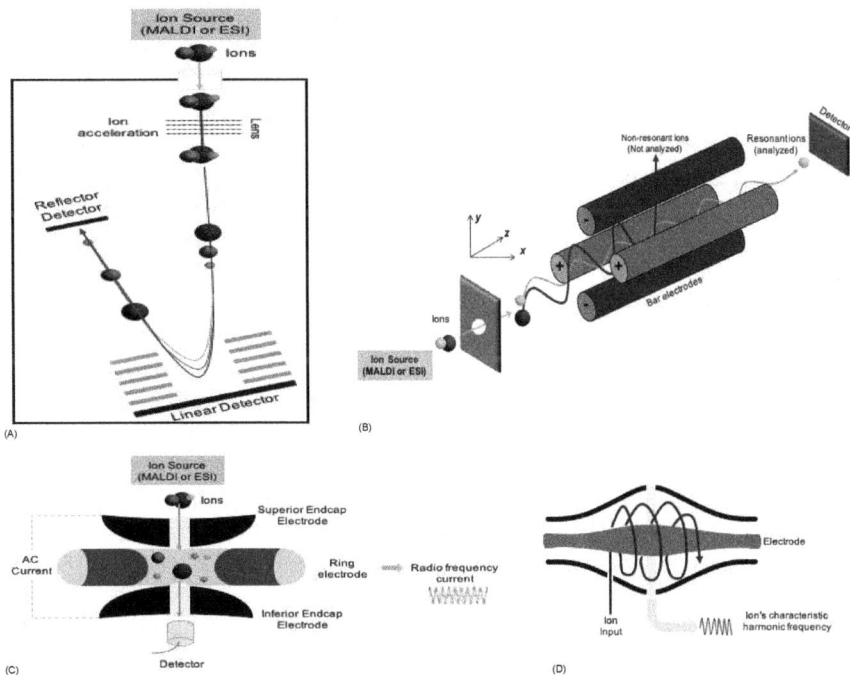

Figure 5. Schematic of the four main mass analyzers used in proteomics. (A) time-of-flight (TOF), whose principle is the separation of ions according to the flight capacity of each ion in a tube; (B) linear quadrupole, in which only the ions that are resonant at a given voltage and frequency are submitted to the detector; (C) ion-trap quadrupole, wherein the ions are trapped in a trap generated by a certain voltage and radiofrequency, where only a few ions are subjected to the detector; and (D) Orbitrap, where the ions present a specific harmonic oscillation, which generates a frequency signal detected by the equipment.

the quadrupole. The most successful use of the linear quadrupole is in the triple quadrupole mass spectrometer, where the second quadrupole is used as a collision cell for fragmentation, allowing for data-dependent MS2 acquisition.

Electric fields with constant voltage and variations in radiofrequency (RF) voltage that vary with time are applied to these axes. When an ion enters a quadrupole analyzer, if it is within a desired range of m/z, it will travel along a z-axis (along the length of the four rods) without hitting the quadrupole rods and then reach the detector. However, ions that are outside this m/z range will oscillate inside the sticks and eventually collide with them, thus not being detected. Changing the RF voltage will allow another ion to have less interference in its z path, which will then be detected (Gross 2006, Siuzdak 2006, Lovric 2011).

The ion trap (Figure 5C) is considered to be a three-dimensional quadrupole mass analyzer. It captures the ions for a very short period in an electrostatic ion trap system. There are quadrupole ion traps (QIT) and linear ion traps (LIT). These analyzers are generally used in hybrid MS and are widely used in proteomics studies because they provide high efficiency in the capture of ions that have a very accelerated movement and high sensitivity when compared with other quadrupoles (Gross 2006, Siuzdak 2006, Lovric 2011).

The Orbitrap (Figure 5D) is a Fourier transform-based instrument that can provide high-resolution and accurate mass measurements. In its earlier form, it was typically coupled with a quadrupole or linear ion trap. Newer versions include dual linear ion traps, quadrupoles, and ion routing multipoles that have enhanced the system's capabilities with regard to bottom-up and top-down tandem MS analysis.

The Orbitrap design is comprised of an inner central spindle electrode elongated on one axis and an outer electrode surrounding the spindle. A high electrostatic field is generated between the electrodes when the outer electrode is held at ground potential. The outer electrode is electrically separated into two halves, so that detection of the ions can be performed. Ions are injected into the Orbitrap using a separate curved linear ion trap (C-trap). The C-trap reduces the kinetic energy of the ions and bunches them into a packet for focusing into the entrance of the Orbitrap. As the ions enter the Orbitrap, they experience axial and radial electrostatic fields that make the ions begin to orbit the central spindle. When the radial field voltage is ramped, the ion packet moves closer to the spindle, which reduces the loss of ions to the outer electrode.

After the stabilization step is completed, mass analysis begins with monitoring the current generated when the ions orbit around the central spindle in complex orbits governed by a quadro-logarithmic electrostatic field. An induced "image current" consisting of many different frequencies produced by the orbiting ions is recorded and mathematically processed using a fast Fourier transform to convert the signal from a frequency to a mass spectrum. The highest frequency signals are produced from the lowest m/z ions. The high mass accuracy (< 1 ppm) and resolution (1,000,000 at m/z 200) allow for the monoisotopic mass to be determined, which greatly facilitates peptide sequencing and protein identification. The parallel acquisition can be programmed to record a mass spectrum (MS1), while collecting several tens of tandem mass spectra, thus protein molecular mass can be determined (Figure 5D) (Hu et al. 2005, Gross 2006, Siuzdak 2006, Lovric 2011).

Most currently available MS instruments are hybrid systems that combine more than one mass analyzer. Some systems consist of a quadrupole followed by a TOF (q-TOF), others with three quadrupoles (QQQ or triple-quadrupole) or two TOF (TOF/TOF), or a quadrupole followed by an ion trap (Q-Trap), or even a linear trap-quadrupole added to an Orbitrap LTQ-Orbitrap. These combinations are crucial for the fast acquisition of tandem MS data (known as MS/MS), essential for sequence characterization and determination of analyzed peptides and proteins, which will be described in the following sections (Gross 2006, Siuzdak 2006, Lovric 2011).

Detectors

The last part of a mass spectrometer is the detector. The detector generates secondary electrons from the ions that strike the detector's surface, making it possible to convert and amplify the signal by generating an electric current. The two main types of detectors in modern MS instruments are the electron multiplier (EM) and microchannel plates (MCP). EM detectors contain a series of electrodes (dynodes) or one continuous dynode (channel electron multiplier, or Channeltron). Ions strike the surface of the dynode and release electrons. These electrons strike another dynode surface within the EM, releasing more electrons. The process continues amplifying the initial signal by 1E6. In MCP detectors, as in EM detectors, an ion strikes the surface of the dynode, and electrons are released. However, MCP consists of a thin plate (2 mm) with 10-micron channels each separated by 10 microns. These plates are staked to provide amplification of the electrons generated from a channel in the first plate to successive channels in the additional stacked plates. EM detectors are mainly associated with electrospray instruments, whereas MCP detectors are used commonly with MALDI sources. One drawback of the MCP is its lower dynamic range when compared with that of the EM. The electrons are then represented as graphics displaying *m/z* values and signal strength of that ion, through applications available on the computers that control the equipment. More information or details about detectors can be found in specific MS books (Gross 2006, Siuzdak 2006, Cole 2011, Lovric 2011).

Peptide Identification and Amino Acid Sequence Determination

This section focuses on the bottom-up strategy for peptide identification and analysis. Proteins are digested and the resulting peptides are analyzed by MS. The *m/z* ratios of ions are measured, and these *m/z* ratios correspond to a certain peptide mass. However, different peptides can have the same *m/z* ratio, making it necessary to analyze the fragmentation of the peptide itself to determine the amino acid sequence.

For this purpose, MS/MS type analyzers (in tandem MS) are used. After detecting the mass of the peptide (MS), known as the parent ion or precursor ion, this ion is fragmented and the ions resulting from this fragmentation are subjected to the analyzer to determine the *m/z* ratio (MS) of each fragment.

This fragmentation usually occurs in a collision cell. Although there are different types of fragmentation, collision-induced dissociation (CID) is widely used in proteomics. In (CID), ions are generated in an atmosphere of an inert gas (usually argon). The precursor ions collide with this gas until reaching the minimum energy required for the fragmentation to occur, generating ions that are capable of being analyzed and detected.

For proteomic analysis, the main ions that result from the breakdown of peptide bonds are b-ions and y-ions, resulting from the breakdown between the carbon (C) of the carboxy-terminal region and nitrogen (N) of the amino-terminal region (Figure 6A). For instance, b-ions are generated when the charge (H^+) is retained from the C-terminal region of the peptide, whereas y-ions are generated when the charge (H^+) is in the N-terminal region of the peptide (Figure 6A). As the random fragmentation of a variable number of the same precursor ions (or parent ions) occurs, b-ions and y-ions of different masses are generated, making it possible to determine the amino acids that make up the peptide (Figure 6B).

Identification of Proteins Using MS/MS Spectra

A significant number of variables must be considered for the generation of MS data. They include the proteomic approach to be used, the origin of the biological sample, the method of protein separation, the type of ionization, the type of mass analyzer to be used, and other variables. After mass spectra are generated, subsequent steps are necessary for data analysis, especially for the determination of the amino acid peptide sequence using MS/MS spectra, protein identification and validation, and further biological characterization of the identified proteins.

To properly identify the proteins, we must first answer an important question: is there a predicted amino acid sequence deposited in a publicly available or privately owned protein database or is there a sequenced genome for the proteome being analyzed? This question is fundamental for the subsequent steps. If amino acid sequences are not available, we will need to analyze each MS/MS spectrum to determine the sequence of each protein, applying *de novo* sequencing (Hughes et al. 2010). However, if genome or protein sequences are available, then search engines can be applied to compare the mass spectra obtained in the experiment with theoretical mass spectra from the database (Eng et al. 2011). Software that has been used to perform such a task includes SEQUEST (Eng et al. 1994), X! Tandem (Craig and Beavis 2004), Byonic (Protein Metrics), OMSSA (Geer et al. 2004), Comet (Eng et al. 2013), Mascot (Perkins et al. 1999), Peaks (Zhang et al. 2012), and Andromeda (Cox et al. 2011), which are among the most frequently used.

Although available software uses different algorithms for processing experimentally generated mass spectra using databases, they all share some basic premises for such identification:

- The endopeptidase used for protein digestion at the beginning of the experiment, such as trypsin, will be disclosed, which is very important for the generation of the theoretical cleavage products and their mass spectra.
- The enzymes might not have their full capacity to function in experimental tests, so failures in protein cleavage (missed cleavages) might occur.

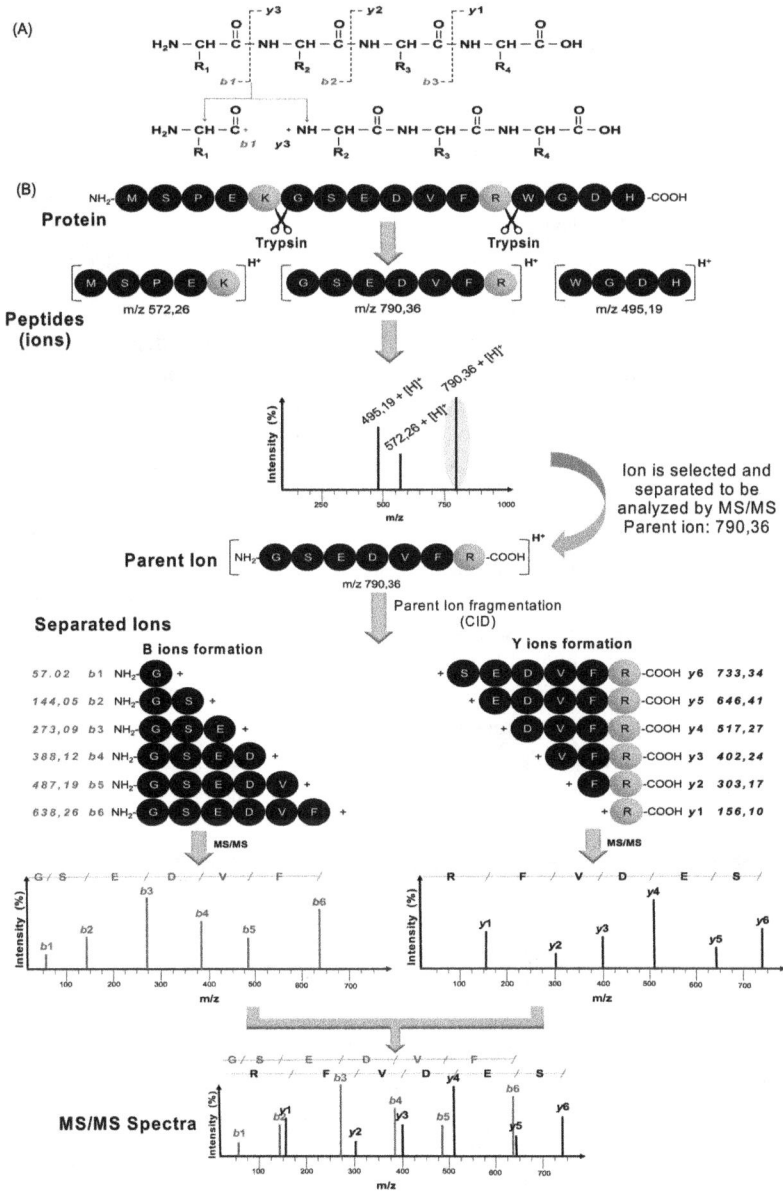

Figure 6. Representative schematic of ion fragmentation and generation of the mass spectrum of b-ions and y-ions. (A) Scheme of the formation of b-ions and y-ions based on the breaking of peptide bonds between residue 1 (R1) and residue 2 (R2). When the ions maintain their charge in the C-terminal region it is named b-ion, and when it remains in the N-terminal region it is named y-ion. (B) A hypothetical protein is subjected to trypsin digestion and generates three peptides that are analyzed in a mass spectrometer. In the first MS analysis, three ions (1H+) are analyzed, which results in three peaks with their respective m/z ratio. The most intense peak (referring to the precursor ion of 790.63) is subjected to fragmentation in collision-induced dissociation, generating the different b-ions and y-ions. When these ions are analyzed, the mass spectrum generated contains all these ions, which allows for the identification and order of the amino acids of the precursor ion.

- If, during the experiment, the cysteines were alkylated using iodoacetamide, then these residues might have their molecular mass changed (from 103.01 Da to 160.03 Da), through carboxymethylation of these residues.
- Following the same logic, if the proteomic study aimed to analyze post-translational changes, these changes must be considered.
- Mass tolerance also should be defined, allowing small variations in the masses (1 to 2 Da) in the spectra of precursor ions and fragments.
- The input data format is dependent on the mass spectrometer used (Cottrell 2011).

Based on these criteria, the software promotes *in silico* digestion of all proteins in a database, generates the theoretical spectra for each peptide, compares those spectra with the spectra experimentally identified, gives an identification score, and then determines which protein corresponds to a determined MS/MS spectrum.

After the first *in silico* analysis, the results must be validated. We can use probabilistic values or other score values, such as the false discovery rate (FDR) (Käll et al. 2008), or the protein prophet (Nesvizhskii et al. 2003) and the peptide prophet (Keller et al. 2002), to assess the chance of error in the identification of peptides and proteins. This step can be performed using software such as Scaffold®,[1] PatternLab,[2] or ProteoIQ®,[3] among others. These software programs provide effective ways to visualize the results. In some cases, they can provide the relative quantification of each protein (Lundgren et al. 2010, Nahnsen et al. 2013).

After the protein identification process is complete, further analyses are needed to determine the functional characteristics and biological significance of each protein. Different bioinformatics tools can be used to do that, including ExPASy,[4] MS-Utils,[5] and OMICTools.[6]

Biomedical Applications of Microorganism Proteomics

Technological advances in MS and bioinformatics have enabled novel applications of clinical proteomics in biomarker discovery, drug development, and disease etiology. Proteomics tools and applications have been applied for understanding and the characterization of several proteins in various species of organisms. Since the middle of the 20th century, MS has been used to characterize organic molecules, which include lipids, sugars, and other organism metabolites. However, the characterization of microorganism proteins by MS dates from the beginning of the 21st century (Cohen et al. 2002) and has proved to be very useful for the discovery of new targets for diagnosis, vaccines, and drugs (Fairlamb 1999, Barret et al. 2000).

---

[1] Scaffold® site http://www.proteomesoftware.com/products/scaffold.
[2] PatternLab site http://www.patternlabforproteomics.org.
[3] ProteoIQ® site http://www.premierbiosoft.com/protein_quantification_software.
[4] ExPASy site http://www.expasy.org/.
[5] MS-Utils site http://www.ms-utils.org/.
[6] OMICTools site https://omictools.com/.

Among these proteomics studies in microbiology and parasitology, some present indirect clinical applications, especially in the search for marker proteins for the diagnosis of different organisms, such as the following:

- *Bacillus* spp., *Burkholderia* spp., *Francisella tularensis*, and *Brucella* spp. (Khan et al. 2019, Malovichko et al. 2019, Chang et al. 2020, Doellinger et al. 2020, Terán et al. 2020, Wang et al. 2020d, Wang et al. 2020b, Wareth et al. 2020).
- *Klebsiella* spp., *Salmonella typhimurium*, *Staphylococcus aureus*, and *Acinetobacter baumannii* (Elhosseiny et al. 2019, Wang et al. 2019c, Iftikhar et al. 2020, Wang et al. 2020a).
- *Plasmodium* spp., *Babesia microti*, and *Toxoplasma gondii* (Yeng et al. 2010, Huang et al. 2012, Thézénas et al. 2013, Mathema and Na-Bangchang 2015, Cornillot et al. 2016, Krause et al. 2017).
- *Trypanosoma* spp., and *Leishmania* spp. (Singh 2012, Duarte et al. 2015, Lima et al. 2017, Singh and Sundar 2017).
- *Entamoeba* spp. (Ujang et al. 2016) and free-living amoebae (Moura et al. 2015).
- *Taenia solium* (Esquivel-Velázquez et al. 2011).
- *Schistosooma* spp. (Driguez et al. 2016; Kardoush et al. 2017).

Although such studies point to the potential use of proteomics for the diagnosis of microorganisms, a direct approach to bacterial identification has been widely used (Shah and Gharbia 2010). This approach uses protein mass fingerprinting (PMF). PMF is based on the identification of microorganisms to the genus and species level, based on standard mass spectra profiles of each organism. Such profiles are obtained by analyzing the MS of the most abundant intact proteins of the cell and generating a protein fingerprint (phenotype) characteristic of each cell. This approach was first described in 1996 for bacteria (Holland et al. 1996) and was later shown to be useful in routine clinical applications (Seng et al. 2009) and after approval of two systems intended exclusively for this purpose: Bruker Biotyper® (Bruker Daltonics) and VITEK MS® (bioMérieux) (Patel 2015).

Despite the increasing use of the PMF approach (Dingle and Butler-Wu 2013) for bacteria and fungi identification, few studies demonstrate the application of this technology in the clinical parasitology routine (Singhal et al. 2016, Murugaiyan and Roesler 2017). Until August 2017, few studies demonstrated the possibility of differentiating species such as *Leishmania* through the PMF profile from promastigote forms grown *in vitro* (Cassagne et al. 2014, Culha et al. 2014, Mouri et al. 2014) or differentiation of *Trypanosoma cruzi* from *Trypanosoma brucei* (Avila et al. 2016). The possibility of differentiating between *Entamoeba histolytica* and *Entamoeba dispar*, obtained from clinical isolates and grown in an axenic medium (Calderaro et al. 2015), was also shown demonstrating that this methodology has potential use in the clinical routine to differentiate these species. Similarly, Martiny and collaborators (Martiny et al. 2014) demonstrated that MALDI-TOF MS can be an efficient approach for the differentiating of *Blastocystis* subtypes. This approach was also used to identify and characterize species and isolates of free-living amoebae such as *Naegleria fowleri* (Moura 2015) and *Acanthamoeba* spp. (Chierico et al. 2016).

A few studies have demonstrated the use of this approach to characterize helminths. In one study, *Schistosoma japonicum* was detected based on the presence of peptides expressed in the serum of mice infected by this parasite (Huang et al. 2016). Another work used MALDI-TOF MS to identify *Trichinella* helminths by species, based on the PMF obtained from larval forms of five species of this genus (Mayer-Scholl et al. 2016).

As noted, PMF technology presents itself as a potential low-cost tool to characterize parasites, especially for laboratories that already have equipment for MALDI-TOF MS for the identification of bacteria. However, to definitively apply this technique in the clinical routine, methodological improvements are needed to increase the sensitivity of the technique, mainly for the identification of parasites, without the need for cultivation or with as little time in culture as possible.

Conclusion

An array of complex technologies has been developed and applied in the area of functional genomics to study protein expression within cells or tissues, which gave rise to what we now call proteomics. Proteomics is an area of great interest, with potential applications in gene expression and function, characterization of proteins, diagnosis of infectious agents, toxins screening, and drug resistance studies. In this review, we have presented and discussed the most important steps to help non-specialists better understand proteomic analysis. We also suggest supplementary references for further exploration of some of these subjects.

The four main steps for a typical proteomic analysis have been introduced and discussed, including (1) protein preparation and extraction; (2) peptide separation; (3) measurement of the *m/z* ratio of peptides; and (4) protein identification. Considering that the study of proteomics aims to identify proteins in a biological sample, regardless of the origin of the proteins or peptides, MS is applied in many basic and clinical studies. In this context, we have also reviewed the essential components of such systems, such as ionization sources, mass spectrometers, and detectors.

A century of technological advances in MS and the consolidation of bioinformatics have enabled novel applications of clinical proteomics. Proteomics presents itself as a technology with a relatively low cost of analysis, increased sensitivity and specificity, and short analysis time. Because of this, these methods have become the preferred approach to detect and identify compounds otherwise difficult to analyze by other methods.

Acknowledgments

The content is solely the responsibility of the authors and does not necessarily represent the official position of the Centers for Disease Control and Prevention.

Use of trade names is for identification only and does not imply endorsement by the Centers for Disease Control and Prevention, the Public Health Service, or the U.S. Department of Health and Human Services.

The Universidade Federal de Santa Catarina (Brazil) group is supported by the CAPES (Coordination for the Improvement of Higher Education Personnel)/Program of Internalization Project (project number 88881.310783/2018-01). Guilherme Augusto Maia has a scholarship from CAPES (Coordination for the Improvement of Higher Education Personnel).

References

Alcolea, P. J., A. Alonso and V. Larraga. (2011_. Proteome profiling of *Leishmania infantum* promastigotes. J. Eukaryot. Microbiol. 58 (4): 352–58. https://doi.org/10.1111/j.1550–7408.2011.00549.x.

Andrade, H. M., S. M. F. Murta, A. Chapeaurouge, J. Perales, P. Nirdé and A. J. Romanha. (2008). Proteomic analysis of *Trypanosoma cruzi* resistance to benznidazole. J. Proteome Res. 7(6): 2357–67. https://doi.org/10.1021/pr700659m.

Atyame Nten, C. M., N. Sommerer, V. Rofidal, C. Hirtz, M. Rossignol, G. Cuny et al. (2010). Excreted/secreted proteins from *Trypanosome procyclic* strains. J. Biomed. Biotechnol. 2010: 1–8. https://doi.org/10.1155/2010/212817.

Avila, C. C., F. G. Almeida and G. Palmisano. (2016_. Direct identification of trypanosomatids by matrix-assisted laser desorption ionization–time of flight mass spectrometry (DIT MALDI-TOF MS). J. Mass Spectrom. 51(8): 549–57. https://doi.org/10.1002/jms.3763.

Ayub, M. J., J. Atwood, A. Nuccio, R. Tarleton and M. J. Levin. (2009). Proteomic analysis of the *Trypanosoma cruzi* ribosomal proteins. Biochem. Biophys. Res. Commun. 382 (1): 30–34. https://doi.org/10.1016/j.bbrc.2009.02.095.

Bantscheff, M., S. Lemeer, M. M. Savitski and B. Kuster. (2012). Quantitative mass spectrometry in proteomics: Critical review update from 2007 to the present. Anal. Bioanal. Chem. https://doi.org/10.1007/s00216–012–6203–4.

Barret, J., J. R. Jefferies and P. M. Brophy. (2000). Parasite proteomics. Parasitol. Today 16(9): 400–403. http://www.sanger.ac.uk/.

Bjellqvist, B., K. Ek, P. G. Righetti, E. Gianazza, A. Gorg, R. Westermeier et al. (1982). Isoelectric focusing in immobilized pH gradients principle, methodology and some applications. J. Biochem. Biophys. Methods 6(4): 317–39.

Brunoro, G. V. F., V. M. Faça, M. A. Caminha, A. T. S. Ferreira, M. Trugilho, K. C. G. Moura et al. (2016). Differential gel electrophoresis (DIGE) evaluation of naphthoimidazoles mode of action: A study in *Trypanosoma cruzi* bloodstream trypomastigotes. PLOS Negl. Trop. Dis. 10(8). https://doi.org/10.1371/journal.pntd.0004951.

Calderaro, A., M. Piergianni, M. Buttrini, S. Montecchini, G. Piccolo, C. Gorrini et al. (2015). MALDI-TOF mass spectrometry for the detection and differentiation of *Entamoeba histolytica* and *Entamoeba dispar*. PLoS One 10(4). https://doi.org/10.1371/journal.pone.0122448.

Campos, J. M., L. X. Neves, N. C. N. Paiva, R. A. O. Castro, A. H. Casé, C. M. Carneiro et al. (2017). Understanding global changes of the liver proteome during murine schistosomiasis using a label-free shotgun approach. J. Proteom. 151(January): 193–203. https://doi.org/10.1016/j.jprot.2016.07.013.

Cassagne, C., F. Pratlong, F. Jeddi, R. Benikhlef, K. Aoun, A. C. Normand et al. (2014). Identification of *Leishmania* at the species level with matrix-assisted laser desorption ionization time-of-flight mass spectrometry. Clin. Microbiol. Infect. 20(6): 551–57. https://doi.org/10.1111/1469–0691.12387.

Chang, Y., D. M. Duong, J. B. Goll, D. C. Wood, T. L. Jensen, L. Yin et al. (2020). Proteomic analysis of human immune responses to live-attenuated tularemia vaccine. Vaccines 8(3): 413. https://doi.org/10.3390/vaccines8030413.

Chierico, F. D., D. D. Cave, C. Accardi, M. Santoro, A. Masotti, R. D'Alfonso et al. (2016). Identification and typing of free-living *Acanthamoeba* spp. by MALDI-TOF MS biotyper. Exp. Parasitol. 170(November): 82–89. https://doi.org/10.1016/j.exppara.2016.09.007.

Cohen, A. M., K. Rumpel, G. H. Coombs and J. M. Wastling. (2002). Characterisation of global protein expression by two-dimensional electrophoresis and mass spectrometry: Proteomics of *Toxoplasma gondii*. Int. J. Parasitol. 32(1): 39–51.

Cole, R. B. (2011). Electrospray and MALDI Mass Spectrometry: Fundamentals, Instrumentation, Practicalities, and Biological Applications. John Wiley & Sons, Ltd. Hoboken, New Jersey.

Cordero, E. M., E. S. Nakayasu, L. G. Gentil, N. Yoshida, I. C. Almeida and J. F. Silveira. (2009). Proteomic analysis of detergent-solubilized membrane proteins from insect-developmental forms of *Trypanosoma cruzi*. J. Proteome Res. 8(7): 3642–52. https://doi.org/10.1021/pr800887u.

Cornillot, E., A. Dassouli, N. Pachikara, L. Lawres, I. Renard, C. Francois et al. (2016). A targeted immunomic approach identifies diagnostic antigens in the human pathogen *Babesia microti*. Transfusion 56(8): 2085–99. https://doi.org/10.1111/trf.13640.

Cottrell, J. S. (2011). Protein identification using MS/MS data. J. Proteom. 74(10): 1842–51. https://doi.org/10.1016/j.jprot.2011.05.014.

Cox, J., N. Neuhauser, A. Michalski, R. A. Scheltema, J. V. Olsen and M. Mann. (2011). Andromeda: A peptide search engine integrated into the maxquant environment. J. Proteome Res. 10(4): 1794–1805. https://doi.org/10.1021/pr101065j.

Craig, R. and R. C. Beavis. (2004). TANDEM: Matching proteins with tandem mass spectra. Bioinformatics 20(9): 1466–67. https://doi.org/10.1093/bioinformatics/bth092.

Cuervo, P., J. B. Jesus, M. Junqueira, L. Mendonça-Lima, L. J. González, L. Betancourt et al. (2007). Proteome analysis of *Leishmania* (Viannia) *braziliensis* by two-dimensional gel electrophoresis and mass spectrometry. Mol. Biochem. Parasitol. 154(1): 6–21. https://doi.org/10.1016/j.molbiopara.2007.03.013.

Culha, G., I. Akyar, F. Y. Zeyrek, Ö. Kurt, C. Gündüz, S. Ö. Töz et al. (2014). Leishmaniasis in Turkey: Determination of *Leishmania* species by matrix-assisted laser desorption ionization time-of-flight mass spectrometry (MALDI-TOF MS). Iran. J. Parasitol. 9(2): 239–48. http://ijpa.tums.ac.ir.

Dingle, T. C. and S. M. Butler-Wu. (2013). MALDI-TOF mass spectrometry for microorganism identification. Clin. Lab. Med. 33(3): 589–609. https://doi.org/10.1016/j.cll.2013.03.001.

Doellinger, J., A. Schneider, M. Hoeller and P. Lasch. (2020). Sample preparation by easy extraction and digestion (SPEED)—A universal, rapid, and detergent-free protocol for proteomics based on acid extraction. Mol. Cell. Proteom. 19(1): 209–22. https://doi.org/10.1074/mcp.TIR119.001616.

Driguez, P., D. P. McManus and G. N. Gobert. (2016). Clinical implications of recent findings in schistosome proteomics. Expert. Rev. Proteom. 13(1): 19–33. https://doi.org/10.1586/14789450.2016.1116390.

Duarte, M. C., D. C. Pimenta, D. Menezes-Souza, R. D. M. Magalhães, J. L. C. P. Diniz, L. E. Costa et al. (2015). Proteins selected in *Leishmania* (Viannia) *braziliensis* by an immunoproteomic approach with potential serodiagnosis applications for tegumentary leishmaniasis. Clin. Vaccine Immunol. 22(11): 1187–96. https://doi.org/10.1128/CVI.00465–15.

Duncan, M. W., A. L. Yergey and S. D. Patterson. (2009). Quantifying proteins by mass spectrometry: The selectivity of SRM is only part of the problem. Proteomics 9(5): 1124–27. https://doi.org/10.1002/pmic.200800739.

Eidhammer, I., K. Flikka, L. Martens and S. Mikalsen. (2007). Computational Methods for Mass Spectrometry Proteomics. Chichester, UK: John Wiley & Sons, Ltd. https://doi.org/10.1002/9780470724309.

Elhosseiny, N. M., N. B. Elhezawy and A. S. Attia. (2019). Comparative proteomics analyses of *Acinetobacter baumannii* strains atcc 17978 and ab5075 reveal the differential role of type II secretion system secretomes in lung colonization and ciprofloxacin resistance. Microb. Pathog. 128(3): 20–27. https://doi.org/10.1016/j.micpath.2018.12.039.

Eng, J. K., T. A. Jahan and M. R. Hoopmann. (2013). Comet: An open-source ms/ms sequence database search tool. Proteomics 13(1): 22–24. https://doi.org/10.1002/pmic.201200439.

Eng, J. K., B. C. Searle, K. R. Clauser and D. L. Tabb. (2011). A face in the crowd: Recognizing peptides through database search. Mol. Cell. Proteom. 10(11). https://doi.org/10.1074/mcp.R111.009522.

Eng, J. K., A. L. Mccormack and J. R. Yates. (1994). An approach to correlate tandem mass spectral data of peptides with amino acid sequences in a protein database. J. Am. Soc. Mass Spectrom. 5(11): 976–89.

Esquivel-Velázquez, M., C. Larralde, J. Morales and P. Ostoa-Saloma. (2011). Protein and antigen diversity in the vesicular fluid of *Taenia solium* cys-ticerci dissected from naturally infected pigs. Int. J. Biol. Sci. 7(9): 1287–97. http://www.biolsci.org.

Eyford, B. A., R. Ahmad, J. C. Enyaru, S. A. Carr and T. W. Pearson. (2013). Identification of trypanosome proteins in plasma from african sleeping sickness patients infected with T. b. rhodesiense. PLoS One 8(8). https://doi.org/10.1371/journal.pone.0071463.

Fairlamb, Alan H. (1999). Future prospects for the chemotherapy of chagas' disease. Future Prospects for Chagas' Disease Chemotherapy 179: 179–87.

Geer, L. Y., S. P. Markey, J. A. Kowalak, L. Wagner, M. Xu, D. M. Maynard et al. (2004). Open mass spectrometry search algorithm. J. Proteome Res. 3(5): 958–64. https://doi.org/10.1021/pr0499491.

Gerber, S. A., J. Rush, O. Stemman, M. W. Kirschner and S. P. Gygi. (2003). Absolute quantification of proteins and phosphoproteins from cell lysates by tandem MS. Proc. Natl. Acad. Sci. U.S.A. 100(12): 6940–45. www.pnas.org.

Goos, C., M. Dejung, C. J. Janzen, F. Butter and S. Kramer. (2017). The nuclear proteome of *Trypanosoma brucei*. PLoS One 12(7). https://doi.org/10.1371/journal.pone.0181884.

Görg, A., W. Weiss and M. J. Dunn. (2004). Current two-dimensional electrophoresis technology for proteomics. Proteomics 4(12): 3665–85. https://doi.org/10.1002/pmic.200401031.

Gross, J. H. (2006). Mass Spectrometry: A Textbook. Springer Science & Business Media. Heidelberg, Berlin.

Han, X., A. Aslanian and J. R. Yates. (2008). Mass spectrometry for proteomics. Curr. Opin. Chem. Biol. https://doi.org/10.1016/j.cbpa.2008.07.024.

Hao, R., C. Adoligbe, B. Jiang, X. Zhao, L. Gui, K. Qu et al. (2015). An optimized trichloroacetic acid/ acetone precipitation method for two-dimensional gel electrophoresis analysis of Qinchuan cattle longissimus dorsi muscle containing high proportion of marbling. PLoS One 10(4). https://doi.org/10.1371/journal.pone.0124723.

Hillenkamp, F., M. Karas, D. Holtkamp and P. Klusener. (1986). Energy deposition in ultraviolet laser desorption mass spectrometry of biomolecules. Int. J. Mass Spectrom. 69(3): 265–76.

Hoffman, E. and V. Stroobant. (2007). Mass Spectrometry: Principles and Applications - 3rd ed. John Wiley & Sons, Ltd. Chichester, West Sussex.

Holland, R. D., J. G. Wilkes, F. Ralli, J. B. Sutherland, C. C. Persons, K. J. Voorhees et al. (1996). Rapid identification of intact whole bacteria based on spectral patterns using matrix-assisted laser desorption/ionization with time-of-flight mass spectrometry. Rapid Commun. Mass Spectrom. 10: 1227–32.

Hong, Y., A. Sun, M. Zhang, F. Gao, Y. Han, Z. Fu et al. (2013). Proteomics analysis of differentially expressed proteins in schistosomula and adult worms of *Schistosoma japonicum*. Acta Trop. 126(1): 1–10. https://doi.org/10.1016/j.actatropica.2012.12.009.

Hu, Q., R. J. Noll, H. Li, A. Makarov, M. Hardman and R. G. Cooks. (2005). The Orbitrap: A new mass spectrometer. J. Mass Spectrom. 40(4): 430–43. https://doi.org/10.1002/jms.856.

Huang, H., M. M. MacKeen, M. Cook, E. Oriero, E. Locke, M. L. Thézénas et al. (2012). Proteomic identification of host and parasite biomarkers in saliva from patients with uncomplicated *Plasmodium falciparum* malaria. Malar. J. 11(1): 1–9. https://doi.org/10.1186/1475-2875-11-178.

Huang, Y., W. Li, K. Liu, C. Xiong, P. Cao and J. Tao. (2016). New detection method in experimental mice for schistosomiasis: ClinProTool and matrix-assisted laser desorption/ionization time-of-flight mass spectrometry. Parasitol. Res. 115(11): 4173–81. https://doi.org/10.1007/s00436-016-5193-0.

Hughes, C., B. Ma and G. A. Lajoie. (2010). *De novo* sequencing methods in proteomics. Methods Mol. Biol. 604: 105–21. https://doi.org/10.1007/978-1-60761-444-9_8.

Iftikhar, R., M. Rizwan, S. Khan, A. Mehmood and A. Munir. (2020). Subtractive proteome mining approach towards unique putative drug targets identification for *Salmonella typhimurium*. Infect. Disord. Drug Targets 20(6): 884–92. https://doi.org/10.2174/1871526519666191211142758.

Jesus, T. C. L., S. G. Calderano, F. N. L. Vitorino, R. P. Llanos, M. C. Lopes, C. B. Araújo et al. (2017). Quantitative proteomic analysis of replicative and nonreplicative forms reveals important insights into chromatin biology of *Trypanosoma cruzi*. Mol. Cell. Proteom. 16(1): 23–38. https://doi.org/10.1074/mcp.M116.061200.

Käll, L., J. D. Storey, M. J. MacCoss and W. S. Noble. (2008). Assigning significance to peptides identified by tandem mass spectrometry using decoy databases. J. Proteome Res. 7(1): 29–34. https://doi.org/10.1021/pr700600n.

Kamali, A. N., P. Marín-García, I. G. Azcárate, A. Diez, A. Puyet and J. M. Bautista. (2012). *Plasmodium yoelii* blood-stage antigens newly identified by immunoaffinity using purified igg antibodies from malaria-resistant mice. Immunobiology 217(8): 823–30. https://doi.org/10.1016/j.imbio.2012.05.002.

Karas, M., D. Bachmann and F. Hillenkamp. (1985). Influence of the wavelength in high-irradiance ultraviolet laser desorption mass spectrometry of organic molecules. Anal. Chem. 57(14): 2935–39. https://pubs.acs.org/sharingguidelines.

Kardoush, M. I., B. J. Ward and M. Ndao. (2017). Serum carbonic anhydrase 1 is a biomarker for diagnosis of human *Schistosoma mansoni* infection. Am. J. Trop. Med. Hyg. 96(4): 842–49. https://doi.org/10.4269/ajtmh.16–0021.

Keller, A., A. I. Nesvizhskii, E. Kolker and R. Aebersold. (2002). Empirical statistical model to estimate the accuracy of peptide identifications made by MS/MS and database search. Anal. Chem. 74(20): 5383–92. https://doi.org/10.1021/ac025747h.

Khan, M. M., S. Chattagul, B. Q. Tran, J. A. Freiberg, A. Nita-Lazar, M. E. Shirtliff et al. (2019). Temporal proteomic profiling reveals changes that support *Burkholderia* biofilms. Pathog. Dis. 77(2). https://doi.org/10.1093/femspd/ftz005.

Krause, R. G. E., R. Hurdayal, D. Choveaux, J. M. Przyborski, T. H. T. Coetzer and J. P. D. Goldring. (2017). *Plasmodium* glyceraldehyde-3-phosphate dehydrogenase: A potential malaria diagnostic target. Exp. Parasitol. 179(August): 7–19. https://doi.org/10.1016/j.exppara.2017.05.007.

Laemmli, U. K. (1970). Cleavage of structural proteins during the assembly of the head of bacteriophage t4. Nature 227(5259): 680–85.

Li, P., M. Kaslan, S. H. Lee, J. Yao and Z. Gao. (2017). Progress in exosome isolation techniques. Theranostics 7(3): 789–804. https://doi.org/10.7150/thno.18133.

Lima, B. S. S., S. F. Pires, L. C. Fialho, E. J. Oliveira, R. A. Machado-de-Avila, C. Chávez-Olórtegui et al. (2017). A proteomic road to acquire an accurate serological diagnosis for human tegumentary leishmaniasis. J. Proteom. 151(January): 174–81. https://doi.org/10.1016/j.jprot.2016.05.017.

Lovric, J. (2011). Introducing Proteomics: From Concepts to Sample Separation, Mass Spectrometry and Data Analysis. John Wiley & Sons, Ltd. Chichester, West Sussex.

Lundgren, D. H., S. Hwang, L. Wu and D. K. Han. (2010). Role of spectral counting in quantitative proteomics. Expert. Rev. Proteom. 7(1): 39–53. https://doi.org/10.1586/epr.09.69.

Machida, M., H. Kosako, K. Shirakabe, M. Kobayashi, M. Ushiyama, J. Inagawa et al. (2007). Purification of phosphoproteins by immobilized metal affinity chromatography and its application to phosphoproteome analysis. FEBS J. 274(6): 1576–87. https://doi.org/10.1111/j.1742–4658.2007.05705.x.

Malovichko, Y. V., A. A. Nizhnikov and K. S. Antonets. (2019). Repertoire of the *Bacillus thuringiensis* virulence factors unrelated to major classes of protein toxins and its role in specificity of host-pathogen interactions. Toxins 11(6): 347. https://doi.org/10.3390/toxins11060347.

Marcilla, A., M. Trelis, A. Cortés, J. Sotillo, F. Cantalapiedra, M. T. Minguez et al. (2012). Extracellular vesicles from parasitic helminths contain specific excretory/secretory proteins and are internalized in intestinal host cells. PLoS One 7(9). https://doi.org/10.1371/journal.pone.0045974.

Martiny, D., A. Bart, O. Vandenberg, N. Verhaar, E. Wentink-Bonnema, C. Moens et al. (2014). Subtype determination of blastocystis isolates by matrix-assisted laser desorption/ionisation time-of-flight mass spectrometry (MALDI-TOF MS). Eur. J. Clin. Microbiol. Infect. Dis. 33(4): 529–36. https://doi.org/10.1007/s10096–013–1980-z.

Mathema, V. B. and K. Na-Bangchang. (2015). A brief review on biomarkers and proteomic approach for malaria research. Asian Pac. J. Trop. Med. 8(4): 253–62. https://doi.org/10.1016/S1995–7645(14)60327–8.

Mayer-Scholl, A., J. Murugaiyan, J. Neumann, P. Bahn, S. Reckinger and K. Nöckler. (2016). Rapid identification of the foodborne pathogen *Trichinella* spp. by matrix-assisted laser desorption/ionization mass spectrometry. PLoS One 11(3). https://doi.org/10.1371/journal.pone.0152062.

McMaster, M. C. (2007). HPLC: A Practical User's Guide. John Wiley & Sons, Ltd. Hoboken, New Jersey.

Meevissen, M. H. J., C. I. A. Balog, C. A. M. Koeleman, M. J. Doenhoff, G. Schramm, H. Haas et al. (2011). Targeted glycoproteomic analysis reveals that kappa-5 is a major, uniquely glycosylated component of *Schistosoma mansoni* egg antigens. Mol. Cell. Proteom. 10(5). https://doi.org/10.1074/mcp.M110.005710.

Moura, H., F. Izquierdo, A. R. Woolfitt, G. Wagner, T. Pinto, C. D. Aguila et al. (2015). Detection of biomarkers of pathogenic *Naegleria fowleri* through mass spectrometry and proteomics. J. Eukaryot. Microbiol. 62(1): 12–20. https://doi.org/10.1111/jeu.12178.

Mouri, O., G. Morizot, G. V. Auwera, C. Ravel, M. Passet, N. Chartrel et al. (2014). Easy identification of *Leishmania* species by mass spectrometry. PLOS Negl. Trop. Dis. 8(6). https://doi.org/10.1371/journal.pntd.0002841.

Murugaiyan, J. and U. Roesler. (2017). MALDI-TOF MS profiling-advances in species identification of pests, parasites, and vectors. Front. Cell. Infect. Microbiol. 7(May): 184–184. https://doi.org/10.3389/fcimb.2017.00184.

Nahnsen, S., C. Bielow, K. Reinert and O. Kohlbacher. (2013). Tools for label-free peptide quantification. Mol. Cell. Proteom. 12(3): 549–56. https://doi.org/10.1074/mcp.R112.025163.

Nakayasu, E. S., M. R. Gaynor, T. J. P. Sobreira, J. A. Ross and I. C. Almeida. (2009). Phosphoproteomic analysis of the human pathogen *Trypanosoma cruzi* at the epimastigote stage. Proteomics 9(13): 3489–3506. https://doi.org/10.1002/pmic.200800874.

Nakayasu, E. S., T. J. P. Sobreira, R. Torres, L. Ganiko, P. S. L. Oliveira, A. F. Marques et al. (2012). Improved proteomic approach for the discovery of potential vaccine targets in *Trypanosoma cruzi*. J. Proteome Res. 11(1): 237–46. https://doi.org/10.1021/pr200806s.

Ndao, M., T. W. Spithill, R. Caffrey, H. Li, V. N. Podust, R. Perichon et al. (2010). Identification of novel diagnostic serum biomarkers for Chagas' disease in asymptomatic subjects by mass spectrometric profiling. J. Clin. Microbiol. 48(4): 1139–49. https://doi.org/10.1128/JCM.02207–09.

Nesvizhskii, A. I., A. Keller, E. Kolker and R. Aebersold. (2003). A statistical model for identifying proteins by tandem mass spectrometry. Anal. Chem. 75(17): 4646–58. https://doi.org/10.1021/ac0341261.

Ong, S., L. J. Foster and M. Mann. (2003). Mass spectrometric-based approaches in quantitative proteomics. Methods 29(2): 124–30. www.elsevier.com/locate/ymeth.

Ong, S. and M. Mann. (2007). A practical recipe for stable isotope labeling by amino acids in cell culture (SILAC). Nat. Protoc. 1(6): 2650–60. https://doi.org/10.1038/nprot.2006.427.

Ongay, S., A. Boichenko, N. Govorukhina and R. Bischoff. (2012). Glycopeptide enrichment and separation for protein glycosylation analysis. J. Sep. Sci. 35(18): 2341–72. https://doi.org/10.1002/jssc.201200434.

Paba, J., J. M. Santana, A. R. L. Teixeira, W. Fontes, M. V. Sousa and C. A. O. Ricart. (2004). Proteomic analysis of the human pathogen *Trypanosoma cruzi*. Proteomics 4(4): 1052–59. https://doi.org/10.1002/pmic.200300637.

Parodi-Talice, A., R. Durán, N. Arrambide, V. Prieto, M. D. Piñeyro, O. Pritsch et al. (2004). Proteome analysis of the causative agent of Chagas disease: *Trypanosoma cruzi*. Int. J. Parasitol. 34(8): 881–86. https://doi.org/10.1016/j.ijpara.2004.05.002.

Patel, R. (2015). MALDI-TOF MS for the diagnosis of infectious diseases. Clin. Chem. 61(1): 100–111. https://doi.org/10.1373/clinchem.2014.221770.

Perkins, D. N., D. J. C. Pappin, D. M. Creasy and J. S. Cottrell. (1999). Probability-based protein identification by searching sequence databases using mass spectrometry data. Electrophoresis 20(18): 3551–67. https://doi.org/10.1002/(SICI)1522–2683(19991201)20:18<3551::AID-ELPS3551>3.0.CO;2–2.

Pillay, D., A. F. V. Boulangé, V. Coustou, T. Baltz and T. H. T. Coetzer. (2013). Recombinant expression and biochemical characterisation of two alanyl aminopeptidases of *Trypanosoma congolense*. Exp. Parasitol. 135(4): 675–84. https://doi.org/10.1016/j.exppara.2013.10.005.

Pollo-Oliveira, L., H. Post, M. L. Acencio, N. Lemke, H. V. D. Toorn, V. Tragante et al. (2013). Unravelling the *Neospora caninum* secretome through the secreted fraction (ESA) and quantification of the discharged tachyzoite using high-resolution mass spectrometry-based proteomics. Parasites Vectors 6(1): 1–14. http://www.parasitesandvectors.com/content/6/1/335.

Price, P. (2011). Standard definitions of terms relating to mass spectrometry a report from the committee on measurements and standards of the american society for mass spectrometry. J. Am. Soc. Mass Spectrom. 2(4): 336–48.

Rainer, M. and G. K. Bonn. (2015). Enrichment of phosphorylated peptides and proteins by selective precipitation methods. Bioanalysis 7(2): 243–52. https://doi.org/10.4155/bio.14.281.

Seng, P., M. Drancourt, F. Gouriet, B. L. Scola, P. E. Fournier, J. M. Rolain et al. (2009). Ongoing revolution in bacteriology: Routine identification of bacteria by matrix-assisted laser desorption ionization time-of-flight mass spectrometry. Clin. Infect. Dis. 49(4): 543–51. https://doi.org/10.1086/600885.

Shah, H. N. and S. E. Gharbia. (2010). Mass Spectrometry for Microbial Proteomics. John Wiley & Sons, Ltd. Chichester, West Sussex.

Singh, A. K., R. K. Pandey, J. L. Siqueira-Neto, Y. J. Kwon, L. H. Freitas-Junior, C. Shaha et al. (2015). Proteomic-based approach to gain insight into reprogramming of thp-1 cells exposed to *Leishmania donovani* over an early temporal window. Infect. Immun. 83(5): 1853–68. https://doi.org/10.1128/IAI.02833–14.

Singh, N. and S. Sundar. (2017). Integrating genomics and proteomics permits identification of immunodominant antigens associated with drug resistance in human visceral leishmaniasis in India. Exp. Parasitol. 176(May): 30–45. https://doi.org/10.1016/j.exppara.2017.02.019.

Singh, O. P. (2012). Analysis of total urine proteins: Towards a non-invasive approach for diagnosis of visceral leishmaniasis. J. Mol. Biomark. Diagn. 03(04). https://doi.org/10.4172/2155–9929.1000131.

Singhal, N., M. Kumar and J. S. Virdi. (2016). MALDI-TOF MS in clinical parasitology: Applications, constraints and prospects. Parasitology 143(12): 1491–1500. https://doi.org/10.1017/S0031182016001189.

Siuzdak, G. (2006). The Expanding Role of Mass Spectrometry in Biotechnology. MCC Press. San Diego, California.

Sodré, C. L., A. D. Chapeaurouge, D. E. Kalume, L. M. Lima, J. Perales and O. Fernandes. (2009). Proteomic map of *Trypanosoma cruzi* CL Brener: The reference strain of the genome project. Arch. Microbiol. 191(2): 177–84. https://doi.org/10.1007/s00203–008–0439–6.

Switzar, L., M. Giera and W. M. A. Niessen. (2013). Protein digestion: an overview of the available techniques and recent developments. J. Proteome Res. 12(3): 1067–77. https://doi.org/10.1021/pr301201x.

Terán, L. C., M. Distefano, B. Bellich, S. Petrosino, P. Bertoncin, P. Cescutti et al. (2020). Proteomic studies of the biofilm matrix including outer membrane vesicles of *Burkholderia multivorans* c1576, a strain of clinical importance for cystic fibrosis. Microorganisms 8(11): 1826. https://doi.org/10.3390/microorganisms8111826.

Théry, C., S. Amigorena, G. Raposo and A. Clayton. (2006). Isolation and characterization of exosomes from cell culture supernatants and biological fluids. Curr. Protoc. Cell. Biol. 30(1). https://doi.org/10.1002/0471143030.cb0322s30.

Thézénas, M. L., H. Huang, M. Njie, A. Ramaprasad, D. C. Nwakanma, R. Fischer et al. (2013). PfHPRT: A new biomarker candidate of acute *Plasmodium falciparum* infection. J. Proteome Res. 12(3): 1211–22. https://doi.org/10.1021/pr300858g.

Ujang, J. A., S. H. Kwan, M. N. Ismail, B. H. Lim, R. Noordin and N. Othman. (2016). Proteome analysis of excretory-secretory proteins of *Entamoeba histolytica* HM1:IMSS via LC-ESI-MS/MS and LC-MALDI-TOF/TOF. Clin. Proteom. 13(1): 1–10. https://doi.org/10.1186/s12014–016–9135–8.

Venter, A., P. E. Sojka and R. G. Cooks. (2006). Droplet dynamics and ionization mechanisms in desorption electrospray ionization mass spectrometry. Anal. Chem. 78(24): 8549–55. https://doi.org/10.1021/ac0615807.

Verissimo da Costa, G. C., L. M. S. Lery, M. L. Silva, H. Moura, R. H. S. Peralta, W. M. A. Krüger et al. (2013). The identification and characterization of epitopes in the 30–34 kDa *Trypanosoma cruzi* proteins recognized by antibodies in the serum samples of chagasic patients. J. Proteom. 80(March): 34–42. https://doi.org/10.1016/j.jprot.2012.11.001.

Wagner, G., L. E. Yamanaka, H. Moura, D. D. Lückemeyer, A. D. Schlindwein, P. H. Stoco et al. (2013). The *Trypanosoma rangeli* trypomastigote surfaceome reveals novel proteins and targets for specific diagnosis. J. Proteom. 82(April): 52–63. https://doi.org/10.1016/j.jprot.2013.02.011.

Walker, J. M. (2002). SDS polyacrylamide gel electrophoresis of proteins. In The Protein Protocols Handbook, 61–67. Humana Press Inc. Totowa, New Jersey.

Wang, G., G. Zhao, X. Chao, L. Xie and H. Wang. (2020a). The characteristic of virulence, biofilm and antibiotic resistance of *Klebsiella pneumoniae*. Int. J. Environ. Res. Public Health 17(17): 6278. https://doi.org/10.3390/ijerph17176278.

Wang, H., O. H. Cissé, T. Bolig, S. K. Drake, Y. Chen, J. R. Strich et al. (2020b). A phylogeny-informed proteomics approach for species identification within the *Burkholderia cepacia* complex. J. Clin. Microbiol. 58(11). https://doi.org/10.1128/JCM.01741-20.

Wang, J., J. Wang, Y. Wang, P. Sun, X. Zou, L. Ren et al. (2019c). Protein expression profiles in methicillin-resistant *Staphylococcus aureus* (MRSA) under effects of subminimal inhibitory concentrations of imipenem. FEMS Microbiol. Lett. 366(15). https://doi.org/10.1093/femsle/fnz195.

Wang, Y., N. Jiang, B. Wang, H. Tao, X. Zhang, Q. Guan et al. (2020d). Integrated transcriptomic and proteomic analyses reveal the role of NprR in *Bacillus anthracis* extracellular protease expression regulation and oxidative stress responses. Front. Microbiol. 11(12). https://doi.org/10.3389/fmicb.2020.590851.

Wareth, G., M. W. Pletz, H. Neubauer and J. Murugaiyan. (2020). Proteomics of *Brucella*: Technologies and their applications for basic research and medical microbiology. Microorganisms 8(5): 766. https://doi.org/10.3390/microorganisms8050766.

Washburn, M. P., D. Wolters and J. R. Yates III. (2001). Large-scale analysis of the yeast proteome by multidimensional protein identification technology. Nat. Biotechnol. 19(3): 242–47. http://biotech.nature.com.

Washburn, M. P., R. Ulaszek, C. Deciu, D. M. Schieltz and J. R. Yates. (2002). Analysis of quantitative proteomic data generated via multidimensional protein identification technology. Anal. Chem. 74(7): 1650–57. https://doi.org/10.1021/ac0157041.

Wiese, S., K. A. Reidegeld, H. E. Meyer and B. Warscheid. (2007). Protein labeling by ITRAQ: A new tool for quantitative mass spectrometry in proteome research. Proteomics 7(3): 340–50. https://doi.org/10.1002/pmic.200600422.

Wilkins, M. R., J. C. Sanchez, A. A. Gooley, R. D. Appel, I. Humphery-Smith, D. F. Hochstrasser et al. (1996). Progress with proteome projects: Why all proteins expressed by a genome should be identified and how to do it. Biotechnol. Genet. Eng. Rev. 13(1): 19–50. https://doi.org/10.1080/02648725.1996.10647923.

Wu, C. C. and M. J. Maccoss. (2002). Shotgun proteomics: Tools for the analysis of complex biological systems. Curr. Opin. Pharmacol. 4(3): 242–50.

Wu, Y. and A. Craig. (2006). Comparative proteomic analysis of metabolically labelled proteins from *Plasmodium falciparum* isolates with different adhesion properties. Malar. J. 5(1): 1–13. https://doi.org/10.1186/1475-2875-5-67.

Wuhrer, M., A. M. Deelder and Y. E. M. Van Der Burgt. (2011). Mass spectrometric glycan rearrangements. Mass Spectrom. Rev. 30(4): 664–80. https://doi.org/10.1002/mas.20337.

Yadav, S. C., R. Kumar, J. Kumar, M. Singh, B. C. Bera, R. Kumar et al. (2017). Antigenic characterization of 52–55 KDa protein isolated from *Trypanosoma evansi* and its application in detection of equine trypanosomosis. Vet. Sci. Res. J. 114(October): 455–60. https://doi.org/10.1016/j.rvsc.2017.07.034.

Yamashita, M. and J. B. Fenn. (1984). Negative ion production with the electrospray ion source. Am. J. Phys. Chem. 88(20): 4671–75. https://pubs.acs.org/sharingguidelines.

Yamashita, M. and J. B. Fenn. (1984). Electrospray ion source. another variation on the free-jet theme. Am. J. Phys. Chem. 88(20): 4451–59. https://pubs.acs.org/sharingguidelines.

Yeng, C., E. Osman, Z. Mohamed and R. Noordin. (2010). Detection of immunogenic parasite and host-specific proteins in the sera of active and chronic individuals infected with *Toxoplasma gondii*. Electrophoresis 31(23-24): 3843–49. https://doi.org/10.1002/elps.201000038.

Yu, Y. Q., M. Gilar, P. J. Lee, E. S. P. Bouvier and J. C. Gebler. (2003). Enzyme-friendly, mass spectrometry-compatible surfactant for in-solution enzymatic digestion of proteins. Anal. Chem. 75(21): 6023–28. https://doi.org/10.1021/ac0346196.

Zarean, M., S. Maraghi, H. Hajjaran, M. Mohebali, M. H. Feiz-Hadad and M. A. Assarehzadegan. (2015). Comparison of proteome profiling of two sensitive and resistant field iranian isolates of *Leishmania major* to glucantime® by 2-dimensional electrophoresis. Iran. J. Parasitol. 10(1): 19–19. http://ijpa.tums.ac.ir.

Zhang, J., L. Xin, B. Shan, W. Chen, M. Xie, D. Yuen et al. (2012). PEAKS DB: *de novo* sequencing assisted database search for sensitive and accurate peptide identification. Mol. Cell. Proteom. 11(4): M111.010587. https://doi.org/10.1074/mcp.M111.010587.

Zhou, C. X., X. Q. Zhu, H. M. Elsheikha, S. He, Q. Li, D. H. Zhou et al. (2016). Global ITRAQ-based proteomic profiling of *Toxoplasma gondii* oocysts during sporulation. J. Proteom. 148(October): 12–19. https://doi.org/10.1016/j.jprot.2016.07.010.

Zhou, D. H., F. R. Zhao, A. J. Nisbet, M. J. Xu, H. Q. Song, R. Q. Lin et al. (2014). Comparative proteomic analysis of different *Toxoplasma gondii* genotypes by two-dimensional fluorescence difference gel electrophoresis combined with mass spectrometry. Electrophoresis 35(4): 533–45. https://doi.org/10.1002/elps.201300044.

Zhu, W., J. W. Smith and C. M. Huang. (2010). Mass spectrometry-based label-free quantitative proteomics. J. Biomed. Biotechnol. 2010. https://doi.org/10.1155/2010/840518.

Zilberstein, D. (2015). Proteomic analysis of posttranslational modifications using ITRAQ in *Leishmania*. Methods Mol. Biol. 1201: 261–68. https://doi.org/10.1007/978–1–4939–1438–8_16.

Chapter 8

Methods for Multiplex Real-Time PCR Melting Curve Assays for Pathogen Detection

Prashant Singh* and Frank J. Velez

Introduction

Initially, melt curve analysis served to check the specificity and presence of primer-dimer artifacts in an intercalating dye-based real-time PCR reaction. However, with the diversification of real-time PCR applications, melt curve-based multiplex real-time PCR assays were proposed. Multiplex real-time PCR melting curve assays are now commonly used to detect multiple gene targets in a single PCR reaction and are an alternative to dual-labeled probe-based multiplex real-time PCR assays. In multiplex real-time PCR melting curve assays, after completion of the amplification cycles, all amplicons generated in the PCR reaction are bound to an intercalating dye and emit maximum fluorescence. A melt curve is then performed, wherein amplified PCR products are gradually heated. This gradual heating process results in the denaturation of the amplicons. Depending on the GC content and secondary structures, each amplicon denatures at a specific temperature. The denaturation at specific temperature results in the dissociation of the intercalating dye, resulting in a decrease in the fluorescence signal, which is recorded with a sequential increase (i.e., 0.02–3°C/s) in the temperature. A melt curve is plotted using the decrease in the fluorescence signal value (negative first derivative of the fluorescence) versus an increase in temperature (–df/dT). A single amplicon in a PCR reaction generates a melt curve with one peak, whereas a multiplex PCR reaction with multiple amplicons

Department of Nutrition and Integrative Physiology, Florida State University, Tallahassee, FL 32306.
* Corresponding author: psingh2@fsu.edu

generates a melt curve with multiple peaks, where each peak corresponds to a specific amplicon.

Melting curve multiplex assays can be used for the development of real-time PCR-based diagnostic assays with various applications, e.g., foodborne pathogen detection (Forghani et al. 2016, Liu et al. 2018a, 2018b, Singh et al. 2019, Singh and Mustapha 2014, 2015), identification of antibiotic resistance genes (Geyer and Hanson 2014, Monteiro et al. 2012, Singh and Mustapha 2014), detection of viruses (Yeh et al. 2004) and food authentication (Sharma et al. 2020). Our research group has extensively worked on the standardizing of the multiplex melting curve and high-resolution melting real-time PCR assays. In this chapter, we will discuss important factors that should be taken into consideration for the standardization of these assays.

Primer Design

Primer design is the first and foremost step for successfully standardizing a multiplex real-time PCR melting curve assay. Currently, several free as well as licensed programs are available for designing PCR primers. The Primer3 software (Untergasser et al. 2012) is one of the most user-friendly and freely available software that can be used for designing primers for these assays. When designing primers for a melting curve real-time PCR assay, the following factors are recommended:

(1) Designing multiple primers that amplify the same target: Designing three to five primer-pairs for the amplification of each gene target facilitates flexibility in selecting the best primer suitable for multiplexing. An attempt should be made to design primers generating amplicons T_m in the range of 70–87°C. This can be achieved by using the "Product Tm" function of Primer3 software. Additionally, primer pairs with different primer-binding sites and generating amplicons with various GC content should be designed.

(2) Amplicon size: PCR products in the size range of 70–250 bp are more suitable for a multiplex melting curve assay. Amplicons shorter than 60 bp generate melt peaks that can be smaller in height (–df/dT) and are prone to false-positive (high primer concentration) and false-negative (low primer concentration) results. Additionally, in the case when results of a PCR reaction with a small amplicon size need to be validated by either agarose gel electrophoresis or Sanger sequencing, these shorter amplicons are challenging to work with. On the contrary, amplicons longer than 300 bp may have a lower amplification efficiency and possess more than one melt domain (due to secondary structures), leading to the dissociation of the same product more than one time, which can result in defects in the final melt curve data.

(3) NCBI/Primer-BLAST tool: The specificity of the designed PCR primers must be tested using the NCBI/Primer-BLAST tool. Degenerated bases can be introduced in the primer pair to accommodate gene variants.

(4) Selection of amplicon T_m estimation tool: Bioinformatics tools can be used to estimate the melting temperature of amplicons. Several bioinformatics tools are available for calculating the T_m of the amplicon. Based on the prediction model used by the program, the predicted T_m values for the same amplicon can significantly vary when the same amplicon sequence is analyzed by multiple bioinformatics tools. An additional challenge with the estimation of the melting temperature of amplicons apart from the GC content of the amplicons is that the Tm values are also affected by the composition of the real-time PCR master mix i.e., intercalating dye, $MgCl_2$ concentration and other additives. All these factors result in variations in the estimated and experimentally obtained amplicon Tm values. Based on our experience, BioEdit (Hall 1999) is a reliable tool that can be used for calculating Tm of the amplicons at different $MgCl_2$ concentrations.

Master Mix

Although a large number of SYBR Green dye-based multiplex real-time PCR melting curve assays have been previously reported, this dye has some limitations. For instance, when the SYBR Green dye is used at a higher concentration, which is preferred for melting curve assays, it can inhibit PCR amplification (Nath et al. 2000). Moreover, the degradation product of SYBR Green generated during a denaturation step of the PCR cycle has been reported to be inhibitory to the PCR reaction (Karsai et al. 2002). Besides, SYBR Green dye shows preferential binding to PCR amplicon with higher T_m or higher GC content in a multiplex reaction. Due to this preferential binding of SYBR Green dye, out of multiple targets amplified in a multiplex real-time PCR reaction, only a limited number of amplicons can be detected by the melting curve assay using SYBR Green dye (Forghani et al. 2016, Giglio et al. 2003, Singh and Mustapha 2014). Further, the SYBR Green has been reported to show the dye-jumping phenomenon resulting in a variation in the melting behavior of the same amplicon (Reed et al. 2007).

Saturating intercalating dyes are an alternative to SYBR Green dye-based master mixes. Saturating dyes are a class of intercalating dyes that can be used at a much higher concentration without inhibiting the PCR reaction, e.g. LCGreen (Idaho Technology Inc., Salt Lake City, UT), Syto9 (Invitrogen, Carlsbad, CA), and EvaGreen (Biotum, Hayward, CA). These dyes do not show preferential intercalation and bind equally to all the amplicons, completely saturating them, which results in the generation of a melt curve of much higher resolution. Multiplexing using high-resolution dye-based master mixes, such as the Meltdoctor HRM master mix, LightCycler 480 High-Resolution Melting Master Mix, or LCGREEN, facilitates easier assay standardizing with assay with a greater number of multiplex targets (Monis et al. 2005). In the past, our research group has extensively worked with Meltdoctor HRM master mix and standardized 4–6 target multiplex melting curve real-time PCR assays (Forghani et al. 2016, Singh et al. 2016, 2019, Singh and Mustapha 2014).

Assay Standardization

The first step toward developing a multiplex melting curve assay is the standardization of the PCR amplification conditions for each primer pair. Primer pairs specifically amplify the target can be used, and primer-pair with non-specific amplicons can be discarded. In the next step, the T_m of each amplicon generated in the real-time PCR reaction in singleplex format can be estimated (Figure 1). Based on the obtained T_m values of the amplicons, a multiplex PCR reaction can be standardized in a stepwise manner. PCR primers generating low T_m (e.g., 70°C) amplicons should first be tested for their ability to work in a multiplex reaction with primer pairs of another gene target generating amplicons with T_m values 2–3°C higher. Other gene targets with increasingly higher T_m are subsequently tested in a stepwise manner (Figure 2). Several primer pairs can be designed for the amplification of each gene target, out of which more than one primer pair may work for the multiplex assay. A standard curve for those primers can be constructed with a serially diluted DNA sample, which can be used to calculate the PCR reaction efficiency, and a primer pair with higher PCR amplification efficiency can be chosen. Although a high amplification efficiency in a singleplex reaction is not proof of equally high efficiency in a multiplex reaction, it can be considered a good elimination criterion. The final set of primer pairs for a multiplex assay can be selected based on the following criteria: (1) at least a 2–3°C melting temperature difference between neighboring peaks; (2) a larger melt peak formed on the melt curve plot; (3) high PCR amplification efficiency in the singleplex reaction, and (4) smaller amplicon size (Singh et al. 2016; Singh and Mustapha 2014).

Optimization of the primer and $MgCl_2$ concentrations is vital for any PCR reaction. However, in a multiplex melting curve assay, this step plays additional roles. In some PCR reactions, the melt peak height is dependent on the primer concentration. A higher primer concentration of one primer-pair in the multiplex assay can result in the formation of a larger melt peak, making all other peaks appear smaller. On the other hand, a lower primer concentration will result in the formation of a smaller melt peak, which might look like noise on the melt peak plot. Melt

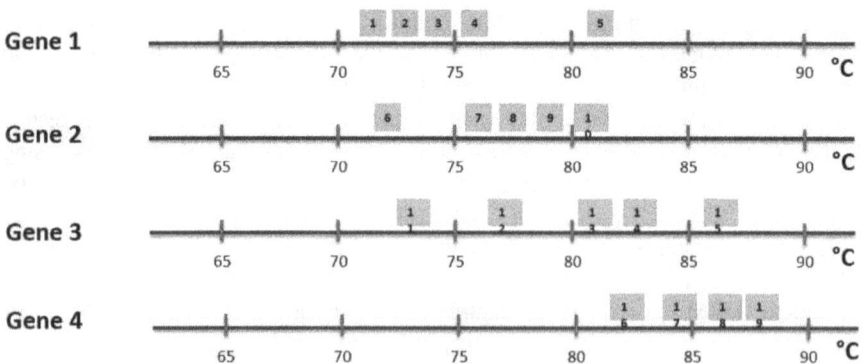

Figure 1. Representation of the actual T_m values of amplicons generated in a real-time PCR reaction in singleplex format by different primer pairs designed for the amplification of a gene.

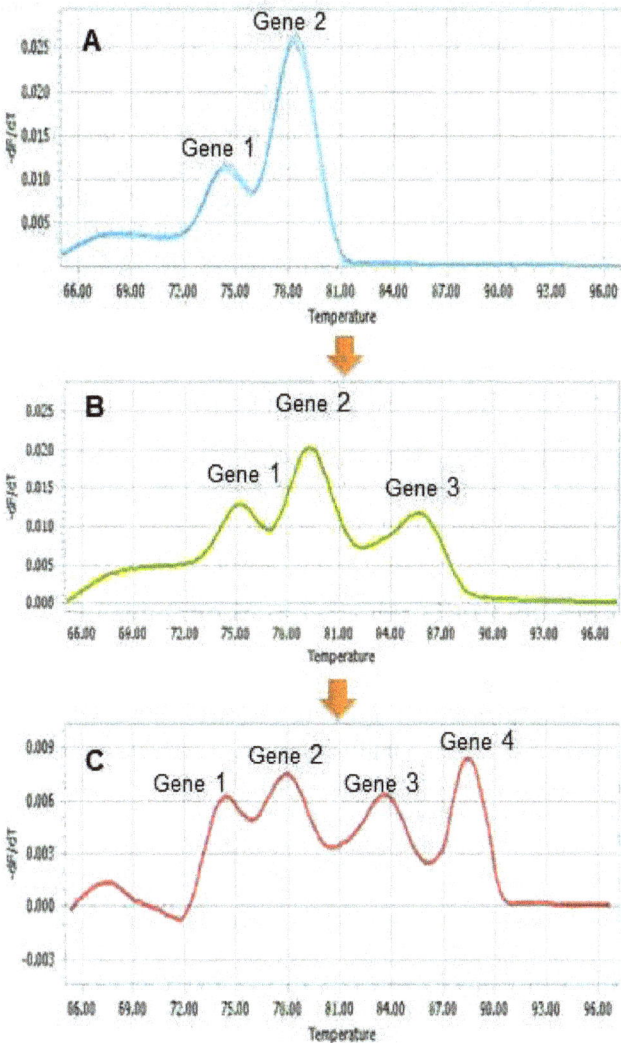

Figure 2. Standardization of multiplex real-time PCR melting curve assays. The primer pairs tested for multiplexing with increasing T_m values. Primer pairs for gene one that generated amplicons of the lowest T_m value were tested for multiplex capabilities with gene two primer pairs followed by genes 3 and 4 primer pairs.

peak height is dependent on several factors, and primer concentration is one factor that can be optimized. Magnesium concentration is another crucial factor for the standardization of any multiplex assay. Real-time PCR master mixes are already optimized for $MgCl_2$ concentration to maintain reproducibility between experiments. However, additional $MgCl_2$ can be added to the PCR reaction. Based on data generated by our research group, increasing $MgCl_2$ concentration has been shown to improve separation between melting peaks and facilitate assay standardization (Sharma et al. 2020).

The total amount of template DNA used in a PCR reaction is another essential factor. PCR assays are generally standardized using a fixed amount of DNA (10–20 ng per reaction). However, the DNA concentration in different samples can greatly vary, and these values are especially higher for DNA isolated from an enriched food sample, i.e., enriched ground beef or enriched ground poultry. A DNA sample isolated from ground beef samples that have been enriched for 12 hours can be in the range of 500–800 ng/µl. Adding an excessive amount of DNA to a PCR reaction can completely inhibit the Taq polymerase enzyme, subsequently inhibiting the PCR amplification. Based on our experience, 50–100 ng of DNA can be added to a real-time PCR reaction. Nevertheless, this value can vary based on each real-time master mix.

Internal Amplification Control (IAC)

An IAC is a separate PCR target that is amplified in the same PCR reaction tube. It is considered the most crucial part of a PCR-based diagnostic assay. It helps to avoid any false-negative PCR results due to reaction failure. Primers targeting 16S rDNA, plasmid DNA, phage DNA, and 16S rRNA gene of gammaproteobacteria are commonly used as IAC. Alternatively, a single-stranded oligonucleotide can be designed and employed as an IAC in a multiplex real-time PCR assay. This oligonucleotide can be co-amplified by one of the primer pairs of a multiplex assay and, in the process, can generate an amplicon, whose melt peak (T_m) either fits an empty area in the melt curve plot or can be detected using a specific dual-labeled probe (Singh et al. 2019, Singh and Mustapha 2013). The advantage of using a single-stranded oligonucleotide-based IAC is that it is much easier to standardize and cheaper to use when compared to other commonly used approaches to add IAC in the PCR reaction. The following points can be considered while designing the IAC using this approach:

(1) Designing IAC oligonucleotide: Designing an IAC oligonucleotide should be performed after the standardization of the multiplex assay is complete. Usually, PCR amplicon T_m varies in the range of 72–85°C depending on the type of master mix or intercalating dye used. In the case of a highly multiplexed assay, a single-stranded IAC oligonucleotide can be designed with either a low or high GC content, which will eventually generate an amplicon of low T_m (68–70°C) or high T_m (85–87°C) value. This approach facilitates maximum space for the targets on the melt curve plot for multiplexing a higher number of targets. Alternatively, for a multiplex PCR with fewer targets, an IAC oligonucleotide can be designed to target any empty space left on the melt curve. An easier way of designing an IAC oligonucleotide with the desired T_m value is to select an amplicon with a known T_m value. Out of the multiple primers tested for developing a multiplex assay, any primer generating an amplicon of the desired T_m can be modified for this purpose.

(2) Primer-binding site: Following the selection of amplicon with desired amplicon T_m, primer-binding sites can be added to the oligonucleotide. Any primer pair with

4-10 bp
overhang

4-10 bp
overhang

| Forward primer sequence | DNA sequence with known T_m | Reverse complement of |

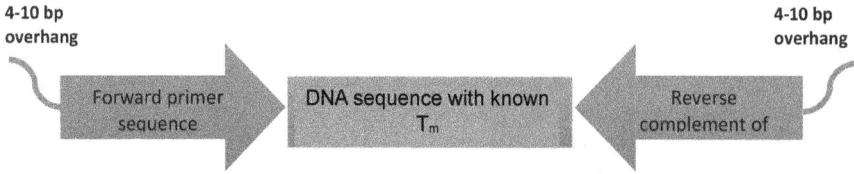

Figure 3. Schematic representation of IAC design. The DNA sequence of the desired T_m is flanked by the forward primer binding and reverse primer binding sites. The primer-binding sites are followed by 4–10 bp overhangs, which facilitate proper primer hybridization.

a high amplification efficiency can be added to the oligonucleotide. A four to ten-base pair overhang before the primer-binding site in the designed oligonucleotide is recommended (Figure 3). This approach to designing IACs reduces the total number of primer-pair used for the multiplex assay, thus reducing the complexity of the assay.

(3) IAC concentration: The optimum concentration of IAC oligonucleotides in the multiplex assay should be carefully standardized. Primer pairs amplifying a single-stranded IAC oligonucleotide in a multiplex reaction amplify at a high amplification efficiency (> 100%). If an IAC oligonucleotide is added at a higher concentration in a PCR reaction (i.e., 5–10 ng), it will amplify much faster compared to any other amplicons in the PCR reaction, consuming all the PCR reagents and forming a higher peak on the melt curve. If the IAC is co-amplified using one of the target gene primer-pair, the concentration of IAC oligonucleotide should be kept as low as possible to prevent any possible competition for primers, facilitating the preferential amplification of the target genes.

Depending on the complexity of the multiplex assay, we recommend IACs oligonucleotide concentration range of 10–100 fg per 10 µL of reaction volume. Another way to reduce the high amplification efficiency of an IAC is to introduce 2–3 bp variations in the central region of the primer-binding sites of the IAC oligonucleotides. In our experience, the working solution of these oligonucleotides tends to degrade during long storage, necessitating the use of higher amounts. Therefore, working with freshly dissolved IAC oligonucleotides helps to avoid any inter-assay variations (Singh et al. 2016, 2019, Singh and Mustapha 2013).

Real-Time PCR Instrument and Analysis Software

There is a wide range of real-time PCR instruments presently available, and each instrument has its own set of capabilities and limitations. The data collection rate during the melt curve analysis step is one of the most important factors for standardizing a highly multiplexed melt curve assay. Different instruments come with different data collection rates during melt curve analysis, e.g., ABI StepOnePlus Real-Time PCR System: 0.1°C/sec, Roche LightCycler96: 0.04°C/sec, Bio-Rad CFX Connect Real-Time PCR Detection System: 0.1°C/sec, and Rotor-Gene Real-

Time PCR: 0.02°C/sec. More data collected during the melting step (25 reading/°C) generates much richer data, leading to a melt curve of higher resolution and facilitating the separation of two amplicons with close T_m values. This allows for the multiplexing of a higher number of targets.

Most real-time PCR-based experiments are performed in a singleplex format using a high-fidelity master mix, which does not require a touchdown PCR amplification. However, the touchdown capabilities in real-time PCR instrument is a useful feature for standardizing or performing multiplex melt curve assays. Only a limited number of instruments have touchdown PCR capabilities. When performing a highly multiplexed melting curve real-time PCR assay, a touchdown PCR protocol can generate more specific amplicons, resulting in an assay with higher specificity.

The data collection time is another important aspect of the real-time PCR instrument. Although it does not directly influence the assay, the data collection time is directly related to the total time required by the instrument for the completion of the assay. Each real-time PCR instrument manufacturing company uses its proprietary technology for recording the fluorescent data generated in the melt curve. Based on the technology used by the instrument, the data collection time at the lowest melting ramp rate can vary from 10 minutes to 2 hours, which has an impact on assay completion.

Besides real-time PCR hardware specifications and capabilities, the data analysis software further plays a vital role in analyzing the data generated by a multiplex melting curve assay. The instrument software analyzes minute variations in the fluorescence data and converts them into melt peaks. Real-time PCR software for analyzing dual-labeled probe-based multiplex assays is more evolved and automated. Hence, each target is automatically identified and quantified. However, for multiplex melting curve assays, each peak needs to be manually analyzed for each sample, which is a very time-consuming process. Computational software, such as MATLAB® and ORIGIN, can also be used for analyzing melt curve data, but they require a user license, which is expensive. To bridge this gap, a software tool needs to be developed that can analyze the melt curve data, automatically annotate each peak based on the standard values, and generate a report for the presence and absence of targets in the sample. Therefore, instrument selection based on hardware and software capabilities is a very crucial factor for standardizing as well as for performing a real-time melting curve assay.

Multiplex real-time melting curve assays are useful and are one of the most economical real-time PCR-based assays. With careful assay design, up to five to six target multiplex melting curve assays can easily be standardized without any overlapping peaks and can be performed on a basic one-channel real-time PCR machine. A higher number of targets can be multiplexed using two-dimensional melting curve assays. To get a better separation of melt peaks, the melting behavior of amplicons generated in the multiplex assay can also be manipulated by incorporating locked nucleic acid bases in the oligonucleotides. Future researchers should investigate the development of an open-source analytical software tool that can be used for batch analysis of data from 96 well plates melt curve data into a report.

References

Forghani, F., P. Singh, K. -H. Seo and D. -H. Oh. (2016). A novel pentaplex real-time (RT)- PCR high resolution melt curve assay for simultaneous detection of emetic and enterotoxin producing *Bacillus cereus* in food. Food Control 60: 560–568. https://doi.org/10.1016/j.foodcont.2015.08.030

Geyer, C. N. and N. D. Hanson. (2014). Multiplex high-resolution melting analysis as a diagnostic tool for detection of plasmid-mediated AmpC β-lactamase genes. Journal of Clinical Microbiology 52(4): 1262–1265. https://doi.org/10.1128/JCM.00214–14.

Giglio, S., P. T. Monis and C. P. Saint. (2003). Demonstration of preferential binding of SYBR Green I to specific DNA fragments in real-time multiplex PCR. Nucleic Acids Research 31(22): e136. https://doi.org/10.1093/nar/gng135.

Hall, T. (1999). BioEdit: A user-friendly biological sequence alignment editor and analysis program for Windows 95/98/NT. Nucleic Acids Symposium Series 41: 95–98.

Karsai, A., S. Müller, S. Platz and M. -T. Hauser. (2002). Evaluation of a Homemade SYBR® Green I reaction mixture for real-time pcr quantification of gene expression. BioTechniques 32(4): 790–796. https://doi.org/10.2144/02324st05.

Liu, Y., P. Singh and A. Mustapha. (2018a). High-resolution melt curve PCR assay for specific detection of *E. coli* O157:H7 in beef. Food Control 86: 275–282. https://doi.org/10.1016/j.foodcont.2017.11.025.

Liu, Y., P. Singh and A. Mustapha. (2018b). Multiplex high resolution melt-curve real-time PCR assay for reliable detection of Salmonella. Food Control 91: 225–230. https://doi.org/10.1016/j.foodcont.2018.03.043.

Monis, P. T., S. Giglio and C. P. Saint. (2005). Comparison of SYTO9 and SYBR Green I for real-time polymerase chain reaction and investigation of the effect of dye concentration on amplification and DNA melting curve analysis. Analytical Biochemistry 340(1): 24–34. https://doi.org/10.1016/j.ab.2005.01.046.

Monteiro, J., R. H. Widen, A. C. C. Pignatari, C. Kubasek and S. Silbert. (2012). Rapid detection of carbapenemase genes by multiplex real-time PCR. Journal of Antimicrobial Chemotherapy 67(4): 906–909. https://doi.org/10.1093/jac/dkr563.

Nath, K., J. W. Sarosy, J. Hahn and C. J. Di Como. (2000). Effects of ethidium bromide and SYBR® Green I on different polymerase chain reaction systems. Journal of Biochemical and Biophysical Methods 42(1): 15–29. https://doi.org/10.1016/S0165–022X(99)00033–0.

Reed, G. H., J. O. Kent and C. T. Wittwer. (2007). High-resolution DNA melting analysis for simple and efficient molecular diagnostics. Pharmacogenomics 8(6): 597–608. https://doi.org/10.2217/14622416.8.6.597.

Sharma, L., E. Watts and P. Singh. (2020). High resolution real-time PCR melting curve assay for identification of top five Penaeidae shrimp species. LWT 133: 109983. https://doi.org/10.1016/j.lwt.2020.109983.

Singh, P., Y. Liu, J. M. Bosilevac and A. Mustapha. (2019). Detection of Shiga toxin-producing Escherichia coli, stx1, stx2 and Salmonella by two high resolution melt curve multiplex real-time PCR. Food Control 96: 251–259. https://doi.org/10.1016/j.foodcont.2018.09.024.

Singh, P. and A. Mustapha. (2013). Multiplex TaqMan® detection of pathogenic and multi-drug resistant Salmonella. International Journal of Food Microbiology 166(2): 213–218. https://doi.org/10.1016/j.ijfoodmicro.2013.07.023.

Singh, P. and A. Mustapha. (2014). Development of a real-time PCR melt curve assay for simultaneous detection of virulent and antibiotic resistant Salmonella. Food Microbiology 44: 6–14. https://doi.org/10.1016/j.fm.2014.04.014.

Singh, P. and A. Mustapha. (2015). Multiplex real-time PCR assays for detection of eight Shiga toxin-producing Escherichia coli in food samples by melting curve analysis. International Journal of Food Microbiology 215: 101–108. https://doi.org/10.1016/j.ijfoodmicro.2015.08.022.

Singh, P., Y. Pfeifer and A. Mustapha. (2016). Multiplex real-time PCR assay for the detection of extended-spectrum β-lactamase and carbapenemase genes using melting curve analysis. Journal of Microbiological Methods 124: 72–78. https://doi.org/10.1016/j.mimet.2016.03.014.

Untergasser, A., I. Cutcutache, T. Koressaar, J. Ye, B. C. Faircloth, M. Remm et al. (2012). Primer3—new capabilities and interfaces. Nucleic Acids Research 40(15): e115–e115.

Yeh, S. -H., C. -Y. Tsai, J. -H. Kao, C. -J. Liu, T. -J. Kuo, M. -W. Lin et al. (2004). Quantification and genotyping of hepatitis B virus in a single reaction by real-time PCR and melting curve analysis. Journal of Hepatology 41(4): 659–666. https://doi.org/10.1016/j.jhep.2004.06.031.

Chapter 9

Persistence and Biofilm Formation of Foodborne Bacterial Pathogens on Fresh Produce and Equipment Surfaces

Hsin-Bai Yin[#] and Jitendra Patel*

Introduction

Consumption of fresh fruit and vegetables has been encouraged by many countries and government health agencies as they are considered an as healthy and balanced diet. As a major ingredient of leafy salads, the U.S. per capita annual consumption of lettuce has increased to 12.0 kg in the last decade (ERS-USDA 2018). Moreover, the yearly sale of bagged salads has increased in the U.S., reaching $3.7 billion in 2015 (Cook 2016), which represents an important change in consumers' behavior toward ready-to-eat products. However, fruits and vegetables, especially salad mix and leafy greens that are often consumed raw or only minimally processed, are increasingly being recognized as important vehicles for transmission of foodborne bacterial pathogens, such as enterohemorrhagic *Escherichia coli*, *Salmonella enterica*, and *Listeria monocytogenes* (Berger et al. 2010, CDC 2011).

During the last two decades, the number, severity, and distribution of outbreaks associated with the consumption of fresh fruits and vegetables contaminated with foodborne bacterial pathogens have attracted the attention of farmers, consumers, scientists, and the food industry (Martinez-Vaz et al. 2014). According to data reported to the U.S. Centers for Disease Control and Prevention's Foodborne Disease Outbreak Surveillance System from 1998 and 2013, there were 972 raw produce-associated outbreaks reported, which accounted for 34,674 illnesses, 2,315 hospitalizations, and 72 deaths in the U.S. (Bennett et al. 2018). Specific types of

U.S. Department of Agriculture, Environmental and Food Safety Microbiology Laboratory, Beltsville, MD 20705, USA.

[#] Current affiliation: U.S. Food and Drug Administration, Center for Food Safety and Applied Nutrition, Division of Produce Safety, College Park, MD 20740, USA.

* Corresponding author: jitu.patel@usda.gov

fresh foods that have been identified as common sources in fresh produce-associated outbreaks include sprouts, leafy greens such as lettuce and spinach, and fruits and vegetables like melons and tomatoes (Doyle and Erickson 2008, Yaron 2014, CDC 2020). *Salmonella enterica* is more frequent in outbreaks caused by fruits, seeds, and sprouts, whereas *E. coli* O157:H7 is more frequent in leafy greens (Brandl 2006, CDC 2020).

Fresh produce is susceptible to contamination by foodborne bacterial pathogens from diverse sources during field production, storage, transport, packaging, and processing (Barak and Schroeder 2012, Sapers and Doyle 2014). Foodborne bacterial pathogens are more hazardous when they attach and form biofilms on fresh produce and equipment surfaces (Shi and Zhu 2009). Bacteria in biofilms can survive for an extended period on the attached biotic and abiotic surfaces, become resistant to disinfectants such as chlorine, and may cause illness due to contaminated foods (Ibusquiza et al. 2011). As some of the largest outbreaks of foodborne illnesses have been linked to contaminated leafy greens, fresh fruits, and vegetables (Sivapalasingam et al. 2004), understanding the persistence and biofilm formation of foodborne bacterial pathogens is important to improve produce safety and protect public health.

At the pre-harvest level, vegetables could be contaminated by bacterial pathogens through irrigation water, manure soil amendments, and wild animal intrusion (Solomon et al. 2002, Islam et al. 2004). In addition, the plant tissue damaged by insects promotes the internalization of bacterial pathogens through natural wound openings (Brandl 2008). During the colonization of bacterial pathogens on vegetable plants, bacteria can attach, form aggregates, and develop biofilms in order to epiphytically survive in the phyllosphere (Yaron and Römling 2014). Vegetable plants are commonly considered to be harsh environments for foodborne bacterial pathogens; however, the biofilm-forming ability of these pathogens could be a fascinating strategy to gain fitness against the challenging conditions of the plants. Microbial biofilms can be formed on leaves, root surfaces, and within intercellular spaces of plant tissues (Yaron and Römling 2014). Bacteria in biofilms are protected from the plant immune responses and antimicrobial compounds produced by the plants or by indigenous microorganisms (Yaron and Römling 2014). Contamination of fresh produce by foodborne bacterial pathogens at the pre-harvest level could be a serious public health concern as these pathogens could survive on the produce in the field for long periods (Brandl 2006, Kisluk and Yaron 2012). *Salmonella* enterica and *E. coli* O157:H7 were reported to be able to survive on produce leaves for at least 100 days (Islam et al. 2004, Kisluk and Yaron 2012, Kisluk et al. 2013).

At the post-harvest level, bacteria such as *S. enterica*, *E. coli* O157:H7, *L. monocytogenes*, *Staphylococcus aureus*, *Bacillus cereus*, *Clostridium perfringens*, and *Yersinia* spp. have been reported to be present in the fresh produce processing facilities and these bacteria could adhere to the plant tissues where they can form biofilms (Beuchat 2002, Felicio et al. 2015). Contaminated equipment surfaces in food-processing facilities have been frequently found to be responsible for foodborne illness outbreaks associated with the consumption of contaminated fresh and processed food products worldwide (Balaban and Rasooly 2000, Braga et al.

2005, Oulahal et al. 2008). Cross-contamination of food through direct contact with the contaminated surface or contaminated wash water has been considered to be one of the factors in the process of pathogen transmission in the food-processing facility (Allende et al. 2004, Delaquis et al. 2007). Once bacteria reach fresh produce through cross-contamination, they rapidly attach to different parts of plants such as stomata, veins, lenticels, and cut edges, and then persist for longer periods that finally lead to biofilm formation, which are much more complex for antimicrobial treatments to remove them (Warning and Datta 2013). It has been suggested that biofilms might facilitate cross-contamination by harboring pathogens and thus protecting them from cleaning and sanitation operations (Pérez-Rodríguez et al. 2008). Besides the presence of biofilms, the effectiveness of sanitizers for decontaminating produce products could vary based on the types of the vegetables, some intrinsic structures of vegetables could protect bacteria from direct contact with the disinfectants (López-Gálvez et al. 2010).

In this review, we describe the current knowledge on the persistence and biofilm formation of foodborne bacterial pathogens on fresh vegetables and the equipment surfaces at both the pre-harvest level and in the food-processing facilities. To begin with, the biofilm formation processes and the factors that affect bacterial persistence and biofilm formation have been discussed. In the next section, the persistence and biofilm formation on specific vegetables and surface materials are summarized. Finally, recent approaches to develop strategies for preventing and combating biofilms on fresh produce and equipment surfaces are described in the current review.

Biofilm Formation Processes

Biofilm formation is a series of responses by bacteria to the environments, including the initial attachment, microcolony, and extracellular polymeric substances (EPS) production, and finally, the maturation process (Davey and O'Toole 2000) (Figure 1). Biofilm formation at the food-processing facility may be different from the natural ecosystem where nutrients are generally low as compared to the nutrient-rich environment in the food industry. In the fresh produce processing facility, bacteria could exist in liquid food products as planktonic bacteria cells, whereas in solid or viscous food, bacteria can adhere to the surface of food materials, food-processing equipment, and the surface of pipelines. The transition of bacterial cells from planktonic to the sessile state is also triggered by environmental signals. In the food-processing industry, organic materials from food are deposited on the equipment surface, and then biologically active microorganisms are attached to the conditioned surfaces. Finally, bacteria attached to such surfaces resist cleaning and sanitation, initiate growth, and form biofilms (Shi and Zhu 2009).

Attachment

The attachment of bacteria to surfaces begins with a reversible attachment, which often occurs within 5 to 30 seconds (Mittelman 1998). At this stage, bacterial cells are loosely attached to surfaces with the involvement of van der Waals, electrostatic

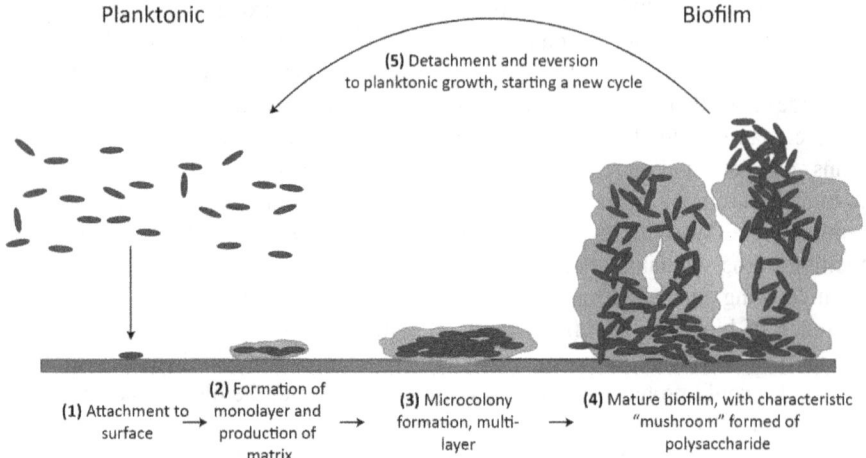

Figure 1. Biofilm formation stages. Biofilm formation on surfaces is a dynamic and complex process influenced by several factors. Factors that are known to play roles in biofilm formations on fresh produce and equipment surfaces include bacterial characteristics, types of fresh produce, equipment surfaces, and environmental factors such as nutrient composition, temperature, pH, and osmotic pressure. Biofilm formation occurs in five stages: attachment, formation of monolayer and microcolony, maturation, and dispersion.

forces, and hydrophobic interactions and are often characterized by polarly attached cells (Hinsa et al. 2003, Caiazza and O'Toole 2004). During the reversible attachment, bacterial cells easily return to the planktonic lifestyle and can be removed by the application of mild shear force. From the stage of reversible attachment to irreversible attachment, the time is as short as several minutes (Palmer et al. 2007). In the stage of irreversible attachments, bacterial cells secrete EPS and enhance cell-to-surface adhesion. The removal of irreversibly attached bacterial cells requires the application of strong shear forces, detergents, surfactants, or heat (Chmielewski and Frank 2003, Armbruster and Parsek 2018). At the irreversible stage, genes responsible for surface protein expression, attachment, and EPS production are activated in response to external stimuli such as population density, stress, or nutrient limitation and the downstream products such as SadB or LapA and EPS proteins assist the adhesion between the cell and surface (Pratt and Kolter 1998, Hinsa et al. 2003, Caiazza and O'Toole 2004). Intracellular second messengers, bis-(3'-5')-cyclic dimeric guanosine monophosphate (c-di-GMP), and (3'-5')-cyclic adenosine monophosphate (cAMP) are released by bacteria, which are involved in the transition from reversible to irreversible bacterial attachment (Ono et al. 2014).

The attachment of microorganisms to surfaces and the subsequent biofilm development are very complex processes and are affected by several variables, including the physicochemical interactions between the contact surfaces and cell-surface properties (Tang et al. 2007). The physical characteristics of solid surfaces in the food-processing industry are critical for biofilm formation; attachment of microorganisms to surfaces occurs mostly on surfaces with rougher conditions (Chae et al. 2006). Stainless steel, Teflon, and other plastics are commonly used for equipment, gaskets, and accessories of instruments and these surfaces become rough or crevice with continuous reuse and form a harborage to protect bacterial from shear forces in the food fluid (Jones et al. 1999, Shi and Zhu 2009).

Microcolony Formation

Following irreversible attachment, cells multiply with the production of biofilm matrix components, such as EPS, and form small aggregates of bacterial called microcolonies. Microcolonies grow via cell proliferation and the production of extracellular polymers. One of the major components of biofilms is EPS, which constitutes about 50–90% of the total organic matter in a biofilm (Saini et al. 2015). Bacterial cells are embedded in EPS composed of polysaccharides, extracellular DNA (eDNA), lipids, and proteins (Flemming et al. 2007). The EPS surrounding the biofilms protects the bacterial cells against various external stresses, such as sanitizers. Inside the biofilms, EPS retains quorum-sensing signaling molecules, extracellular enzymes, and metabolic products, supporting cell-cell communication (Flemming et al. 2010). Quorum sensing occurs mainly in the microcolony formation stage and works in a density-dependent manner that bacteria use autoinducers as signaling molecules (Schauder and Bassler 2001). When the bacterial populations reach a certain threshold level, autoinducers that gather on the outside of the cells regulate the expression of genes related to virulence and biofilm formation (Bordi and de Bentzmann 2011). The N-acyl homoserine lactones and oligopeptides act as autoinducers for Gram-negative and Gram-positive bacteria, respectively.

Maturation

When conditions are suitable for sufficient growth of microcolonies, biofilms start to develop an organized three-dimensional structure called the maturation process. The attachment between the cells-to-surfaces and cells-to-cells, mainly relies on the EPS, in which the colonies could withstand a certain degree of mechanical pressure to prevent shedding from the surfaces. At the food-processing facility, microcolonies in biofilms commonly consist of diverse microbial communities and form relatively complex multispecies biofilms. The successful adaptation of bacteria to changing natural conditions is dependent on their ability to sense and respond to the external environment and modulate gene expression accordingly (Daniels et al. 2004, Yawata et al. 2008). The eDNA released from the bacterial cells is also an important matrix component in biofilm maturation. It has been reported that eDNA is responsible for cellular communication and stabilization of *Pseudomonas aeruginosa* biofilms (Gloag et al. 2013). The mature biofilms are composed of three layers: (1) the inner layer is a regulating film that forms a network structure without completely covering the attached surface; (2) the middle layer is a compact microbial basement membrane; and (3) the outermost surface is inhabited by planktonic cells.

Dispersion

The final stage in the biofilm formation is dispersion, which marks the shedding of the biofilm and the return of sessile cells to the motile form (Hall-Stoodley et al.

2004). In this stage, bacteria inside the biofilms produce enzymes such as alginate lyase in *P. aeruginosa* biofilms, N-acetyl-heparosan lyase for *E. coli* biofilms, and hyaluronidase in *Streptococcus equi* biofilms (Sutherland 1999). These enzymes break the polysaccharides that stabilize the biofilm structure and thereby releasing surface bacteria residing on the top of the biofilm structure. Subsequently, the released bacteria then spread and colonize the new surfaces. Environmental factors including increased shear stress and a lack of nutrient supply could also cause biofilm separation (Sauer et al. 2004). At this stage, microorganisms upregulate the expression of the flagella proteins so that the organisms become motile and bacteria can translocate to a new site for biofilm formation.

Factors Affecting Biofilm Formation

Bacterial Characteristics

Surface properties of bacteria such as flagella, pili, adhesin protein, capsules, surface charge, and hydrophobicity affect the initial steps of cell adhesion (Kumar et al. 1998, Pagedar et al. 2010). The hydrophobicity and surface charge of bacteria are different between bacterial species, bacterial serotypes, or strains, and can change with variations in growth conditions, physiological state of cells, and composition of suspension media (Chavant et al. 2002, Giovannacci et al. 2000). Wang et al. (2013) reported a positive correlation between the cell hydrophobicity of *S. enterica* strains and the biofilm levels formed on polystyrene surface; however, cell hydrophobicity of *L. monocytogenes* and *Campylobacter jejuni* did not affect the biofilm formation of these bacteria on the glass surface (Dykes et al. 2003, Chae et al. 2006).

Bacterial strain variations have been identified to affect biofilm formation on fresh vegetables. Plant-associated bacterial isolates could be phenotypically and phylogenetically different from strains isolated from humans and mammals. Méric et al. (2013) reported that plant-associated *E. coli* isolates displayed higher biofilm and extracellular matrix production than a group of strains isolated from human and other mammalian hosts. A strong association between phenotypes and *E. coli* phylogenetic groups has been observed; strains belonging to phylogroup B1 were more likely to harbor traits indicative of a higher ability to colonize plants, whereas phylogroup A and B2 isolates were mostly of animal origin (Méric et al. 2013). Macarisin et al. (2013) reported that the persistence of *E. coli* O157:H7 on the spinach leaves varied depending on the strain's phenotypic characteristics, specifically the expression of curli. It has been well discussed that curli-producing bacteria could exhibit greater persistence than non-curliated bacteria on produce surfaces (Jeter et al. 2005, Patel et al. 2011b, Saldaña et al. 2011, Macarisin et al. 2012, Macarisin et al. 2013, Macarisin et al. 2014).

Differences in the adhesion of *Salmonella* serotypes including *S. Sofia*, *S. Typhimurium*, *S. Infantis*, and *S. Virchow* to Teflon, stainless steel, glass, rubber, and polyurethane were reported by Chia et al. (2009). They reported that *S. Sofia* isolates containing more fimbriae adhered to all material surfaces in significantly higher populations as compared to other serotypes. Wang et al. (2013) investigated the attachment and biofilm formation of 17 strains of *S. enterica* on polystyrene surfaces and the results indicated that the biofilms formed by *S. enterica* were significantly influenced by serotypes. In their study, *S.* London, *S.* Indiana, and *S. Typhimurium* produced greater biofilms regardless of the tested conditions compared with other strains examined.

Serotype-dependent differences in the attachment of *S. enterica* serotypes have also been reported on cucumber; the persistence of *S. Javiana* on cucumber was significantly higher than *S.* Newport after 24 hours of storage (Challahan and Micallef 2019). *Salmonella enterica* attachment to basil, lettuce, or spinach leaves varied with serotypes; *S.* Senftenberg and *S. Typhimurium* showed higher attachment compared with *S.* Agona or *S.* Arizonae (Berger et al. 2009). The fate of *S. enterica* on the produce seedlings was also reported to be influenced by bacterial strains; among 43 *Salmonella* strains tested for their persistence on lettuce and tomato seedlings, 26 strains showed increased populations, whereas the population of other strains remained unchanged or declined during 5-day storage at 21°C (Wong et al. 2019). The ability of attachment or biofilm formation on polypropylene and glass surfaces under the same environmental conditions varied among *S. enterica* strains; among five *S. enterica* serotypes tested; *S. Typhimurium* showed the highest ability to attach and *S. Infantis* showed the highest ability to form biofilms on these surfaces after 3 days of incubation at 25°C (Moraes et al. 2019). However, contradicting results have also been reported in other studies. The findings of a study conducted by Agarwal et al. (2011) showed no serotype-specific effects on the biofilm-forming ability of 151 *S. enterica* strains belonging to 69 serotypes in microplates. Likewise, the biofilm-forming ability of 60 S. enterica strains in polystyrene microtiter plates did not appear to be related to the *Salmonella* serotypes (Lianou and Koutsoumanis 2012). Keelara et al. (2016) examined the biofilm formation of 15 environmental isolates of *S. enterica* on microplates and reported that the biofilm-forming ability of *S. enterica* serovars may be associated with curli expression and strain hydrophobicity. The cell hydrophobicity of 99 non-0157 Shigatoxigenic *E. coli* strains affected their attachment rather than biofilm formation on stainless steel, glass, and polystyrene at various temperatures (Nesse et al. 2014).

Kalmokoff et al. (2001) investigated the differences in biofilm formation on the stainless steel surface among 36 food or environmental isolates of *L. monocytogenes*. Results of their study revealed marked variances among strains including the density of the attached cells, the presence of extracellular fibrils, and the biofilm formation ability. Di Bonaventura et al. (2008) tested the biofilm formation of 44 strains of *L. monocytogenes* that were isolated from food and food environments on equipment surfaces (polystyrene, glass, and stainless steel). The results of their study showed no significant difference in biofilm formation due to the source of origin (environmental or food), but it varied with serotypes. *L. monocytogenes* serotype 1/2c formed greater levels of biofilms on stainless steel surfaces and serotypes 1/2a and 4b on the glass surface (Di Bonaventura et al. 2008). The relationship between biofilm formation ability and *Listeria* serotype was also reported by Kadam et al. (2013), who showed that *L. monocytogenes* serotypes 1/2b and 1/2a formed stronger biofilms than serotype 4b in the nutrient-rich medium at 20°C, 30°C, and 37°C, whereas serotypes 1/2a and 4b produced levels of biofilms similar to serotype 1/2b strains in the nutrient-poor medium.

Type of Fresh Produce

It has been known that fresh produce such as lettuce exhibits a degree of cultivar resistance to several plant pathogens, which is driven by the genotype of the plant; however, the resistant characteristic of one cultivar is not universal for all types of plant pathogens (Quilliam et al. 2012). Variations in produce leaf traits have been shown to facilitate or hamper the leaf attachment of foodborne bacterial pathogens (Golberg et al. 2011, Kroupitski et al. 2011, Macarisin et al. 2013, Hunter et al. 2015). Different lettuce genotypes may have different microenvironments including the content of surface phenolics, proteins, wax, sugars, and stomatal density (Hunter et al. 2015). Several studies have examined the effects of these cultivar-specific properties on colonization and biofilm formation by foodborne pathogens. Mitra et al. (2009) reported that the interactions between *E. coli* O157:H7 and spinach were influenced by leaf topography by comparing the bacterial colonization on three spinach cultivars including Tyee (savoy-leaf), Space (hybrid smooth-leaf), and Bordeaux (delicate cordate-leaf). The highest populations of *E. coli* O157:H7 were observed on cultivar Tyee, suggesting that the leaf niches of this cultivar may protect the attached pathogens or promote stronger bacterial adherence (Mitra et al. 2009). Likewise, Macarisin et al. (2013) found differential persistence of *E. coli* O157:H7 on the leaves of spinach cultivars (Emilia, Lazio, Space, and Waitiki) in which cultivar Waitiki leaves that had the greatest leaf roughness supported significantly higher bacterial population than other cultivars.

Quilliam et al. (2012) determined the cultivar-specific effects on *E. coli* O157:H7 colonization on 12 lettuce cultivars, where the metabolic activity of pathogens in different types of lettuce has been proposed to influence their colonization potential in agricultural environments. The cultivar-specific factors including root exudate, root architecture, or differences in microbial communities have been found to affect the *E. coli* O157:H7 persistence and activity in the rhizosphere (Nicola et al. 2004, Klerks et al. 2007, Someya et al. 2008). Carter et al. (2019) reported that spinach indigenous microflora significantly inhibited the growth of *E. coli* O157:H7 and the subsequent biofilm formation on stainless steel surface for 10-day storage at 26°C in an incubation time-dependent manner. *E. coli* O157:H7 cells that have been internalized or very firmly attached to the lettuce leaf exerted greater metabolic activity as compared to the cells loosely attached on the leaves' surface, indicating that these cells not only persisted on the phyllosphere and rhizosphere of lettuce but also actively metabolized plant-derived nutrients (Quilliam et al. 2012). Indigenous microbial communities associated with different cultivars affected the colonization of S. enterica and *E. coli* O157:H7 to lettuce seedlings (Cooley et al. 2003). Wong et al. (2019) investigated the fate of 43 strains of *S. enterica* from 29 serotypes on seedlings of lettuce and tomato cultivars and reported that *S. enterica* colonization on lettuce and tomato seedlings was linked to the plant species and cultivars.

Equipment Surfaces

Stainless steel is one of the most commonly used materials in food-processing facilities that can be easily cleaned with resistance against chemical disinfectants. Polypropylene and glass are used in food-processing facilities such as cutting boards, jars, and tubs (Fink et al. 2017). However, these materials could be damaged by mechanical cleaning, and organic residues could stick to the cracks and scratches on the damaged surfaces (Wirtanen et al. 1996, Di Ciccio et al. 2015). The initial adhesion phase during biofilm formation on surfaces is primarily controlled by the physicochemical properties of the interacting surfaces (Prokopovich and Perni 2009, Lorite et al. 2011). Surface properties such as electrostatic charges, hydrophobicity, and roughness influence biofilm development (Poortinga et al. 2001, Tang et al. 2007). For instance, hydrophilic surfaces are more quickly colonized by *L. monocytogenes*, whereas there was no difference between hydrophobic and hydrophilic surfaces for *S. aureus* attachment (Chavant et al. 2002, da Silva Meria et al. 2012). Zhang et al. (2020) reported that the biofilm formation ability by *L. monocytogenes* on the nylon surface was the strongest, followed by stainless steel and glass because the hydrophobic surface is conducive to microbial adhesion. Further, *S. enterica* adhered to a greater extent on more hydrophobic materials than hydrophilic surfaces (Sinde and Carballo 2000, Joseph et al. 2001). The chemical composition of the surface can also influence bacterial attachment. *E. coli* attached at lower numbers to copper alloy and killed by antimicrobial properties of copper surface than to stainless steel (Noyce et al. 2006).

Surface roughness could be another factor that affected the adhesion of microorganisms by protecting the attached bacteria from shear forces and providing more available surface area (Vadillo-Rodríguez et al. 2018, Park et al. 2019). The formation of biofilms by *S. aureus* occurred preferentially on the polystyrene surface as compared to the stainless steel surface at 37°C (Di Ciccio et al. 2015). Chia et al. (2009) reported the adhesion of *Salmonella* isolates to different surface materials and found that isolates attached in significantly higher populations to Teflon® compared to glass, rubber, and polyurethane surfaces. Biofilm formation by *Acinetobacter* spp. and *Pseudomonas* spp. was affected more by the roughness of the contact surface than the surface hydrophobicity, as greater biofilm was formed on the rougher stainless steel surface as compared to a smoother sol-gel coated surface (Tang et al. 2011).

Environmental Factors

Food-related environmental factors including nutrient compositions, temperatures, and osmotic pressure are known to be involved in the process of biofilm formation by bacteria. Bacteria are exposed to various levels of nutrients in the fresh produce processing facility, and these environmental conditions affect the attachment and biofilm formations (Djordjevic et al. 2002). Understanding the effect of environmental factors on biofilm formation by bacterial pathogens is important to prevent biofilm formation (Wang et al. 2013b, Pilchova et al. 2014).

Nutrient Composition

Nutrient compositions could have a significant impact on biofilm-forming capability; numerous studies have focused on the effect of nutrient levels on the biofilm-formation ability of bacterial pathogens in laboratory-based conditions. An earlier study suggested that the adherence and biofilm formation of *E. coli* could increase under low-nutrient conditions in the growth media with lower osmolarity (Dewanti and Wong 1995, Stepanović et al. 2004, Reisner et al. 2006). However, a poor correlation between biofilm formation by *E. coli* strains in different growth media was reported by Reisner et al. (2006), indicating that *E. coli* isolates responded differently under different growth conditions. Hasan and Frank (2003) observed a stronger attachment of *E. coli* O157:H7 to lettuce and apple surfaces when grown in tryptic soy broth (TSB) compared to the nutrient broth. They attributed a stronger attachment of TSB-grown bacteria to capsule production in TSB and not in nutrient broth. Biofilm formation of *S. enterica* was reported to be enhanced in the nutrient-poor medium than nutrient-rich medium (Stepanović et al. 2004, Govaert et al. 2018). Higher biofilms formed by *S. Typhimurium* were observed when incubated with 20-fold diluted TSB compared to the full-strength TSB during 24 hours of incubation at 25°C (Govaert et al. 2018). A study conducted by Kadam et al. (2013) demonstrated rapid biofilm formation by *L. monocytogenes* and early biofilm maturation in a nutrient-poor medium rather than in a nutrient-rich medium. However, other studies have reported that nutrient-rich mediums such as brain heart infusion broth (BHI) favored the biofilm productions by *L. monocytogenes* as compared to nutrient-poor medium (Tomičić et al. 2016, Govaert et al. 2018). Kim and Frank (1995) have suggested that the low levels of phosphates initially stimulated *Listeria* biofilm formation. Glucose is another essential nutrient in terms of biofilm formation because it is required during the production of extracellular matrix components (Ammendolia et al. 1999); therefore, the presence of glucose was found to increase the biofilm formation of *S. aureus* in a dose-dependent manner (Rode et al. 2007, Khalil et al. 2014, Lee et al. 2015).

Temperature

The effect of environmental temperatures on the biofilm formation by microorganisms has been extensively studied and the temperatures that are commonly researched include the refrigerated temperatures (4°C–15°C) that represent the routine and storage conditions at the food-processing plants, the room temperature (20–25°C) that mimics the standard processing conditions, and the optimum temperatures (37°C) for the growth of bacteria in the laboratory-based conditions (Karaca et al. 2013). Biofilm formation by *S. enterica* Poona on different food-contact surfaces including stainless steel, nitrile buna-n rubber, and thermoplastic polyethylene was reduced by at least 1 log CFU/cm2 at 10°C as compared to 22°C during a 7-day incubation period (Abeysundara et al. 2018). Persistence of bacterial pathogens on vegetables was affected by storage temperature; populations of *E. coli* O157:H7 and *S. Typhimurium* slowly declined on fresh lettuce, cucumber, and parsley at 10°C, while the growth of these bacteria was observed on all three vegetables at 30°C (Likotrafiti et al. 2014). The ability of foodborne bacterial pathogens to colonize and form biofilms on the surfaces at low temperatures might increase the likelihood of cross-contamination in the produce facility during processing and storage. *L. monocytogenes* in biofilms could survive at 4°C for a least 5 days (Somers and Wong 2004). Di Ciccio et al. (2015) found *S. aureus* strain isolated from the food-handler showed the ability to form biofilm on polystyrene and stainless steel at 12°C.

The biofilm formation by *L. monocytogenes* was influenced by the environmental temperatures; greater biofilm formation was found at 37°C than at 30°C (Kadam et al. 2013). As reported by Di Bonaventura and coworkers (2008), the biomass of *L. monocytogenes* biofilms was significantly higher on glass at the lower environmental temperatures (4°C, 12°C, and 22°C) as compared to polystyrene and stainless steel surfaces; however, biofilm production by *L. monocytogenes* was comparable on glass and stainless steel surfaces at 37°C. Another study delineated the biofilm formation of *S. enterica* isolated from the food-processing plants under various temperatures (4°C to 42°C) and the strongest biofilm formation of *S. enterica* serotypes Agona, Senftenberg, Kottbus, Calabar, Kingston, and Typhimurium was formed at 25°C (Yin et al. 2018). Similarly, Govaert et al. (2018) reported that *S. Typhimurium* biofilm formation capacity was significantly increased at 25°C compared to 37°C. Pagedar et al. (2010) reported that *S. aureus* formed stronger biofilms on stainless steel surfaces at 25°C than at 37°C after 48 hours of incubation in TSB.

pH

Environmental pH is an important factor that affects the development of biofilms by microorganisms. Tilahun et al. (2016) reported that the optimal pH for *Vibrio cholerae* multiplication was 8.2 and the ability of this bacterium to form a biofilm was limited if the pH of the environmental was at pH 7. Weak acidic pH conditions promoted the formation of biofilms in *S. aureus*, but neither a highly acidic (pH 3) nor a strong alkaline (pH 12) condition could support biofilm formation by *S. aureus* (Arce et al. 2011, Khalil and Sonbol 2014).

The most optimal pH value for biofilm formation by *S. enterica* varied depending on the serotype and the environmental temperatures. Lianou et al. (2012) evaluated the biofilm formation by 60 strains of *S. enterica* that belonged to 9 serotypes under various environmental conditions, and the results showed that most of the *S. enterica* strains formed the highest amount of biofilm mass at pH 5.5 (35 out of 60 strains), whereas 3 of the 60 strains exhibited their highest biofilm-forming ability under stressful environmental conditions at pH 4.5. Yin et al. (2018) reported that *S. enterica* strains isolated from the food-processing plants produced the highest biofilm at pH 7 as compared to other pH tested (4.5–8). Another study by Karaca et al. (2013) showed that pH 6.5–7.4 was the optimal range of pH values for *S. enterica* adhesion and biofilm production. For L. monocytogenes, significantly increased biofilm formation was observed under highly acidic (pH 4.7) and alkaline (pH 8.5) culture conditions after 48 hours of incubation on stainless steel (Nilson et al. 2011).

Osmotic Pressure

The osmotic pressure has been reported to affect the ability of microorganisms to form biofilms (Liu et al. 2020). Ions in the medium could influence the biofilm formation by *S. aureus* due to the moderate hydrophobic property of staphylococcal cells. The presence of NaCl in the food matrix and food-contact surfaces may enhance the adhesion and biofilm maturation (Møretrø et al. 2003, Jensen et al. 2007, Rode et al. 2007), especially during seafood processing. Vázquez-Sánchez et al. (2013) demonstrated the electrostatic interactions between the *S. aureus* and polystyrene surface in which significantly stronger attachment of *S. aureus* to the abiotic surfaces was found when the ionic strength conditions of the growth medium increased from 1.5 mM NaCl to 150 mM NaCl. It was reported that NaCl-enhanced biofilm formation was more prevalent in methicillin-sensitive *S. aureus* strains than in methicillin-resistant strains (O'Neill et al. 2007). The effect of NaCl concentrations on the biofilm formation of 99 strains of *S. enterica* belonging to 18 serotypes was investigated by Karaca et al. (2013). In their study, NaCl concentration at 0.5% gave the highest biofilm production and an increase in NaCl concentrations from 0.5% to 10.5% resulted in complete inhibition of bacterial adhesion to microplate wells. *E. coli* O157:H7 was unable to grow in TSB containing greater than 6.5% NaCl (Glass et al. 1992). The production of EPS comprised of colonic acid by *E. coli* O157:H7 was found to play a role in protecting this pathogen from osmotic stress (Chen et al. 2004).

Genetic Basis in Biofilm Formation

Biofilm formation of microorganisms on fresh produce and the equipment surfaces is controlled by a series of genetic regulations by microorganisms. It has been reported that 1–10% of bacterial transcripts are differentially regulated between planktonic and sessile bacteria, and the gene expression profile of microorganisms also changes during the development of biofilms (Schembri et al. 2003, Beloin and Ghigo 2005). In *L. monocytogenes*, several genes have been identified to be related to biofilm formation including genes associated with flagella synthesis (*degU*), flagella structure (*flaA* and *flgL*), and motility (*motB*) (Lemon et al. 2007, Gueriri et al. 2008, Todhanakasem et al. 2008, Tresse et al. 2009). At the attachment stage, flagella play important role in early biofilm formation for surface adhesion and motility. The motility of *E. coli* O157:H7 is regulated by at least 50 flagellar genes; *Hha*, a nucleoid-associated protein, and *QseBC*, encoding a two-component signal transduction system, activate *E. coli* O157:H7 motility by up-regulating *flhDC* expression (Madrid et al. 2007). Sharma and Casey (2014) demonstrated that the motility of the *Hha* deletion mutant was significantly more compromised than that of the *qseC* deletion mutant strains, suggesting that Hha exerted a greater regulatory effect on motility compared to QseBC. A previous study reported that flagellated *L. monocytogenes* cells attached more rapidly to a stainless steel surface than flagellum-minus cells (Vatanyoopaisarn et al. 2000). In-frame deletion of the flagellin gene in *L. monocytogenes* was defective in surface-adhered biofilm formation as compared to the wild-type strain on the polyvinyl chloride surfaces (Lemon et al. 2007). Similarly, mutation of the *fliC* flagellin gene in *E. coli* O157:H7 strain EDL993 significantly reduced its attachment to spinach and lettuce leaf surface, suggesting the role of flagella in the bacteria-leaf interaction (Xicohtencatl-Cortes et al. 2009). Enterohemorrhagic *E. coli* O157 and O26 strains used filamentous type III secretion systems for attachment to salad leaves (Shaw et al. 2008). Another study reported by Tremoulet et al. (2002) showed that the flagellin protein (FlaA) was suppressed during the development of biofilms in L. monocytogenes, suggesting that flagellin may be synthesized at the initial attachment stage, but inhibited during the biofilm formation process. Sharma and Bearson (2013) demonstrated that Hha, a bacterial motility-related protein, is a negative regulator of biofilm production, where *Hha* mutant showed a significant reduction in bacterial motility but produced significant greater quantities of biofilms as compared to the wild-type *E. coli* O157:H7 strain at 30°C and 37°C. In the irreversible attachment phase, *Staphylococcus epidermidis* produces polysaccharide intercellular adhesin (PIA), which is encoded by the *icaADBC* locus, as the main component mediating intercellular adhesion (Qin et al. 2007). RelA and Hpt proteins are involved in synthesizing guanosine pentaphosphate which is required in bacterial growth and biofilm formation after adhesion. Taylor et al. (2002) reported that both *L. monocytogenes* relA and hpt mutants could not grow and form mature biofilm after adhering to the microtiter plate surface.

After the initial attachment, bacteria sense the environment by receiving signals that are transmitted to the cells through the mechanism of phosphorylation and dephosphorylation and regulate the expression of related genes in bacterial cells (Abee et al. 2011). The signal molecules of the bacteria quorum-sensing system are mainly autoinducing peptides. Sine autoinducing peptides cannot pass through the cytoderm by themselves, quorum sensing plays a role in the ATP-binding cassette transporter delivery system or other membrane channel protein transport to the extracellular systems (Lewis et al. 2012). The LuxS/2 autoinducer 2 (AI-2) quorum-sensing system is widely present in Gram-positive and Gram-negative bacteria, known as the interspecies quorum-sensing system. LuxS system was reported to be negatively related to biofilm formation as the deletion of *luxS* gene led to a denser biofilm by *L. monocytogenes* (Belval et al. 2006, Sela et al. 2006). AI-2 is considered to be a universal signal molecule and is involved in regulating the biofilm of many bacteria. AI-2 increasingly accumulates in the extracellular membrane with more bacterial growth (Guo et al. 2011). The extracellular AI-2 enters bacterial cells by LsrACB, resulting in the expression of the *lsrACDB* gene relevant to biofilm formation as the accumulation of AI-2 reaches a certain threshold. The 4,5-dihydroxy-2,3-pentanedione (DPD), a product of the *LuxS* enzyme in the catabolism of S-ribosylhomocysteine act as a precursor to AI-2. Since the intramolecular cyclization of DPD in organisms may generate different AI-2 molecules, different AI-2 signals are produced by different kinds of bacteria. The peptide-mediated quorum-sensing system auxiliary gene regulator (Agr) controls the expression of several virulence factors and is also involved in the early stage of biofilm formation in *L. monocytogenes* (Rieu et al. 2007). In-frame deletion of *agrA* and *agrD* genes resulted in an altered biofilm formation on abiotic surfaces (Rieu et al. 2007). Additionally, the concentrations of two enzymes for carbon metabolism, pyruvate dehydrogenase (PdhD) and 6-phosphofructokinase, increased in biofilm cells, indicating that the central metabolism of *L. monocytogenes* is also affected by the biofilm development (Tremoulet et al. 2002).

Curli and cellulose are two important components in biofilms; curli are amyloid fibers, which are involved in adhesion to surfaces, cell aggregation, environmental persistence, and biofilm development (Collinson et al. 1993, White et al. 2006). Plant symbiotic and pathogenic bacteria utilize curli and cellulose to persist on plant surfaces (Teplitski et al. 2009). Enteric bacterial pathogens are suggested to behave similarly to plant-associated bacteria during the colonization of plant tissues. Lapidot et al. (2006) reported that the transfer of *S. Typhimurium* from the contaminated water to the edible parts of parsley was closely linked to cellulose and curli. The synthesis of curli and cellulose is regulated by a complex regulatory network, which is the LuxR-type regulator CsgD (Zogaj et al. 2001, Solano et al. 2002, Abdallah et al. 2014). The production of curli is stimulated by the LuxR type regulator CsgD protein through transcriptional activation of the *csgBAC* and *csgDEFG* operons (Römling et al. 2000, Gerstel and Römling 2003). An insertion mutant in the *csgB-csgD* intergenic region showed a reduced attachment of *S. enterica* on the alfalfa sprouts (Barak et al. 2005). Grantcharova et al. (2010) reported that *csgD* is required for *S. Typhimurium* biofilm maturation on the glass surface in a flow cell-based experimental setting. Latasa et al. (2005) also found that BapA (biofilm-associated protein), a large cell-surface protein was required for the biofilm formation of *S. enterica*. The expression of *bapA* gene was demonstrated to be coordinated with the expression of curli and cellulose through the action of CsgD (Latasa et al. 2005). Ryu et al. (2004) reported that curli-producing *E. coli* O157:H7 strains did not affect bacterial attachment on stainless steel but these strains formed better biofilms. Saldaña et al. (2009) reported that overexpression of *csgD* resulted in increased attachment and biofilm formation of *E. coli* O157:H7. The results suggested that curli and cellulose acted together to support attachment and biofilm formation. However, the curli production by *E. coli* O157:H7 did not result in increased attachment of these pathogens on stainless steel, glass, or Teflon® surface (Goulter et al. 2010). Strong curli-expressing *E. coli* O157:H7 strains were reported to attach at significantly higher levels to cabbage and iceberg lettuce than other weak curli-expressing strains (Patel et al. 2011). Similarly, curli-expressing *E. coli* O157:H7 strains developed a stronger association with spinach leaf surface, whereas curli-deficient mutants (*csgA* and *csgD* mutants) attached to spinach at significantly lower levels (Macarisin et al. 2012). The findings by Nesse et al. (2014) revealed that non-O157 Shiga toxigenic *E. coli* isolates expressing eae genes produced fewer biofilms on abiotic surfaces than isolates without eae genes.

Cellulose, a β-1-4-D-glucose polymer, encoded by the *bcsABZC-bcsEFG* genes, is an important biofilm-associated EPS. As a matrix component in the bacterial biofilms, *S. enterica* produces cellulose to support long-range cell-cell interactions responsible for sticky texture (Römling et al. 2000). Fimbriae imparted *Salmonella* attachment to polystyrene and glass surfaces and cellulose expression enhanced biofilm formation of *Salmonella* on these surfaces (Jain and Chen 2007). Barak et al. (2007) reported the role of cellulose for *S. Enteritidis* and *S.* Newport attachment and colonization of alfalfa sprouts by using *bcsA* mutant strains. The genome of *S. Typhimurium* encodes five proteins with GGDEF domain and seven with EAL domain, while seven proteins harbor both domains. The GGDEF domain protein AdrA was identified to be important in *S. enterica* biofilm formation due to its effect on the *bcs* genes, responsible for cellulose biosynthesis, through the production of secondary messenger c-di-GMP (Römling et al. 2000, Zogaj et al. 2001, Simm et al. 2004). It has also been confirmed that besides the close relationship with cellulose biosynthesis, the increased c-di-GMP concentrations increased curli production by enhancing transcriptional and post-transcriptional CsgA and CsgD expression. Kader et al. (2006) reported a positive feedback loop as higher *csgD* expression resulted in higher AdrA levels, leading to elevated cytoplasmic c-di-GMP levels, whereby the elevated cytoplasmic c-di-GMP in turn caused the activation of CsgD.

The regulation of the two-component (BarA/SirA) system was found to be involved in the biofilm formation and virulence of *S. enterica* (Teplitski et al. 2006). SirA is a response regulator of the FixJ family (as is CsgD) that is phosphorylated by its cognate sensor kinase BarA (Teplitski et al. 2003). SirA regulates the *fim* operon that encodes a type I fimbriae, which is an important factor for *S. enterica* biofilm formation (Boddicker et al. 2002). Teplitski et al. (2006) showed that a *sirA* mutant and a *fimI* mutant were defective in biofilm formation by *S. Typhimurium* on polystyrene surfaces. Likewise, the deletion of *sirA* impaired surface attachment and survival of *S. enterica* on spinach leaves during post-harvest processing (Salazar et al. 2013).

Besides the genes with known functions as described above, the uncharacterized genes in the biofilm-forming bacteria may also play roles during biofilm development. Barak et al. (2009) studied two *S. enterica* genes with unknown functions, STM0278 (a putative periplasmic protein) and STM0650 (a putative protein with a hydrolase in the C-terminus), and found that these genes might be important for colonization on alfalfa seeds. Both STM0278 and STM0650 mutants showed a reduction in initial attachment and colonization of alfalfa seedlings at 24 hours, but the STM0278 mutant also showed reduced alfalfa seedling colonization at 48 hours compared to the wild-type strain of *S. enterica* (Barak et al. 2009). Another gene with unknown function, namely *yigG*, was found to be associated with biofilm formation in *S. enterica*; in-frame deletion of this gene resulted in a reduced bacterial attachment to equipment surfaces including glass and polystyrene as well as fresh produce surfaces including spinach and grape tomato for *Salmonella* serotypes Typhimurium and Saintpaul as compared to the wild-type strains (Salazar et al. 2013).

Environmental factors associated with biofilm formation by bacterial pathogens may also affect the gene expression profile of microorganisms during biofilm development (Wolfe et al. 2003, Cue et al. 2009). It has been reported that transcriptomic changes of *E. coli* and *S. enterica* during colonization on fresh produce were associated with the phyllosphere of intact and damaged tissues (Fink et al. 2012). At the produce processing facility, foodborne pathogens could adapt to the harsh environment by utilizing the nutrients released by the damaged plant tissues during post-harvest processing. Kyle et al. (2010) showed the transcriptional profile of *E. coli* O157:H7 after exposure to lettuce lysates, in which genes encoding proteins for carbohydrate transport and utilization systems such as *malE* and *malZ* were up-regulated in bacterial cells that were exposed to lettuce lysates. On the lettuce leaf surfaces, bacterial genes responsible for energy metabolism and transport processes, including *tnaA* (encoding tryptophanase), were down-regulated due to the stress responses triggered by the lack of nutrients, whereas genes that were involved in biofilm modulation (*bhsA* and *ybiM*) and curli production (*csgA* and *csgB*) were up-regulated in *E. coli* K12 and *E. coli* O157:H7 under these conditions (Fink et al. 2012).

Additionally, the osmotic pressure of nutrient media is reported to be associated with regulations of genes responsible for biofilm modulation including *icaA*, *scarA*, *rbf*, and *sigmaB* (Cramton et al. 1999, Cerca et al. 2008, Cue et al. 2009). Mirani et al. (2012) reported that an addition of 7% of NaCl could increase the biofilm formation by *S. aureus* strains that harbor *icaA* gene. However, Lim et al. (2004) claimed that NaCl may repress the biofilm formation for some *S. aureus* strains by inducing over-production of the Sigma B factor. These various findings suggest that the response of the osmotic pressure during biofilm formation is a complicated regulatory pathway. In addition, oxygen concentrations could be an important parameter in controlling different gene expressions; two gene clusters (*cydAB* and b2997-*hybABC*) were up-regulated in *E. coli* during biofilm development as known to be induced under limiting oxygen conditions (Schembri et al. 2003).

Multispecies Biofilms and Subsequent Interactions with Surfaces

Besides the research that focused on the biofilms formed by single-species, microorganisms most likely exist as a complex community consisting of several species on the fresh produce leaves and equipment surfaces at the food-processing facility (Djordjevic et al. 2002, Fagerlund et al. 2017). Several conditions in bacterial biofilms could be altered between the single and multispecies biofilms including the enhanced production of EPS, the differences in the physiological status of the bacteria, the interspecies cross-protection, and the internalization into the foods (Stewart 2015). Bacterial interactions in multispecies biofilms can be competitive, cooperative, or neutral depending on their growth, nutrition requirements, and environmental conditions (Burmølle et al. 2014).

Interactions and competition between the natural microbiota and the bacterial pathogens in fresh produce products and in the processing facility could affect the survival and biofilm formation ability of bacterial pathogens (Heir et al. 2018, Papaioannou et al. 2018). The common competitive interactions include the superior utilization of a given energy source or the production of compounds that directly inhibit the growth of other microorganisms. The production of secondary metabolites or physiological by-products such as bacteriocins, enzymes, hydrogen peroxide, and organic acids, also provides a competitive advantage over neighboring microorganisms within mixed-species biofilms (Rendueles and Ghigo 2012). Results of several research studies have supported the hypothesis that the indigenous microflora has a strong effect on the biofilm formation by *L. monocytogenes* on surfaces in food-processing environments. As previously reported, *L. monocytogenes* was able to establish in mixed bacterial biofilms, but the growth of *L. monocytogenes* was hampered (Guillier et al. 2008, Langsrud et al. 2016). Winkelströter et al. (2015) reported that the biofilm formation of *L. monocytogenes* was suppressed when co-cultured with *Lactobacillus paraplantarum* due to the production of antimicrobials, such as lactic acid and bacteriocins.

Heir et al. (2018) investigated the competitive ability of biofilm formation by *L. monocytogenes* when co-cultured along with *Listeria innocua* and environmental background bacteria including *Pseudomonas fragi, Pseudomonas fluorescens, Serratia liquefaciens, Stenotrophomonas maltophilia*, and *Acinetobacter* spp. on stainless steel surface at 12°C. When both *L. innocua* and the background bacteria were present in the multispecies cultures, the growth of certain *L. monocytogenes* strains that were suppressed by certain *L. innocua* strains was further inhibited by the background microbiota; *Pseudomonas* spp. were the dominant strains in the multispecies biofilms on the stainless steel surface. *Pseudomonas* spp. are commonly associated with spoilage of fresh food products due to their widespread existence in water, soil, and vegetation under both optimal as well as refrigerated temperatures (Patange et al. 2019). *Pseudomonas aeruginosa* and *S. enterica* could coexist on food-contact surfaces; however, the presence of cell-free culture supernatants containing N-acyl-L-homoserine lactones produced by *P. aeruginosa* inhibits biofilm formation of *S. enterica* (Wang et al. 2013).

Fresh produce-associated bacteria could promote the survival of foodborne bacterial pathogens in the produce tissues. For example, *E. coli* O157:H7 survived at significantly higher population levels on the lettuce surfaces in the presence of epiphytic bacteria, *Wausteria paucula* (Cooley et al. 2006). The survival and proliferation of *E. coli* O157:H7 on the lettuce leaves were enhanced when *Dickeya dadantii*, a plant pathogen coexisted, mainly due to the secretion of pectate lyases by plant pathogen (Yamazaki et al. 2011). In a mixed biofilm study, Habimana et al. (2010) demonstrated that the presence of the biofilm formed by *Acinetobacter calcoaceticus* increased the colonization and biofilm formation by *E. coli* O157:H7 under dynamic-flow conditions.

Ralstonia insidiosa is commonly isolated from water bodies, soil, and the water distribution systems in industries (Ryan et al. 2011), and this bacterium was the most represented bacterial species found on food-contact and non-food-contact surfaces (Liu et al. 2013). Liu and others (2014) examined a dual-species biofilm formation by *E. coli* O157:H7 and environmental bacteria isolated from fresh-cut processing facilities and observed a significant increase in biomass and thickening biofilms by *Burkholderia caryophylli* and *R. insidiosa*, when co-cultured with *E. coli* O157:H7. Biofilm formation of foodborne bacterial pathogens including *L. monocytogenes, S. enterica* and *E. coli* was facilitated when co-cultured with *R. insidiosa* as this bacterium is highly efficient in nutrient utilization and proliferates well in oligo-nutrient environments, providing a micro-environment for bacterial accumulation and survival (Liu et al. 2016a).

The interspecies interactions can develop structural and functional dynamics of these communities differently from single-species populations. Recently, multispecies biofilms have gained more attention due to the increased resistance of multispecies biofilms to disinfectants in comparison with single-specie biofilms (Lohse et al. 2017, Pang et al. 2017, Parijs and Steenackers 2018). Ibusquiza et al. (2012) reported a significantly increased resistance to benzalkonium chloride in dual-species biofilm formed by *L. monocytogenes* and *Pseudomonas putida* after 4 days of incubation as compared to that of single-species biofilms. Likewise, dual-species biofilms by *Serratia liquefaciens* and *Serratia putrefaciens* were more resistant to both ethanol and benzalkonium chloride than their single-species counterparts (Liu et al. 2017). Patange et al. (2019) reported that an extended treatment time of the atmospheric cold plasma (ACP) was required to reduce the mixed culture biofilms of *L. monocytogenes* and *P. fluorescens* on lettuce.

The enhanced resistance to disinfectants may occur even when the overall production of biofilm decreased. Pang and Yuk (2018) found that the presence of *P. aeruginosa* has been shown to reduce the cell density of *S. Enteritidis* when mixed in dual-species biofilms, meanwhile protecting *Salmonella* cells form sanitizer treatment. In multispecies biofilm produced by *L. monocytogenes*, *Staphylococcus xylosus* and *P. fragi*, the dominant microorganisms in the multispecies biofilms were *P. fragi* (59%) and *S. xylosus* (39.5%). Despite the populations of *L. monocytogenes* in this multispecies, biofilm significantly declined and an increased protective property of multispecies biofilms, containing *L. monocytogenes* against chlorine, was found as compared with those of single-culture biofilms (Norwood and Gilmour 2000).

The exact mechanisms of enhanced resistance to disinfectants within mixed-species biofilms remain unclear. The alternation of matrix composition and the enhancement of EPS production in mixed-species biofilms have been hypothesized to be relevant for the enhanced resistance to disinfectants (Flemming and Wingender 2010). Puga et al. (2014) reported that the enhanced resistance of multispecies biofilms could be due to the amount of EPS produced by the *P. fluorescens* that protected *L. monocytogenes* in biofilms. The spatial arrangement of certain bacterial species within a biofilm was suggested as another explanation for the enhanced resistance to disinfectants in multispecies biofilms (Lee et al. 2014). Some strains may be protected from a disinfectant by their aggregation with others within the differential three-dimensional structure (Liu et al. 2016b). The structural organization of microorganisms within the multispecies biofilms could be arranged in layers, where one species locates in the lower layers and the other species is in the upper layers. In this type of organization, bacterial interactions could be either cooperative or competitive (An et al. 2006, Habimana et al. 2010). These studies suggest that multispecies in determining the pattern of biofilm formation would be necessary to mimic microbial life on food-processing surfaces where different bacterial species live intermingled.

Persistence and Biofilm Formation of Bacterial Pathogens on Fresh Produce

Due to the increase in the number of foodborne pathogens associated with fresh produce outbreaks in the past years, studies have focused on the contamination routes and the persistence of these bacterial pathogens in vegetables. Laboratory-based experiments focused on the biofilm formation ability of bacteria on different material surfaces with standard systems such as CDC bioreactor and drip flow biofilm reactor assays may provide a suitable prediction model for pathogen-plant interactions (Kroupitski et al. 2009, Patel and Sharma 2010). Some studies have reported that strong *S. enterica* biofilm producers on polystyrene surfaces also attached at higher population levels on lettuce leaves (Kroupitski et al. 2009, Patel aend Sharma 2010). Formation of biofilms by foodborne bacterial pathogens such as Shiga toxigenic *E. coli* on fresh produce enhances the survival of bacterial pathogens (Carter and Brandl 2015). *E. coli* and *S. enterica* strains isolated from fruit and vegetable samples have been reported to have the biofilm-forming ability (Amrutha et al. 2017). Studies that focused on the colonization and biofilm formation of foodborne pathogens in plant tissues are summarized (Table 1).

Pre-harvest Level

At the pre-harvest level, understanding the contamination routes and the persistence of foodborne bacterial pathogens on vegetables could help improve the microbial safety of fresh produce. Barak et al. (2011) inoculated the leaves of four-week-old tomato plants grown in the climate-controlled growth chamber with contaminated water ($\sim$ 8 logs CFU/ml) to simulate overhead sprinkler irrigation. Approximately 3.8 log CFU/cm^2 of *S. enterica* populations were recovered on the tomato leaves 7 days after the inoculation, and bacterial populations were reduced to < 3 log CFU/cm^2 on day 14 (Barak et al. 2011). Although tomato leaves are not edible, data on susceptibility to leaf colonization are relevant since *S. enterica* residing on leaves can be transmitted to fruit (Barak et al. 2011, Gu et al. 2011). When *S. enterica* serotypes were inoculated on the tomato seedling (3.5 log CFU/seedling) at 3 weeks post-germination, populations of *S*. Newport and *S. Typhimurium* recovered at 24 hours post-inoculation were in the range of $\sim$ 6–7 log CFU/seedling and $\sim$ 6.5–7.5 log CFU/seedling, respectively (Han and Micallef 2014).

Post-harvest Level

Studies used vegetables with post-harvest inoculation of foodborne bacterial pathogens to evaluate the attachment of pathogens to plant tissues. Boyer and others (2007) reported that curli-producing *E. coli* O157:H7 strains attached at a significantly higher level on intact and cut lettuces. Irrespective of curli expression, higher bacterial populations were attached to the cut lettuce surface. Similarly, Kroupitski et al. (2009) observed preferential binding of 8 *S. enterica* serovars to the cut edges of the lettuce leaf than the intact leaf. Patel et al. (2011) compared the attachment of several *E. coli* O157:H7 strains on iceberg lettuce, romaine lettuce, and green cabbage by submerging the produce leaves in 11 ml of 6 log CFU/ml bacterial culture. Results of their study showed that *E. coli* attached within 5 minutes post-inoculation to the intact and cut produce leaf surfaces at 3.6–5.0 log CFU/cm^2 for cabbage, 3.8–4.7 log CFU/cm^2 for iceberg lettuce, and 3.8–4.9 log CFU/cm^2 for

Table 1. Attachment and persistence of foodborne pathogens on fresh produce.

Conditions	Bacteria	Fresh Produce	Results	Reference
Pre-harvest persistence	*S. enterica* cocktail of Baildon, Cubana, Enteritidis, Havana, Mbandaka, Newport, Poona, Schwarzengrund	Tomato leaves	*S. enterica* persisted on tomato leaves for 14 days; 3.8 log and 2.9 log CFU/cm² recovered on day 7 and day 14, respectively	Barak et al. 2011
Pre-harvest persistence	*S.* Newport and *S. Typhimurium*	Tomato seedlings	*S.* Newport and Typhimurium populations increased from 3.5 log to 6–7 log and 6.5–7.5 log CFU/seedling, respectively	Han and Micallef 2014
Post-harvest attachment	*E. coli* O157:H7	Lettuce cultivars iceberg and Romaine, and green cabbage	3.6–5.0, 3.8–4.7, and 3.8–4.9 log CFU/cm² of *E. coli* attached to cabbage, iceberg lettuce, and romaine lettuce leaves, respectively, within 5 minutes of exposure to 6 log CFU/ml inoculum	Patel et al. 2011
Post-harvest attachment	*E. coli* O157:H7	Lettuce cultivar Green leaf	More than 1 log CFU/cm² of *E. coli* attached on lettuce leaves within 15 min exposure to 3 log CFU/cm² inoculum	Fink et al. 2012
Post-harvest attachment	*S. Typhimurium* and *S.* saintpaul	Spinach leaf	~ 7 log CFU of *S. enterica* attached on spinach leaves within 10 min exposure to 8 log CFU inoculum	Salazar et al. 2013
Post-harvest attachment	*S. Typhimurium*, *L. monocytogenes*, and *E. coli*	Lettuce cultivar iceberg	6.5, 6.0, and 5.6 log CFU/sample of *Salmonella*, *Listeria*, and *E. coli* attached on lettuce leaves within 2 h exposure to 7 log CFU/ml inoculum	Ziuzina et al. 2015
Post-harvest attachment	*L. monocytogenes*	Lettuce cultivar Buttercrunch	0.77 and 1.5 log CFU/cm² of *L. monocytogenes* attached to lettuce leaves within 1 s and 2 min exposure to 5 log CFU/ml inoculum	Kyere et al. 2019
Post-harvest persistence	*S.* Newport	Tomato	Increase of 1–3 log CFU/fruit within 24 hours at room temperature	Han and Micallef 2014

Table 1 contd. ...

...Table 1 contd.

Conditions	Bacteria	Fresh Produce	Results	Reference
Post-harvest persistence	*S. Typhimurium* and *E. coli* O157:H7	Lettuce, cucumber, and parsley	Decline of 1.8 and 1.4 log CFU in *S. enterica* and *E. coli* O157:H7 populations, respectively, during 7-day storage at 10°C	Likotrafiti et al. 2014
Post-harvest persistence	*S.* Newport	Cucumber	Decline of 2.5 log CFU/6 cm² in *S.* Newport populations during 7-day storage at 22°C	Sharma et al. 2017
Post-harvest persistence	*S.* Newport and *S.* Javiana	Cucumber	Decline of 1.5 and 1.0 log CFU/g in *S.* Newport and *S.* Javiana populations during 24 h storage at 22°C	Callahan and Micallef 2019
Post-harvest persistence	*S. enterica* cocktail of Newport, Poona, and Typhimurium	Cucumber	Increase of 0.7 log CFU/cm² and decline of 0.6 log CFU/cm² during 7-day storage at 22°C and 10°C, respectively	Byun et al. 2019

Romaine lettuce. Fink et al. (2012) examined the attachment of a non-pathogenic strain of wild-type *E. coli* K12 and a pathogenic strain of *E. coli* O157:H7 on the Green leaf lettuce leaves. With an initial inoculum of 3 log CFU/cm² of either *E. coli* K12 or O157:H7, more than 1 log CFU/cm² was attached to the lettuce leaves within 15 minutes post-inoculation and a further 15 minutes increased an additional 0.5 log CFU/cm² of attached bacteria. Salazar et al. (2013) immersed spinach leaves in 45 ml of inoculum containing 8 log CFU of *S. Typhimurium* and *S.* Saintpaul for 10 min and recovered ~ 7 log CFU of *S. enterica* cells that were attached to the baby spinach leaves. Han and Micallef (2014) reported that a tomato outbreak strain of *S.* Newport was better adapted to colonize and persist on tomato fruit than *S. Typhimurium* strain ATCC 700720. Populations of S. Newport increased from 2.5 log CFU/fruit to 3.5–5.5 log CFU/fruit 24 hours post-inoculation on 13 tomato cultivars, in which the lowest *Salmonella* recovery was found in cultivar Heinz-1706 and the highest recovery in cultivar Nyagous (Han and Micallef 2014). The survival pattern of *E. coli* O157:H7 and *S. Typhimurium* on lettuce, cucumber, and parsley was determined by Likotrafiti et al. (2014) during post-harvest storage. The decline of up to 1.8 and 1.4 log CFU in *S. enterica* and *E. coli* O157:H7 populations, respectively, was observed on all three vegetables during 7-day storage at 10°C (Likotrafiti et al. 2014). Similar persistence of *S. enterica* on the cucumber surfaces was obtained by Sharma et al. (2017), who reported a decline of ~ 2.5 log CFU per 6 cm² inoculated area on cucumber surfaces in *S.* Newport populations stored at 22°C for 7 days. Ziuzina et al. (2015) deep-inoculated fresh iceberg lettuce in 300 ml of 0.85% NaCl containing 7 log CFU/ml foodborne pathogen and within 2 hours; 6.5, 6.0, and

5.6 log CFU per sample of *S. enterica*, *L. monocytogenes*, and *E. coli* were attached on produce leaves, respectively. After 24 hours of storage at 4°C, bacterial populations of *S. enterica*, *L. monocytogenes*, and *E. coli* in biofilms recovered from the lettuce were 7.8, 6.8, and 6.2 log CFU per sample, respectively (Ziuzina et al. 2015). Callahan and Micallef (2019) investigated the persistence of produce-associated outbreak isolates of *S. enterica* on the exocarp of several unwaxed cucumber cultivars. In their study, *S. Newport* and *S. Javiana* populations decreased by 1.5 log CFU/g and 1.0 log CFU/g on all cucumber cultivars after 24 hours of storage at room temperature. They also reported vegetable oil-based wax facilitated the higher attachment of *S. Newport* on cucumbers as a greater decline of *S. Newport* populations was observed on the unwaxed cucumber surface than the waxed cucumber surface during 24 hours of storage at room temperature, regardless of the cucumber cultivar. Populations of a mixture of *S. enterica* Newport, Poona, and Typhimurium declined from 3.6 log CFU/cm² to 3 log CFU/cm² on Persian cucumber surfaces after 7-day storage at 10°C, whereas *Salmonella* populations increased from 2.9 log CFU/cm² to 3.6 log CFU/cm² when stored at 22°C (Byun et al. 2019). Populations of *L. monocytogenes* in biofilms recovered from cucumber and lettuce surfaces after 4 days of storage at 25°C were ~ 6 log and ~ 6.5 log CFU/cm², respectively, with initial inoculum level of 4–5 log CFU/ml (Zhang et al. 2020).

Several studies have described leafy green as unfavorable media for the survival and growth of *L. monocytogenes* (Farber et al. 1998, Jacxsens et al. 1999), whereas others have reported the ability of leafy greens to support *L. monocytogenes* growth (Koseki and Isobe 2005, Omac et al. 2018). Koseki and Isobe (2005) estimated the growth rates of *L. monocytogenes* at 0.021, 0.047, 0.090, 0.156, 0.200 log CFU/h on fresh-cut iceberg lettuce during 20 hours of storage at 5°C, 10°C, 15°C, 20°C, and 25°C, respectively. Kyere et al. (2019) investigated the attachment of fresh produce-associated *L. monocytogenes* strains on soil and hydroponically grown Buttercrunch lettuce with different exposure times (1 s, 10 s, 30 s, 60 s, 2 minutes, and 5 minutes). Results of their study showed that exposure of lettuce to 5 log CFU/ml of *L. monocytogenes* strain O8A08 (cabbage isolate) for just 1 s resulted in at least 0.77 log CFU/cm² attachment, while 2 minutes exposure had increased the attached bacterial population to 1.5 log CFU/cm² (Kyere et al. 2019). In addition, *L. monocytogenes* strain O8A08 also attached at significantly higher levels to the lettuce grown in soil than hydroponically grown lettuce during the exposure times of 60 s, 2 minutes, and 5 minutes, suggesting that the use of cleaner growing techniques for fresh produce may have a lower risk of microbial colonization (Lopez et al. 2014, Kyere et al. 2019).

At the post-harvest level, fresh produce tissues could be damaged by various mechanical processes and it has been previously reported that the growth rate of *E. coli* O157:H7 on lettuce leaves increased with the severity of tissue damage as bacteria may benefit from the nutrients released by the lysed plant cells (Brandl 2008). Kyle et al. (2010) also reported that the populations of *E. coli* O157:H7 remained stable for the first 4–5 h of incubation at ~ 6 log CFU/ml in the Romaine lettuce lysates and reached ~ 9 log CFU/ml after 24 hours of incubation at 28°C. Kyere et al. (2020) found both soil and hydroponically-grown lettuce leaf extracts supported the growth of *L. monocytogenes* at 10°C; bacterial populations were higher in soil-grown leaf extracts than in hydroponic leaf extract, though the difference was not significantly different.

Biofilm Formation of Bacterial Pathogens on Equipment Surfaces

At the pre-harvest level, biofilms produced by foodborne bacterial pathogens in agricultural irrigation system has been reported to be a potential source of contamination to downstream irrigated produce and several ready-to-eat produce outbreaks have been shown to be directly linked with irrigation (Gelting et al. 2011, Yao and Habimana 2019). Common irrigation systems involve either pipes, drippers, or sprinklers that provide the necessary surface for allowing biofilm formation (Yao and Habimana 2019). Bacterial pathogens are capable of prolonged survival in irrigation water and contamination of water sources could transfer pathogens to agricultural commodities (Dandie et al. 2020). Kabir et al. (2020) reported that *S. enterica* survived in surface water at 5°C, 25°C, and 37°C for at least 28 days and these bacteria could form biofilms on rubber and stainless steel surfaces at 25°C and 37°C.

In the fresh produce processing facility, most biofilm-forming microorganisms can form aggregates on the equipment surfaces and at the bottom of containers in liquid media. As previously reported, 76% of pathogenic *E. coli* isolates from farms and packing facilities of tomatoes, jalapeno pepper, and cantaloupe were confirmed as biofilm producers on polystyrene surfaces (Corzo-Ariyama et al. 2019). Similarly, Han et al. (2017) reported the biofilm-producing ability of seven *S. enterica* strains with six serotypes, including Stanley, Cabana, Baildon, Enteritidis, Montevideo, and Michigan of fresh produce origin on the polystyrene surface. Biofilms have been detected on industrial surfaces, such as stainless steel, aluminum, glass, PTFE, Buna-N, and Teflon seals (Cappitelli et al. 2014). Bacteria attach and form biofilms on abiotic surfaces in the processing facility, representing a severe potential health risk to consumers. Contaminated food-contact surfaces could lead to cross-contamination of fresh produce that threatens public health and may result in foodborne infections. Studies have focused on the biofilm formation ability of bacterial strains isolated from various environments on common food-contact surfaces used in the processing facility.

Adetunji and Isola (2011) compared biofilm formation by *L. monocytogenes* on glass, stainless steel, and wooden surfaces and found that biofilm formation was the strongest on wooden surfaces, followed by steel and glass. Similarly, Bang et al. (2014) reported that *E. coli* O157:H7 formed the strongest biofilms on wooden surfaces as compared to other food-contact surfaces. Populations of *E. coli* O157:H7 attached on stainless steel, glass, plastic, and wooden coupons on day 0 were 4.9, 4.3, 4.1, and 5.3 log CFU per coupon, respectively. Within 2 days of incubation in the M9 medium, the bacterial population in biofilms on those coupons increased to 8.6, 7.9, 8.6, and 9.5 log CFU per coupon, and these populations remained stable for an additional 3 days (Bang et al. 2014). Corcoran et al. (2014) observed significantly higher populations of *S. Agona*, *S. Enteritidis*, and *S. Typhimurium* in biofilms after 168 hours as compared to 48 hours biofilms on equipment surfaces including glazed tiles, 316L stainless steel, borosilicate glass, polycarbonate plastic, and concrete coupons.

A greater *L. monocytogenes* biofilm matrix was observed by the microscopic analysis with an incubation period of 48 hours as compared to 24 hours and 72 hours of incubation on the stainless steel surface (Ripolles-Avila et al. 2018). Similarly, Bumunang et al. (2020) reported that the biofilm-forming ability of six non-O157 Shiga toxigenic *E. coli* strains, including O116:H21, wzx-Onovel5:H9, O129:H21, O129:H23, O26:H11, and O154:H10 was the strongest at 22°C after 48 hours of incubation on stainless steel surface than 24 hours and 72 hours incubation periods. For other studies with the age of biofilms, Carpentier and Chassaing (2004) reported the presence of a *Bacillus* spp. strain CCL 9 led to a 3-log decline in *L. monocytogenes* populations of multispecies biofilm on stainless steel surfaces as compared to the single *L. monocytogenes* biofilm. Whereas de Grandi et al. (2018) reported no significant interference of a non-pathogenic *E. coli* strain over the biofilm formation ability of *L. monocytogenes* on the stainless steel surface. Further, populations of four bacterial strains (*Kocuria varians* CCL 73, *Staphylococcus capitis* CCL 54, *Stenotrophomonas maltophilia* CCL 47, and *Comamonas testosteroni* CCL 24) increased from 0.5 to 1 log in this *L. monocytogenes* multispecies biofilm.

Several studies have indicated that the presence of the food residues, such as juice and lysate of fresh produce, during the post-harvest processing could support the attachment and biofilm formations by bacterial pathogens on the equipment surfaces (Leff and Fierer 2013, Kyere et al. 2020). Cantaloupe extracts induced the growth of *L. monocytogenes* and biofilm formation on the stainless steel surfaces. For 50 mg/ml cantaloupe extracts inoculated with 3 log CFU/ml of *L. monocytogenes*, the biofilm formation of *Listeria* on stainless steel surface was ~ 7 log CFU/coupon in 4–7 days of incubation at 22°C (Abeysundara et al. 2017). They also reported that six outbreak strains of *S. enterica* serotypes Poona, Stanley, and Montevideo formed 4–4.5 log CFU/cm^2 biofilms in 4–7 days of incubation at 22°C on stainless steel in 2 mg/ml cantaloupe extracts (Abevsundara et al. 2018). When the concentration of cantaloupe extracts increased to 50 mg/ml, significantly higher populations of *S. enterica* (5–6 log CFU/cm^2) in biofilms were found on stainless steel under the same environmental conditions. Kyere et al. (2020) found that leaf extracts of hydroponic and soil-grown lettuce supported the biofilm formation of *L. monocytogenes* on stainless steel surfaces. The populations of *L. monocytogenes* in biofilms formed on stainless steel in both soil and hydroponic leaf extracts increased from 3 log CFU/cm^2 after 2 days to 6.4–7.2 log CFU/cm^2 and 4.3–4.8 log CFU/cm^2 after 10 days incubation at 10°C and 4°C, respectively (Kyere et al. 2020).

Certain bacteria such as *S. enterica* serotypes, *E. coli*, *P. fluorescens*, and *V. cholerae* produce rigid or fragile pellicle structures at air-liquid interfaces (Rainey and Travisano 1998, Yildiz and Schoolnik 1998, Römling and Rohde 1999, Anriany et al. 2001, Zogaj et al. 2001, Solano et al. 2002, Spiers et al. 2002). Medrano-Félix et al. (2018) confirmed that *S.* Saintpaul strains isolated from river water and animal feces were able to form biofilms at the air-liquid interface. Bumunang et al. (2020)

reported that two non-O157 Shiga toxigenic *E. coli* strains O129:H23 and O154:H10 were able to form biofilms on both the submerged surface and the air-liquid interface of the stainless steel coupons by using crystal violet staining. Biofilm production at the air-liquid interface can facilitate and contribute to gas exchange while enabling the acquisition of nutrients and water from the liquid phase (Spiers et al. 2003). The biofilms at air-liquid and solid-air interfaces can cause serious problems in industrial water systems (Scher et al. 2004).

Control and Removal Strategies

Foodborne pathogenic bacteria cause bacterial food poisoning, which seriously endangers human health and could lead to severe economic losses. The major concern about biofilms is their wide resistance to disinfectants commonly used in food industries, such as quaternary ammonium compounds including benzalkonium chloride (Ibusquiza et al. 2011). The resistance of biofilms to antimicrobials is attributed to several intrinsic biofilm properties such as reduced diffusion, physiological changes of bacterial cells, reduced growth rate, and the production of enzymes that degrade the antimicrobial compounds (Bridier et al. 2011). Generally, the antibiofilm strategies include disinfection to prevent the development of biofilms, the removal of mature biofilms using mechanical or chemical treatments, and the prevention of biofilm dispersion.

Prevention of Biofilm Formation

In the industry, quaternary ammonium compounds, chlorine-based biocides, and peroxides are commonly used as a disinfectant to kill microorganisms. However, bacterial cells in the biofilms could tolerate the presence of biocides much better than planktonic cells. The production of EPS by bacteria after the irreversible attachment on the surfaces makes the traditional surface cleaning procedures insufficient to eliminate mature biofilms (Parker et al. 2004). Effective cleaning and disinfection are the key steps to disrupt the initial attachment of biofilms. In addition, biofilm formation could be simply controlled by treatments that prevent the initial attachment of bacteria on fresh produce and equipment surfaces to inhibit the development of mature biofilms. To prevent biofilm formation, preventive strategies including physical, chemical, and biological treatments have been extensively researched and discussed in this review.

For physical prevention, irradiation, and UV treatments have been reported to effectively reduce populations of foodborne pathogens on fresh produce. Food irradiation can damage microbial DNA without any adverse effect on the sensory or nutritional quality of the food, when an appropriate irradiation dose is applied (Farkas and Mohácsi-Farkas 2011). Treatments with 1.0 kGy X-ray significantly reduced populations of *E. coli* O157:H7, *L. monocytogenes*, and *S. enterica* on shredded iceberg lettuce by 4.4 log, 4.1 log, and 4.8 log CFU/5cm^2 at 22°C, respectively (Mahmoud 2010). Similarly, Kim et al. (2013) reported that UV treatment at 25°C for 1 minutes achieved 1.5, 1.4, and 2.1 log CFU/g reductions of *E. coli* O157:H7, *S. Typhimurium*, and *L. monocytogenes* on fresh-cut iceberg lettuce, respectively, whereas the reductions of these pathogens at 4°C was 0.1, 0.6, and 1.2 log, respectively. Non-fouling coating with polytetrafluoroethylene (PTFE) on stainless steel surface reduced *B. cereus* biofilm by 2 log CFU/cm^2 (Huang et al. 2016). Nanoparticle-encapsulated surfaces have gained attention as antimicrobial surfaces to prevent bacterial adhesion. The chitosan-encapsulated zinc ferrite nanoparticles were evaluated for their antibiofilm efficiency (Sharma et al. 2020). These nanoparticles inhibited biofilm formation of bacterial pathogens by < 65% and removed the biofilm by 50% as demonstrated by minimum inhibition concentration (MIC) assay. Baig and others (2020) have reported the antibiofilm effect of copper oxide-titanium dioxide nanocomposites against methicillin-resistant *S. aureus*.

In addition to the physical treatments, the use of various chemical wash treatments has been suggested to reduce bacterial pathogens on fresh produce; for instance, populations of *L. monocytogenes* and *E. coli* O157:H7 were reduced by 0.61 log and 0.67 CFU/g, respectively, when shredded iceberg lettuce samples were washed with 200 mg/L sodium hypochlorite for 5 min (Baert et al. 2009). Many factors including the type and concentration of disinfectants, exposure time, targeted organisms, types of surfaces, pH, food residues, and temperature could affect the efficiency of disinfectants against biofilms (Cappitelli et al. 2014). Bang et al. (2014) observed that *E. coli* O157:H7 biofilms were more resistant to sanitizers compared to other surfaces including stainless steel, glass, and plastic. Higher resistance of *E. coli* O157:H7 against sodium hypochlorite and chlorine dioxide on wooden surfaces could be attributed to the limited penetration of disinfectants into the crevices and pores on the wooden surface, resulting in protection of bacterial cells from disinfectants.

The use of natural antimicrobial compounds including essential oil, phytochemicals, and antimicrobial peptides to control biofilm formation has also been suggested by researchers. Essential oils and phytochemicals may contain natural antioxidants and antimicrobial compounds, which have been hypothesized to exhibit beneficial health effects and minimize the risk of chronic infections (Yousefi et al. 2019). Algburi et al. (2020) suggested the antibiofilm potential of black cardamom oil against *E. coli* O157:H7 and *S. Typhimurium* through inhibition of bacterial quorum sensing. Black cardamom oil at 0.5% concentration inhibited the biofilm formation of *S. Typhimurium* and *E. coli* O157:H7 by 50.2% and 84.6% in 96-well plates, respectively (Algburi et al. 2020). Antimicrobial peptides are an integral part of innate immunity and are produced by varied living organisms. Anunthawan et al. (2015) designed two antimicrobial peptides containing tryptophan namely KT2 and RT2 and found that these two peptides effectively controlled *E. coli* O157:H7 biofilm formation at the concentration of 1 μmol/L.

Lactic acid bacteria have shown great potential as an alternative and environmentally friendly biological treatment to prevent biofilm formation (Gómez et al. 2016, Camargo et al. 2018). The production of EPS by the lactic acid bacteria *Lactobacillus acidophilus* A4 had been identified as one of the mechanisms of action against the biofilm formation of *E. coli* O157:H7 on polystyrene and PVC surfaces

(Kim and Kim 2009). The adherence of *L. monocytogenes* to stainless steel surface was reduced by 5 log CFU/cm^2 with lactic acid bacteria including *Lactococcus lactis* and *Enterococcus durans* (Zhao et al. 2004). The efficacy of cell-free supernatants obtained from *Lactobacilli* on *S. aureus* biofilm removal was investigated by Koohestani and others (2018). They observed significant biofilm removal of *S. aureus* biofilm on polystyrene and steel surfaces; the effect of *L. acidophilus* supernatant was superior compared to *L. casei*. The cell-free supernatants and exopolysaccharides produced by *Lactobacilli* and *Saccharomyces boulqrdii* were used to remove biofilms produced by bacterial pathogens (Komal and Shilpa 2020). Maximum biofilm removal was observed for *S. aureus* biofilms (86%) whereas 65–75% was *P. aeruginosa* and *Klebsiella pneumoniae*. Hossain et al. (2020) reported that six lactic acid bacteria isolated from kimchi namely *Lactobacillus plantarum*, *Lactobacillus curvatus*, *Lactobacillus sakei*, and *Leuconostoc mesenteroides* effectively inhibited the biofilm formation of *L. monocytogenes* on stainless steel and lettuce. Following co-culture with lactic acid bacteria for 24 hours, *L. monocytogenes* populations in biofilms were significantly inhibited by 2.2 log and 1.6 log CFU/cm^2 on stainless steel and lettuce, respectively (Hossain et al. 2020).

Removal and Eradication of Biofilms

It is difficult to remove a biofilm once formed since bacteria are protected within the biofilms and become resistant to a lot of antimicrobials. To remove mature biofilms, treatments including physical, chemical, and biological strategies have been reported to improve the efficiency of biofilm disruption.

Physical Treatments

Physical treatment could lead to the destruction of biofilm structure. Common physical treatments used in the pipelines of the food-processing facility include heat shock treatment, shear stress, and ultrasound. The benefit of the physical treatments is that there is no residue left over in the removal process. Ultrasound treatment is a nonchemical and environmentally friendly technology to disrupt biofilm structure, which releases bacterial cells in their planktonic state or even inactivates microorganisms (Yu et al. 2020). Bang et al. (2017) reported a synergistic antibiofilm effect of ultrasound and peroxyacetic acid against *Cronobacter sakazakii* on cucumbers in which a combination of 60 minutes of ultrasound (37 kHz; 380 W) and 200 ppm peroxyacetic acid results in 3.5 log reductions of C. sakazaki populations in biofilms. *Bacillus* cereus can form biofilms on the surfaces of fresh leafy green vegetables. A combination of physical and chemical treatments was suggested by Hussain et al. (2019) to remove *B. cereus* biofilm from leafy green vegetables. They reported an additional reduction of ~ 1.5 logs CFU/cm^2 using a combined treatment of acidic electrolyzed water (80 mg/L), mild heat (60°C), and ultrasound (40 kHz; 400 W) for 12 minutes on spinach, beet leaf, and lettuce surfaces. Similarly, ultrasound treatment (75%; 700 W) for 14 minutes reduced more than 3 log *L. monocytogenes* in biofilm formed on brine injection needles (Hamann et al. 2019).

Further, a combination of ultrasound with peracetic acid enhanced the antibiofilm effect against *L. monocytogenes*.

Air bubbles of various sizes have been effective in removing bacterial populations from steel and polypropylene pipe walls by incorporating bubbles into cleaning water (Burfoot et al. 2017). The cavitation process to generate bubbles for removing pathogens from equipment surfaces has also been evaluated to remove pathogens on fresh produce (Lee et al. 2018). The air bubbles generated by cavitation removed ~ 1 log CFU of *L. monocytogenes* and *Salmonella* from submerged tomatoes and cantaloupe. Further, the bacterial removal efficiency of air bubbles increased with an increase in airflow rate. In a recent study, silver nanoparticles were comparable to sodium hypochlorite in removing mature biofilms formed by *P. aeruginosa* (Ismail et al. 2019). The antibiofilm efficiency of nanoparticles increased with an increase in contact time with biofilms. The electrolyzed water has been investigated to remove bacterial pathogen biofilms in liquid media and on equipment surfaces (Li et al. 2017, Moradi and Tajik 2017). The use of electrolyzed water has several advantages such as low cost, environmentally friendly, and fewer health hazards compared to other chemicals. Li et al (2017) reported that acidified electrolyzed water was more efficient than chlorine against *B. cereus* and removed < 99% of *B. cereus* populations in biofilms from the stainless steel surfaces. Khan and others (2016) reported that a submerged dielectric barrier discharge plasma significantly reduced *E. coli* O157:H7, *S. aureus*, and *C. sakazakii* populations from stainless steel surfaces. During plasma exposure, a reduction in the EPS layer of biofilm was also observed. A sequential treatment of the cold nitrogen plasma and phage was effective in reducing *E. coli* O157:H7 biofilms on lettuce, cucumbers, and carrots during storage at 4°C, 12°C, and 25°C for 14 days (Cui et al. 2018). Further, sensory evaluation data showed that sequential treatment of cold nitrogen plasma and phage did not cause significant changes in the surface color of these vegetables (Cui et al. 2018).

Chemical Treatments

Removal of biofilms on equipment surfaces is challenging once the biofilms are formed. Corcoran et al. (2014) reported that treatments with sodium hypochlorite (500 mg/L) or benzalkonium chloride (0.02%) for 10, 45, and 90 minutes reduced only 0.5–1 log CFU populations of S. Typhimurium in 48 hours biofilm formed on concrete surface coupon. Knowles and others (2005) reported that peroxide-based sanitizer was superior to carvacrol in removing the early stage of multispecies biofilm formed by *S. aureus* and *S. enterica* serovar Typhimurium; however, continuous feed of carvacrol helped in preventing mature stage of multispecies biofilms. Ölmez and Temur (2010) reported 3 log reduction of *E. coli* and *L. monocytogenes* populations in biofilms formed on lettuce leaves using ozone (2 ppm), chlorine (100 ppm), or a combination of citric and ascorbic acid. However, none of these treatments were effective in completely removing these bacterial biofilms. Shen and others (2012) used T-128, a fresh produce washing aid, in chlorinated wash solutions to remove *S. enterica* and *P. fluorescens* biofilms on the stainless steel surfaces. They reported significant inactivation of these bacteria using 1–5 ppm free chlorine in combination with 0.1% T-128 compared to free chlorine alone. A combination treatment of 3% Levulinic and 2% SDS was able to remove 7 log CFU/ml of bacterial populations in multispecies biofilm formed by *E. coli* O157:H7 and *S. enterica* compared to < 1 log reduction by 150 ppm quaternary ammonium compounds (Chen et al. 2015). Sanifoam®, a chlorinated alkaline detergent at 4% concentration was superior to 2% peracetic acid in removing *S. enterica* in biofilms formed on polystyrene slides (Ziech et al. 2016). Speranza and others (2017) evaluated the effects of sanitizers, exposure time, and temperature on *S. enterica* biofilms from the stainless steel surface. In their study, peracetic acid and quaternary ammonium salts were more effective than sodium hydroxide in removing biofilms, and the antibiofilm efficacy of these sanitizers varied with temperature. The dual-species biofilms of Serratia liquefaciens and Shewanella putrefaciens showed stronger resistance to ethanol and benzalkonium chloride than the single-species biofilms (Liu et al. 2017). They also reported that the biofilm removal by ethanol was significantly higher than the benzalkonium chloride. Cleaning-in-place (CIP) often used in the dairy industry could achieve only 4.69 log CFU/cm² reduction in *B. cereus* biofilms on stainless steel surfaces (Huang et al. 2019). However, benzalkonium bromide treatment following the CIP regime removed biofilm cells below the detection limit. Papaioannou and others (2018) used two commercial sanitizers, Hypofoam VF6, and Divosan SU319/VT8w, to remove single and multispecies biofilms formed by 5 strains of *Pseudomonas* spp. and 6 *L. monocytogenes* strains on the stainless steel surface. The sanitizers removed mixed-species sessile communities when applied for 15–30 minutes of exposure but were ineffective against *L. monocytogenes* single-species biofilms. Wang and others (2020) investigated a multicomponent sanitizer containing quaternary ammonium compound, hydrogen peroxide, and diacetin for removing *E. coli* O157:H7 and *S. enterica* biofilms under meat processing conditions. They reported 10 minutes of exposure to multicomponent sanitizer reduced these pathogens in biofilms to below the detection limit and dissolved EPS matrix. Fumarate, a weak acid at 25 mM concentration significantly reduced *L. monocytogenes* biofilms on polystyrene surfaces (Barnes and Karatzas 2020). Further, the effect of fumarate was also enhanced when combined with acidic sanitizer.

Essential oils derived from plant materials are alternative biocides that have also been evaluated for the removal of biofilms on various surfaces. Bacterial pathogens could become resistant to chemical disinfectants; the use of essential oils can avoid the concern of disinfectant resistance in microbial films. Essential oils namely thyme oil, oregano oil, and carvacrol at 0.006–0.12% concentrations reduced *Salmonella* biofilm by 2–4 fold on stainless steel surface; high concentration (0.05–0.1%) of these essential oils was needed to reduce 7 log CFU of *Salmonella* on polystyrene and stainless steel surface (Soni et al. 2013). Keelara et al. (2016) reported that 1,000 ppm of cinnamaldehyde and Sporan® significantly reduced *S. enterica* populations in biofilms by 6 log CFU from their initial biofilm populations of 7–7.5 log CFU/cm² on the MBEC biofilm assay. Further, a 24-hour biofilm of *S. aureus* biofilm on stainless steel was reduced from 7 log CFU to 3 log CFU with a treatment of Cinnamomum cassian essential oil microemulsion for 90 minutes (Campana et al. 2017). Yin et al. (2019) used antimicrobial peptide 1018 for inactivating bacterial cells in biofilms on stainless steel and polycarbonate surfaces. In their study, peptide 1018 at 50 µg/ml significantly reduced 3.7–4.6 and 1.0–3.5 log CFU/cm^2 populations of *L. monocytogenes* and Shiga toxigenic *E. coli* in biofilms, respectively, on the stainless steel surfaces. The extracts of turmeric and cinnamon were used to remove Staphylococcus biofilms on glass, steel, and polyvinyl chloride surfaces (Didar and Sani 2019). The antibiofilm effect of these hydrosol extracts was evident in removing *Staphylococcus saprophyticus* biofilms on the glass surfaces. Zhang and others (2020) found that clove oil was able to remove *L. monocytogenes* biofilms on polystyrene surfaces. The oil also down-regulated the expression of agrA, agrC, agrD, and prfA genes, which are important in biofilm formation. Clove oil encapsulated liposome at 0.001% and 0.0015% was reported to significantly reduce *E. coli* O157:H7 biofilms by 96.67% and 99.98% on cucumber skin stored at 25°C for 3 days (Cui et al. 2020). Moreover, the antibiofilm effect was stronger at 4°C; 99.81% and 99.99% of biofilms were reduced by 0.001% and 00015% clove oil solid liposome (Cui et al. 2020).

Biological Treatments

Bacteriophages isolated from a wide range of environments are viruses that can infect bacteria and affect biofilm formation. Bacteriophages have specific host ranges that directly attack bacteria within biofilms instead of targeting EPS. Bacteriophages have been investigated for their potential as an effective strategy for eradicating biofilms of single or multispecies. Certain bacteriophages could produce virion-associated polysaccharide depolymerases, which are enzymes for capsule degradations (Pires et al. 2016). Studies have found that depolymerase-producing bacteriophages exert greater biofilm eradication ability than non-secreting ones. The presence of this enzyme enhances the phage invasion and dispersion process through the biofilm under treatment (Parasion et al. 2014). Sharma and others (2004) reported that bacteriophage reduced *E. coli* O157:H7 attachment on stainless steel; however, it failed to kill cells in the biofilms. Patel et al. (2011b) investigated the efficacy of a phage mixture for the removal of biofilms formed on a spinach harvester blade and found a reduction of 4.5 log of *E. coli* O157:H7 populations in biofilms after 2 hours of phage treatment. Studies have focused on the applications of phages for removing biofilms on equipment surfaces. The treatment with single or mixed phages effectively reduced *L. monocytogenes* biofilms on stainless steel surfaces (Soni and Nannapaneni 2010, Montañez-Izquierdo et al. 2012, Arachchi et al. 2013). Bacteriophage-derived proteins were able to disrupt *S. aureus* biofilms as observed by a real-time cell analyzer (Gutierrez et al. 2017). Commercially available bacteriophage antimicrobials: Listex P100 and ListSield were equally effective in removing 72 hours old *L. monocytogenes* biofilms formed on stainless steel surfaces (Gutierrez et al. 2017). Madurkay and others (2019) were able to decrease Cronobacter spp. biofilm production in liquid medium using bacteriophage cocktail. However, the antibiofilm effect of bacteriophage against *Cronobacter* spp. was limited when used in powdered infant formula. Marine fungal extracts were investigated for their potential to remove *S. aureus, L. monocytogenes,*

E. coli, and *S. typhi* biofilms on stainless steel surfaces (Mahyudin et al. 2018). The antibiofilm activity was affected by the fungal extract, its exposure time, and the test pathogen; an extract from Sarocladium strictum was superior to other fungal extracts and S. typhi was the most sensitive pathogen used in the study. Enzymes specifically proteases have been investigated for removing biofilms on various equipment surfaces (Meireles et al. 2016). Proteolytic and polysaccharidases were evaluated for removing biofilms formed by 25 spoilage or pathogenic bacteria on stainless steel surfaces (Lequette et al. 2010). Serine proteases were more efficient in removing *B. cereus* biofilm and polysaccharidases were superior in removing *P. fluorescens* biofilm. Antimicrobial peptides derived from *B. subtilis* and *Paenibacillus thiaminolyticus* have shown antibiofilm effect against *Shewanella putrifaciens* and *L. monocytogenes*, respectively (Deng et al. 2017, Li et al. 2018). In another study, the enzyme treatment containing proteases was investigated to remove biofilm formed by *L. monocytogenes* on stainless steel surfaces. The effect of the enzyme varied with strains; it reduced up to 7 log CFU/cm^2 for one of the 17 strains used in the study (Mazaheri et al. 2020). Similarly, another proteolytic enzyme, papain at 5 ppm reduced 2 log CFU of *S. aureus* and *C. jejuni* biofilms on stainless steel coupon (Song et al. 2020). Nahar and others (2021) reported that flavourzyme, an industrial peptidase, significantly reduced 72 hours old mature biofilms formed by *S. Typhimurium*, *E. coli*, and *P. aeruginosa* on polyethylene and rubber surfaces.

Conclusion

Biofilms represent a source of foodborne pathogen contamination that has received a great deal of attention. Foodborne bacterial pathogens can attach, produce EPS, and form biofilms on fresh produce surfaces and food-contact surfaces at the pre-harvest and post-harvest levels. Biofilms on food-contact surfaces in the fresh produce processing facility provide a persistent source of contamination. Biofilm formation of foodborne pathogens could either be single-species biofilms or coexist with other environmental microorganisms with potentially enhanced antimicrobial resistant ability against disinfectants commonly used in the industry.

Research studies are conducted to understand the factors that influence the formation and maturation of biofilm and identify novel strategies for biofilm control. The formation of bacterial biofilm is a complex process and depends on several factors such as environmental factors, genetic regulations, as well as properties of fresh produce, equipment surfaces, and bacterial cells. Surface properties of bacteria, the origin of bacterial isolates, and bacterial serotypes have been found to affect the persistence and biofilm formation on abiotic and biotic surfaces. Produce-specific factors could include leaf topography, leaf roughness and number and size of the stoma, and indigenous microflora. As bacterial persistence and biofilm formation are affected by complex variables and regulatory networks, various results have been reported and suggest that assessments of biofilms on surfaces should be analyzed on a case-by-case basis.

The control of bacterial biofilms on fresh produce and equipment surfaces at the pre-harvest and post-harvest levels is important to protect fresh produce safety and public health. Physical, chemical, and biological controls that prevent biofilm formation or eradicate the formed biofilms have been proposed as control and removal strategies against biofilms by foodborne pathogens. The hurdle concept, a combination of physical-chemical or chemical-biological treatments could also be a promising approach, especially for biofilm eradication since the removal of mature biofilms can be very challenging. In summary, the effective prevention and control of biofilm-associated bacterial pathogens on fresh produce and equipment surface demand a greater understanding of the complexity of single- and multispecies biofilms as well as biological, environmental, and genetic factors that influence the persistence and biofilm formation of bacterial pathogens. Expanding knowledge in these areas would be beneficial to the fresh produce industry for improving fresh produce safety, thereby protecting public health.

Declaration of Competing Interest

None

Acknowledgments

The U.S. Department of Agriculture, Agricultural research service, is an equal opportunity provider and employer. Mention of trade names or commercial products in this publication is solely to provide specific information and does not imply recommendation or endorsement by the U.S. Department of Agriculture.

References

Abeysundara, P. D. A., N. Dhowlaghar, R. Nannapaneni, M. W. Schilling, S. Chang, B. Mahmoud et al. (2017). Growth and biofilm formation by *Listeria monocytogenes* in cantaloupe flesh and peel extracts on four food-contact surfaces at 22°C and 10°C. Food Control 80: 131–142.

Abeysundara, P. D. A., N. Dhowlaghar, R. Nannapaneni, M. W. Schilling, B. Mahmoud, C. S. Sharma et al. (2018). *Salmonella enterica* growth and biofilm formation in flesh and peel cantaloupe extracts on four food-contact surfaces. Int. J. Food Microbiol. 280: 17–26.

Abdallah, F. B., R. Lagha, S. A. I. D. Khaled, H. Kallel and J. Gharbi. (2014). Detection of cell surface hydrophobicity, biofilm and fimbirae genes in *Salmonella* isolated from tunisian clinical and poultry meat. Iran. J. Public Health 43: 423–431.

Abee, T., Á. T. Kovács, O. P. Kuipers and S. Van der Veen. (2011). Biofilm formation and dispersal in Gram-positive bacteria. Curr. Opin. Biotechnol. 22: 172–179.

Adetunji, V. O. and T. O. Isola. (2011). Crystal violet binding assay for assessment of biofilm formation by *Listeria monocytogenes* and *Listeria* spp on wood, steel and glass surfaces. Glob. Vet. 6: 6–10.

Agarwal, R. K., S. Singh, K. N. Bhilegaonkar and V. P. Singh. (2011). Optimization of microtitre plate assay for the testing of biofilm formation ability in different *Salmonella* serotypes. Int. Food Res. J. 18: 1493.

Algburi, A., A. Asghar, Q. Huang, W. Mustfa, H. U. Javed, S. Zehm et al. (2020). Black cardamom essential oil prevents *Escherichia coli* O157: H7 and *Salmonella Typhimurium* JSG 1748 biofilm formation through inhibition of quorum sensing. J. Food Sci. Technol. 1–9. https://doi.org/10.1007/s13197–020–04821–8.

Allende, A., E. Aguayo and F. Artés. (2004). Microbial and sensory quality of commercial fresh processed red lettuce throughout the production chain and shelf life. Int. J. Food Microbiol. 91: 109–117.

Ammendolia, M. G., R. Di Rosa, L. Montanaro, C. R. Arciola and L. Baldassarri. (1999). Slime production and expression of the slime-associated antigen by staphylococcal clinical isolates. J. Clin. Microbiol. 37: 3235–3238.

Amrutha, B., K. Sundar and P. H. Shetty. (2017). Study on *E. coli* and *Salmonella* biofilms from fresh fruits and vegetables. J. Food Sci. Technol. 54: 1091–1097.

An, D., T. Danhorn, C. Fuqua and M. R. Parsek. (2006). Quorum sensing and motility mediate interactions between *Pseudomonas aeruginosa* and Agrobacterium tumefaciens in biofilm cocultures. Proc. Natl. Acad. Sci. 103: 3828–3833.

Anunthawan, T., C. De La Fuente-Núñez, R. E. Hancock and S. Klaynongsruang. (2015). Cationic amphipathic peptides KT2 and RT2 are taken up into bacterial cells and kill planktonic and biofilm bacteria. Biochim. Biophys-Acta Biomembr. 1848: 1352–1358.

Anriany, Y. A., R. M. Weiner, J. A. Johnson, C. E. De Rezende and S. W. Joseph. (2001). *Salmonella enterica* serovar Typhimurium DT104 displays a rugose phenotype. Appl. Environ. Microbiol. 67: 4048–4056.

Arachchi, G. J. G., A. G. Cridge, B. M. Dias-Wanigasekera, C. D. Cruz, L. McIntyre, R. Liu et al. (2013). Effectiveness of phages in the decontamination of *Listeria monocytogenes* adhered to clean stainless steel, stainless steel coated with fish protein, and as a biofilm. J. Ind. Microbiol. Biotechnol. 40: 1105–1116.

Arce Miranda, J. E., C. E. Sotomayor, I. Albesa and M. G. Paraje. (2011). Oxidative and nitrosative stress in *Staphylococcus aureus* biofilm. FEMS Microbiol. Lett. 315: 23–29.

Armbruster, C. R. and M. R. Parsek. (2018). New insight into the early stages of biofilm formation. Proc. Natl. Acad. Sci. 115: 4317–4319.

Baert, L., I. Vandekinderen, F. Devlieghere, E. Van Coillie, J. Debevere and M. Uyttendaele. (2009). Efficacy of sodium hypochlorite and peroxyacetic acid to reduce murine norovirus 1, B40–8, *Listeria monocytogenes*, and *Escherichia coli* O157: H7 on shredded iceberg lettuce and in residual wash water. J. Food Prot. 72: 1047–1054.

Baig, U., M. A. Ansari, M. A. Gondal, S. Akhtar, F. A. Khan and W. S. Falath. (2020). Single step production of high-purity copper oxide-titanium dioxide nanocomposites and their effective antibacterial and anti-biofilm activity against drug-resistant bacteria. Materials Sci. Engg. 113: 110992.

Balaban, N. and A. Rasooly. (2000). Staphylococcal enterotoxins. Int. J. Food Microbiol. 61: 1–10.

Bang, J., A. Hong, H. Kim, L. R. Beuchat, S. Rhee, Y. Kim et al. (2014). Inactivation of *Escherichia coli* O157: H7 in biofilm on food-contact surfaces by sequential treatments of aqueous chlorine dioxide and drying. Int. J. Food Microbiol. 191: 129–134.

Bang, H. J., S. Y. Park, S. E. Kim, M. M. F. Rahaman and S. D. Ha. (2017). Synergistic effects of combined ultrasound and peroxyacetic acid treatments against *Cronobacter sakazakii* biofilms on fresh cucumber. LWT-Food Sci. Technol. 84: 91–98.

Barak, J. D., C. E. Jahn, D. L. Gibson and A. O. Charkowski. (2007). The role of cellulose and O-antigen capsule in the colonization of plants by *Salmonella enterica*. Mol. Plant Microbe. Interac. 20: 1083–1091.

Barak, J. D., L. Gorski, P. Naraghi-Arani and A. O. Charkowski. (2005). *Salmonella enterica* virulence genes are required for bacterial attachment to plant tissue. Appl. Environ. Microbiol. 71: 5685–5691.

Barak, J. D., L. Gorski, A. S. Liang and K. E. Narm. (2009). Previously uncharacterized *Salmonella enterica* genes required for swarming play a role in seedling colonization. Microbiol. 155: 3701–3709.

Barak, J. D., L. C. Kramer and L. Y. Hao. (2011). Colonization of tomato plants by *Salmonella enterica* is cultivar dependent, and type 1 trichomes are preferred colonization sites. Appl. Environ. Microbiol. 77: 498–504.

Barak, J. D. and B. K. Schroeder. (2012). Interrelationships of food safety and plant pathology: The life cycle of human pathogens on plants. Annu. Rev. Phytopathol. 50: 241–266.

Barnes, R. H. and K. A. G. Karatzas. (2020). Investigation into the antimicrobial activity of fumarate against *Listeria monocytogenes* and its mode of action under aerobic conditions. Int. J. Food Microbiol. 324: 108614.

Bennett, S. D., S. V. Sodha, T. L. Ayers, M. F. Lynch, L. H. Gould and R. V. Tauxe. (2018). Produce-associated foodborne disease outbreaks, USA, 1998–2013. Epidemiol. Infect. 11: 1397–1406.

Beloin, C. and J. M. Ghigo. (2005). Finding gene-expression patterns in bacterial biofilms. Trends Microbiol. 13: 16–19.

Belval, S. C., L. Gal, S. Margiewes, D. Garmyn, P. Piveteau and J. Guzzo. (2006). Assessment of the roles of LuxS, S-ribosyl homocysteine, and autoinducer 2 in cell attachment during biofilm formation by *Listeria monocytogenes* EGD-e. Appl. Environ. Microbiol. 72: 2644–2650.

Berger, C. N., R. K. Shaw, D. J. Brown, H. Mather, S. Clare, G. Dougan et al. (2009). Interaction of *Salmonella enterica* with basil and other salad leaves. ISME J. 3: 261–265.

Berger, C. N., S. V. Sodha, R. K. Shaw, P. M. Griffin, D. Pink, P. Hand et al. (2010). Fresh fruit and vegetables as vehicles for the transmission of human pathogens. Environ. Microbiol. 12: 2385–2397.

Beuchat, L. R. (2002). Ecological factors influencing survival and growth of human pathogens on raw fruits and vegetables. Microbes Infect. 4: 413–423.

Boddicker, J. D., N. A. Ledeboer, J. Jagnow, B. D. Jones and S. Clegg. (2002). Differential binding to and biofilm formation on, HEp-2 cells by *Salmonella enterica* Serovar Typhimurium is dependent upon allelic variation in the fimH gene of the fim gene cluster. Mol. Microbiol. 45: 1255–1265.

Bordi, C. and S. de Bentzmann. (2011). Hacking into bacterial biofilms: a new therapeutic challenge. Ann. Intensive Care 1: 19. https://doi.org/10.1186/2110–5820–1–19.

Boyer, R. R., S. S. Summer, R. C. Williams, M. D. Pierson, D. L. Popham and K. E. Kniel. (2007). Influence of curli expression by *Escherichia coli* O157: H7 on the cell's overall hydrophobicity, charge, and ability to attach to lettuce. J. Food Protect. 70: 1339–1345.

Braga, L. C., J. W. Shupp, C. Cummings, M. Jett, J. A. Takahashi, L. S. Carmo et al. (2005). Pomegranate extract inhibits *Staphylococcus aureus* growth and subsequent enterotoxin production. J. Ethnopharmacol. 96: 335–339.

Brandl, M. T. (2006). Fitness of human enteric pathogens on plants and implications for food safety. Annu. Rev. Phytopathol. 44: 367–392.

Brandl, M. T. (2008). Plant lesions promote the rapid multiplication of *Escherichia coli* O157: H7 on postharvest lettuce. Appl. Environ. Microbiol. 74: 5285–5289.

Bridier, A., R. Briandet, V. Thomas and F. Dubois-Brissonnet. (2011). Comparative biocidal activity of peracetic acid, benzalkonium chloride and ortho-phthalaldehyde on 77 bacterial strains. J. Hosp. Infect. 78: 208–213.

Bumunang, E. W., C. N. Ateba, K. Stanford, T. A. McAllister and Y. D. Niu. (2020). Biofilm formation by South African non-O157 Shiga toxigenic *Escherichia coli* on stainless steel coupons. Can. J. Microbiol. 66: 328–336.

Burfoot, D., R. Limburn and R. Busby. (2017). Assessing the effects of incorporating bubbles into the water used for cleaning operations relevant to the food industry. Int. J. Food Sci. Technol. 52: 1894–1903.

Burmølle, M., D. Ren, T. Bjarnsholt and S. J. Sørensen. (2014). Interactions in multispecies biofilms: do they actually matter? Trends Microbiol. 22: 84–91.

Byun, S., C. Chen, H. Yin and J. R. Patel. (2019). Antimicrobial effects of natural fruit extracts against *Salmonella* on cucumbers. Int. Association Food Prot. 2: 194.

Caiazza, N. C. and G. A. O'Toole. (2004). SadB is required for the transition from reversible to irreversible attachment during biofilm formation by *Pseudomonas aeruginosa* PA14. J. Bacteriol. 186: 4476–4485.

Callahan, M. T. and S. A. Micallef. (2019). Waxing and cultivar affect *Salmonella enterica* persistence on cucumber (*Cucumis sativus* L.) fruit. Int. J. Food Microbiol. 310: 108359.

Camargo, A. C., S. D. Todorov, N. E. Chihib, D. Drider and L. A. Nero. (2018). Lactic acid bacteria (LAB) and their bacteriocins as alternative biotechnological tools to control *Listeria monocytogenes* biofilms in food processing facilities. Mol. Biotechnol. 60: 712–726.

Campana, R., L. Casettari, L. Fagioli, M. Cespi, G. Bonacucina and W. Baffone. (2017). Activity of essential oil-based microemulsions against *Staphylococcus aureus* biofilms developed on stainless steel surface in different culture media and growth conditions. Int. J. Food Microbiol. 240: 132–140.

Cappitelli, F., A. Polo and F. Villa. (2014). Biofilm formation in food processing environments is still poorly understood and controlled. Food Engineering Rev. 6: 29–42.

Carpentier, B. and D. Chassaing. (2004). Interactions in biofilms between *Listeria monocytogenes* and resident microorganisms from food industry premises. Int. J. Food Microbiol. 97: 111–122.

Carter, M. Q. and M. T. Brandl. (2015). Biofilms in fresh vegetables and fruits. pp. 176–204. *In*: A. L. Pometto III and A. Demirci (eds.). Biofilms in the Food Environment, 2nd edition. Wiley-Blackwell Hoboken, NJ, USA.

Centers for Disease Control and Prevention. (2005). Outbreaks of *Salmonella* infections associated with eating Roma tomatoes—United States and Canada, 2004. Morb. Mortal. Wkly. Rep. 54: 325–328.

Centers for Disease Control and Prevention. (2006). Multistate outbreak of *Salmonella typhimurium* infections linked to tomatoes. https://www.cdc.gov/*salmonella*/2006/tomatoes-11–2006.html.

Centers for Disease Control and Prevention (CDC). (2011). Surveillance for foodborne disease outbreaks—United States, 2008. MMWR. Morb. Mortal. Wkly. Rep. 60: 1197.

Centers for Disease Control and Prevention (CDC). (2020). Foodborne outbreaks. https://www.cdc.gov/foodsafety/outbreaks/index.html.

Cerca, N., J. L. Brooks and K. K. Jefferson. (2008). Regulation of the intercellular adhesin locus regulator (icaR) by SarA, σB, and IcaR in *Staphylococcus aureus*. J. Bacteriol. 190: 6530–6533.

Chae, M. S., H. Schraft, L. T. Hansen and R. Mackereth. (2006). Effects of physicochemical surface characteristics of *Listeria monocytogenes* strains on attachment to glass. Food Microbiol. 23: 250–259.

Chavant, P., B. Martinie, T. Meylheuc, M. N. Bellon-Fontaine and M. Hebraud. (2002). *Listeria monocytogenes* LO28: Surface physicochemical properties and ability to form biofilms at different temperatures and growth phases. Appl. Environ. Microbiol. 68: 728–737.

Chen, J., S. M. Lee and Y. Mao. (2004). Protective effect of exopolysaccharide colanic acid of *Escherichia coli* O157: H7 to osmotic and oxidative stress. Int. J. Food Microbiol. 93: 281–286.

Chen, D., T. Zhao and M. P. Doyle. (2015). Single- and multi-species biofilm formation by *Escherichia coli* O157:H7 and *Salmonella*, and their sensitivity to levulinic acid plus sodium dodecyl sulfate. Food Control 57: 48–53.

Chia, T. W. R., R. W. Goulter, T. McMeekin, G. A. Dykes and N. Fegan. (2009). Attachment of different *Salmonella* serovars to materials commonly used in a poultry processing plant. Food Microbiol. 26: 853–859.

Chmielewski, R. A. N. and J. F. Frank. (2003). Biofilm formation and control in food processing facilities. Compr. Rev. Food Sci. F. 2: 22–32.

Collinson, S. K., P. C. Doig, J. L. Doran, S. Clouthier and W. W. Kay. (1993). Thin, aggregative fimbriae mediate binding of *Salmonella enteritidis* to fibronectin. J. Bacteriol. 175: 12–18.

Cook, R. (2016). Fresh-cut/value-added produce marketing trends. UC Davis fresh cut products workshop: maintaining quality and safety (Davis, CA, USA). https://arefiles.ucdavis.edu/uploads/filer_public/fb/7b/fb7b6380-cdf9-4db5-b5d2–993640bcc1e6/ freshcut2016cook20160926final.pdf.

Cooley, M. B., D. Chao and R. E. Mandrell. (2006). *Escherichia coli* O157: H7 survival and growth on lettuce is altered by the presence of epiphytic bacteria. J. Food Prot. 69: 2329–2335.

Cooley, M. B., W. G. Miller and R. E. Mandrell. (2003). Colonization of Arabidopsis thaliana with *Salmonella enterica* and enterohemorrhagic *Escherichia coli* O157: H7 and competition by Enterobacter asburiae. Appl. Environ. Microbiol. 69: 4915–4926.

Corcoran, M., D. Morris, N. De Lappe, J. O'connor, P. Lalor, P. Dockery et al. (2014). Commonly used disinfectants fail to eradicate *Salmonella enterica* biofilms from food contact surface materials. Appl. Environ. Microbiol. 80: 1507–1514.

Corzo-Ariyama, H. A., A. García-Heredia, N. Heredia, S. García, J. León, L. Jaykus et al. (2019). Phylogroups, pathotypes, biofilm formation and antimicrobial resistance of *Escherichia coli* isolates in farms and packing facilities of tomato, jalapeño pepper and cantaloupe from Northern Mexico. Int. J. Food Microbiol. 290: 96–104.

Cramton, S. E., C. Gerke, N. F. Schnell, W. W. Nichols and F. Götz. (1999). The intercellular adhesion (ica) locus is present in Staphylococcus aureus and is required for biofilm formation. Infect. Immun. 67: 5427–5433.

Cue, D., M. G. Lei, T. T. Luong, L. Kuechenmeister, P. M. Dunman, S. O'Donnell et al. (2009). Rbf promotes biofilm formation by Staphylococcus aureus via repression of icaR, a negative regulator of *icaADBC*. J. Bacteriol. 191: 6363–6373.

Cui, H., M. Bai, L. Yuan, D. Surendhiran and L. Lin. (2018). Sequential effect of phages and cold nitrogen plasma against *Escherichia coli* O157: H7 biofilms on different vegetables. Int. J. Food Microbiol. 268: 1–9.

Cui, H., C. Zhang, C. Li and L. Lin. (2020). Inhibition of *Escherichia coli* O157: H7 biofilm on vegetable surface by solid liposomes of clove oil. LWT-Food Sci. Technol. 117: 108656. Doi: 10.1016/j. lwt.2019.108656.

Dandie, C. E., A. D. Ogunniyi, S. Ferro, B. Hall, B., Drigo, C. W. Chow et al. (2020). Disinfection options for irrigation water: Reducing the risk of fresh produce contamination with human pathogens. Crit. Rev. Environ. Sci. Technol. 50: 2144–2174.

Daniels, R., J. Vanderleyden and J. Michiels. (2004). Quorum sensing and swarming migration in bacteria. FEMS Microbiol. Rev. 28: 261–289.

da Silva Meira, Q. G., I. de Medeiros Barbosa, A. J. A. A. Athayde, J. P. de Siqueira-Júnior and E. L. de Souza. (2012). Influence of temperature and surface kind on biofilm formation by *Staphylococcus aureus* from food-contact surfaces and sensitivity to sanitizers. Food Control 25: 469–475.

Davey, M. E. and G. A. O'toole. (2000). Microbial biofilms: From ecology to molecular genetics. Microbiol. Mol. Biol. Rev. 64: 847–867.

de Grandi, A. Z., U. M. Pinto and M. T. Destro. (2018). Dual-species biofilm of *Listeria monocytogenes* and *Escherichia coli* on stainless steel surface. World J. Microb. Biot. 34: 1–9.

Delaquis, P., S. Bach and L. D. Dinu. (2007). Behavior of *Escherichia coli* O157: H7 in leafy vegetables. J. Food Prot. 70: 1966–1974.

Deng, Q., Y. Pu, L. Sun, Y. Wang, Y. Liu, R. Wang et al. (2017). Antimicrobial peptide AMPNT-6 from Bacillus subtilis inhibits biofilm formation by Shewanella putrefaciens and disrupts its performed biofilms on both abiotic and shrimp cell surfaces. Food Res. Int. 102: 8–13.

Dewanti, R. and A. C. Wong. (1995). Influence of culture conditions on biofilm formation by *Escherichia coli* O157: H7. Int. J. Food Microbiol. 26: 147–164.

Di Bonaventura, G., R. Piccolomini, D. Paludi, V. D'orio, A. Vergara, M. Conter et al. (2008). Influence of temperature on biofilm formation by *Listeria monocytogenes* on various food-contact surfaces: Relationship with motility and cell surface hydrophobicity. J. Appl. Microbiol. 104: 1552–1561.

Di Ciccio, P., A. Vergara, A. R. Festino, D. Paludi, E. Zanardi, S. Ghidini et al. (2015). Biofilm formation by *Staphylococcus aureus* on food contact surfaces: Relationship with temperature and cell surface hydrophobicity. Food Control 50: 930–936.

Didar, Z. and A. M. Sani. (2019). Comparison of the effects of hydrosol extracted from turmeric (Curcuma longa) and cinnamon (Cinnamomum verum) on Staphylococcal biofilm. J. Babol Uni. Med. Sci. 21: 293–298.

Djordjevic, D., M. Wiedmann and L. A. McLandsborough. (2002). Microtiter plate assay for assessment of *Listeria monocytogenes* biofilm formation. Appl. Environ. Microbiol. 68: 2950–2958.

Doyle, M. P. and M. C. Erickson. (2008). Summer meeting 2007–the problems with fresh produce: An overview. J. Appl. Microbiol. 104: 317–330.

Dykes, G. A., B. Sampathkumar and D. R. Korber. (2003). Planktonic or biofilm growth affects survival, hydrophobicity and protein expression patterns of a pathogenic Campylobacter jejuni strain. Int. J. Food Microbiol. 89: 1–10.

Economic Research Service - United States Department of Agriculture (ERS-USDA). (2018). Vegetables and pulses yearbook data. U.S. per capita use of fresh and processing vegetables, dry pulse crops, and potatoes; cash receipts; U.S. vegetable trade. https://www.ers.usda.gov/ data-products/vegetables-and-pulses-data/vegetables-and-pulses-yearbooktables/.

Espina, L., D. Berdejo, P. Alfonso, D. Garcia-Gonzalo and R. Pagan. (2017). Potential use of carvacrol and citral to inactivate biofilm cells and eliminate biofouling. Food Control 82: 256–265.

Fagerlund, A., T. Møretrø, E. Heir, R. Briandet and S. Langsrud. (2017). Cleaning and disinfection of biofilms composed of *Listeria monocytogenes* and background microbiota from meat processing surfaces. Appl. Environ. Microbiol. 83: e01046–17.

Farber, J. M., S. L. Wang, Y. Cai and S. Zhang. (1998). Changes in populations of *Listeria monocytogenes* inoculated on packaged fresh-cut vegetables. J. Food Prot. 61: 192–195.

Farkas, J. and C. Mohácsi-Farkas. (2011). History and future of food irradiation. Trends Food Sci. Technol. 22: 121–126.

Felício, M. D. S., T. Hald, E. Liebana, A. Allende, M. Hugas, C. Nguyen-The et al. (2015). Risk ranking of pathogens in ready-to-eat unprocessed foods of non-animal origin (FoNAO) in the EU: Initial evaluation using outbreak data (2007–2011). Int. J. Food Microbiol. 195: 9–19.

Fink, R. C., E. P. Black, Z. Hou, M. Sugawara, M. J. Sadowsky and F. Diez-Gonzalez. (2012). Transcriptional responses of *Escherichia coli* K-12 and O157: H7 associated with lettuce leaves. Appl. Environ. Microbiol. 78: 1752–1764.

Flemming, H. C. and J. Wingender. (2010). The biofilm matrix. Nature Rev. Microbiol. 8: 623–633.

Flemming, H. C., T. R. Neu and D. J. Wozniak. (2007). The EPS matrix: The "house of biofilm cells". J. Bacteriol. 189: 7945–7947.

Gelting, R. J., M. A. Baloch, M. A. Zarate-Bermudez and C. Selman. (2011). Irrigation water issues potentially related to the 2006 multistate *E. coli* O157: H7 outbreak associated with spinach. Agric. Water Manag. 98: 1395–1402.

Gerstel, U. and U. Römling. (2003). The csgD promoter, a control unit for biofilm formation in *Salmonella typhimurium*. Res. Microbiol. 154: 659–667.

Giovannacci, I., G. Ermel, G. Salvat, J. L. Vendeuvre and M. N. Bellon-Fontaine. (2000). Physicochemical surface properties of five *Listeria monocytogenes* strains from a pork-processing environment in relation to serotypes, genotypes and growth temperature. J. Appl. Microbiol. 88: 992–1000.

Glass, K. A., J. M. Loeffelholz, J. P. Ford and M. P. Doyle. (1992). Fate of *Escherichia coli* O157: H7 as affected by pH or sodium chloride and in fermented, dry sausage. Appl. Environ. Microbiol. 58: 2513–2516.

Gloag, E. S., L. Turnbull, A. Huang, P. Vallotton, H. Wang, L. M. Nolan et al. (2013). Self-organization of bacterial biofilms is facilitated by extracellular DNA. Proc. Natl. Acad. Sci. 110: 11541–11546.

Golberg, D., Y. Kroupitski, E. Belausov, R. Pinto and S. Sela. (2011). *Salmonella Typhimurium* internalization is variable in leafy vegetables and fresh herbs. Int. J. Food Microbiol. 145: 250–257.

Gómez, N. C., J. M. Ramiro, B. X. Quecan and B. D. de Melo Franco. (2016). Use of potential probiotic lactic acid bacteria (LAB) biofilms for the control of *Listeria monocytogenes*, *Salmonella Typhimurium*, and *Escherichia coli* O157: H7 biofilms formation. Front. Microbiol. 7: 863.

Goulter, R. M., I. R. Gentle and G. A. Dykes. (2010). Characterization of curli production, cell surface hydrophobicity, autoaggregation and attachment behaviour of *Escherichia coli* O157. Curr. Microbiol. 61(3):157–162.

Govaert, M., C. Smet, M. Baka, T. Janssens and J. V. Impe. (2018). Influence of incubation conditions on the formation of model biofilms by *Listeria monocytogenes* and *Salmonella Typhimurium* on abiotic surfaces. J. Appl. Microbiol. 125: 1890–1900.

Grantcharova, N., V. Peters, C. Monteiro, K. Zakikhany and U. Römling. (2010). Bistable expression of CsgD in biofilm development of *Salmonella enterica* serovar typhimurium. J Bacteriol. 192: 456–466.

Gu, G., J. Hu, J. M. Cevallos-Cevallos, S. M. Richardson, J. A. Bartz and A. H. Van Bruggen. (2011). Internal colonization of *Salmonella enterica* serovar Typhimurium in tomato plants. PloS One 6: e27340.

Gueriri, I., C. Cyncynatus, S. Dubrac, A. T. Arana, O. Dussurget and T. Msadek. (2008). The *DegU* orphan response regulator of *Listeria monocytogenes* autorepresses its own synthesis and is required for bacterial motility, virulence and biofilm formation. Microbiol. 154: 2251–2264.

Guillier, L., V. Stahl, B. Hezard, E. Notz and R. Briandet. (2008). Modelling the competitive growth between *Listeria monocytogenes* and biofilm microflora of smear cheese wooden shelves. Int. J. Food Microbiol. 128: 51–57.

Guo, S., Y. Li, J. Chu, L. Wang, X. Zhao, N. Zhong et al. (2011). First observation of excision and integration in Class 1 integron in staphylococci. Afr. J Biotechnol. 10: 12847–12851.

Gutierrez, D., L. Fernandez, B. Martinez, P. Ruas-Madiedo, P. Garcia and A. Rodriguez. (2017). Real-time assessment of *Staphylococcus aureus* biofilm disruption by phage-derived proteins. Front. Microbiol. 8: 1632. Doi: 10.3389/fmicb.2017.01632.

Gutierrez, D., L. Rodriguez-Rubio, L. Fernandez, N. Martinez, A. Rodriguez and P. Garcia. (2017). Applicability of commercial page-based products against *Listeria monocytogenes* for improvement of food safety in Spanish dry-cured ham and food contact surfaces. Food Control 73: 1474–1482.

Habimana, O., E. Heir, S. Langsrud, A. W. Åsli and T. Møretrø. (2010). Enhanced surface colonization by *Escherichia coli* O157: H7 in biofilms formed by an *Acinetobacter calcoaceticus* isolate from meat-processing environments. Appl. Environ. Microbiol. 76: 4557–4559.

Hall-Stoodley, L., J. W. Costerton and P. Stoodley. (2004). Bacterial biofilms: From the natural environment to infectious diseases. Nature Rev. Microbiol. 2: 95–108.

Hamann, D., K. F. Tonkiel, A. Matthiense, J. Zeni, E. Valduga, N. Paroul et al. (2018). Ultrasound use for *Listeria monocytogenes* attached cells removal from industrial brine injection needles. Italian J. Food Sci. 30: 662–672.

Han, S., and S. A. Micallef. (2014). *Salmonella* Newport and Typhimurium colonization of fruit differs from leaves in various tomato cultivars. J. Food Prot. 77: 1844–1850.

Han, R., Y. A. K. Klu and J. Chen. (2017). Attachment and biofilm formation by selected strains of *Salmonella enterica* and entrohemorrhagic *Escherichia coli* of fresh produce origin. J. Food Sci. 82: 1461–1466.

Hassan, A. N. and J. F. Frank. (2004). Attachment of *Escherichia coli* O157:H7 grown in tryptic soy broth and nutrient broth to apple and lettuce surfaces as related to cell hydrophobicity, surface charge, and capsule production. Int. J. Food Microbiol. 96(1): 103–109.

Heir, E., T. Møretrø, A. Simensen and S. Langsrud. (2018). *Listeria monocytogenes* strains show large variations in competitive growth in mixed culture biofilms and suspensions with bacteria from food processing environments. Int. J. Food Microbiol. 275: 46–55.

Hinsa, S. M., M. Espinosa-Urgel, J. L. Ramos and G. A. O'Toole. (2003). Transition from reversible to irreversible attachment during biofilm formation by *Pseudomonas fluorescens* WCS365 requires an ABC transporter and a large secreted protein. Mol. Microbiol. 49: 905–918.

Hossain, M. I., M. F. R. Mizan, M. Ashrafudoulla, S. Nahar, H. J. Joo, I. K. Jahid et al. (2020). Inhibitory effects of probiotic potential lactic acid bacteria isolated from kimchi against *Listeria monocytogenes* biofilm on lettuce, stainless-steel surfaces, and MBEC™ biofilm device. LWT-Food Sci. Technol. 118: 108864.

Huang, K., L. A. McLandsborough and J. M. Goddard. (2016). Adhesion and removal kinetics of *Bacillus cereus* biofilms on NI-PTFE modified stainless steel. Biofouling 32: 523–533.

Huang, Z., Y. Lin, F. Ren, S. Song and H. Guo. (2019). Benzalkonium bromide is effective in removing Bacillus cereus biofilm on stainless steel when combined with cleaning-in-place. Food Control. 105: 13–20.

Hunter, P. J., R. K. Shaw, C. N. Berger, G. Frankel, D. Pink and P. Hand. (2015). Older leaves of lettuce (Lactuca spp.) support higher levels of *Salmonella enterica* ser. Senftenberg attachment and show greater variation between plant accessions than do younger leaves. FEMS Microbiol. Lett. 362: fnv077. Doi: 10.1093/femsle/fnv077.

Hussain, M. S., M. Kwon, E. J., Park, K. Seheli, R. Huque and D. H. Oh. (2019). Disinfection of *Bacillus cereus* biofilms on leafy green vegetables with slightly acidic electrolyzed water, ultrasound and mild heat. LWT-Food Sci. Technol. 116: 108582. Doi: 10.1016/j.lwt.2019.108582.

Ibusquiza, P. S., J. J. R. Herrera and M. L. Cabo. (2011). Resistance to benzalkonium chloride, peracetic acid and nisin during formation of mature biofilms by *Listeria monocytogenes*. Food Microbiol. 28: 418–425.

Ibusquiza, P. S., J. J. Herrera, D. Vßzquez-Sßnchez and M. L. Cabo. (2012). Adherence kinetics, resistance to benzalkonium chloride and microscopic analysis of mixed biofilms formed by *Listeria monocytogenes* and *Pseudomonas putida*. Food Control 25: 202–210.

Islam, M., M. P. Doyle, S. C. Phatak, P. Millner and X. Jiang. (2004). Persistence of enterohemorrhagic *Escherichia coli* O157: H7 in soil and on leaf lettuce and parsley grown in fields treated with contaminated manure composts or irrigation water. J. Food Prot. 67: 1365–1370.

Ismail, A. E. M. A., S. A. H. Kotb, I. A. H. Mohamed and H. S. Abdel-Mohsein. (2019). Silver nanoparticles and sodium hypochlorite inhibitory effects on biofilm produced by *Pseudomonas aeruginosa* from poultry farms. J. Adv. Vet. Research 9: 178–186.

Jacxsens, L., F. Devlieghere, P. Falcato and J. Debevere. (1999). Behavior of *Listeria monocytogenes* and Aeromonas spp. on fresh-cut produce packaged under equilibrium-modified atmosphere. J. Food Prot. 62: 1128–1135.

Jain, S. and J. Chen. (2007). Attachment and biofilm formation by various serotypes of *Salmonella* as influenced by cellulose production and thin aggregative fimbriae biosynthesis. J. Food Prot. 70: 2473–2479.

Jensen, A., M. H. Larsen, H. Ingmer, B. F. Vogel and L. Gram. (2007). Sodium chloride enhances adherence and aggregation and strain variation influences invasiveness of *Listeria monocytogenes* strains. J. Food Prot. 70: 592–599.

Jeter, C. and A. G. Matthysse. (2005). Characterization of the binding of diarrheagenic strains of *E. coli* to plant surfaces and the role of curli in the interaction of the bacteria with alfalfa sprouts. Mol. Plant Microbe. Interact. 18: 1235–1242.

Jones, C. R., M. R. Adams, P. A. Zhdan and A. H. L. Chamberlain. (1999). The role of surface physicochemical properties in determining the distribution of the autochthonous microflora in mineral water bottles. J. Appl. Microbiol. 86: 917–927.

Joseph, B., S. K. Otta, I. Karunasagar and I. Karunasagar. (2001). Biofilm formation by *Salmonella* spp. on food contact surfaces and their sensitivity to sanitizers. Int. J. Food Microbiol. 64: 367–372.

Kabir, M. N., S. Aras, S. Wadood, S. Chowdhury and A. C. Fouladkhah. (2020). Fate and biofilm formation of wild-type and pressure-stressed pathogens of public health concern in surface water and on abiotic surfaces. Microorganisms 8: 408. Doi: 10.3390/microorganisms8030408.

Kadam, S. R., H. M. den Besten, S. van der Veen, M. H. Zwietering, R. Moezelaar and T. Abee. (2013). Diversity assessment of *Listeria monocytogenes* biofilm formation: Impact of growth condition, serotype and strain origin. Int. J. Food Microbiol. 165: 259–264.

Kader, A., R. Simm, U. Gerstel, M. Morr and U. Römling. (2006). Hierarchical involvement of various GGDEF domain proteins in rdar morphotype development of *Salmonella enterica* serovar Typhimurium. Mol. Microbiol. 60: 602–616.

Kalmokoff, M. L., J. W. Austin, X. D. Wan, G. Sanders, S. Banerjee and J. M. Farber. (2001). Adsorption, attachment and biofilm formation among isolates of *Listeria monocytogenes* using model conditions. J. Appl. Microbiol. 91: 725–734.

Karaca, B., N. Akcelik and M. Akcelik. (2013). Biofilm-producing abilities of *Salmonella* strains isolated from Turkey. Biologia 68: 1–10.

Keelara, S., S. Thakur and J. Patel. (2016). Biofilm formation by environmental isolates of *Salmonella* and their sensitivity to natural antimicrobials. Foodborne Pathog. Dis. 13: 509–516.

Khalil, M. A. and F. I. Sonbol. (2014). Investigation of biofilm formation on contact eye lenses caused by methicillin resistant *Staphylococcus aureus*. Niger. J. Clin. Pract. 17: 776–784.

Khan, M. S. I., E. -J. Lee and Y. -J. Kim. (2016). A submerged dielectric barrier discharge plasma inactivation mechanism of biofilms produced by *Escherichia coli* O157:H7, *Cronobacter sakazakii* and *Staphylococcus aureus*. Scientific Reports 6: 37072.

Kim, K. Y. and J. F. Frank. (1995). Effect of nutrients on biofilm formation by *Listeria monocytogenes* on stainless steel. J. Food Prot. 58: 24–28.

Kim, Y., and S. H. Kim. (2009). Released exopolysaccharide (r-EPS) produced from probiotic bacteria reduce biofilm formation of enterohemorrhagic *Escherichia coli* O157: H7. Biochem. Bioph. Res. Co. 379: 324–329.

Kisluk, G. and S. Yaron. (2012). Presence and persistence of *Salmonella enterica* serotype Typhimurium in the phyllosphere and rhizosphere of spray-irrigated parsley. Appl. Environ. Microbiol. 78: 4030–4036.

Kisluk, G., E. Kalily and S. Yaron. (2013). Resistance to essential oils affects survival of *Salmonella enterica* serovars in growing and harvested basil. Environ. Microbiol. 15: 2787–2798.

Klerks, M. M., E. Franz, M. van Gent-Pelzer, C. Zijlstra and A.H. Van Bruggen. (2007). Differential interaction of *Salmonella enterica* serovars with lettuce cultivars and plant-microbe factors influencing the colonization efficiency. The ISME J. 1: 620–631.

Knowles, J. R., S. Roller, D. B. Murray and A. S. Naidu. (2005). Antimicrobial action of carvacrol at different stages of dual-species biofilm development by Staphylococcus aureus and *Salmonella enterica* serovar Typhimurium. Appl. Environ. Microbiol. 71: 797–803.

Komal, S. and G. Shilpa. (2020). Postbiotics: A potential approach towards eradication of biofilms of various pathogens. Res. J. Biotechnol. 15: 115–120.

Koohestani, M., M. Moradi, H. Tajik and A. Badali. (2018). Effects of cell-free supernatant of *Lactobacillus acidophilus* LAS and Lactobacillus casei 431 against planktonic form and biofilm of Staphylococcus aureus. Vet. Res. Forum. 9: 301–306.

Koseki, S. and S. Isobe. (2005). Growth of *Listeria monocytogenes* on iceberg lettuce and solid media. Int. J. Food Microbiol. 101: 217–225.

Kroupitski, Y., R. Pinto, E. Belausov and S. Sela. (2011). Distribution of *Salmonella typhimurium* in romaine lettuce leaves. Food Microbiol. 28: 990–997.

Kroupitski, Y., R. Pinto, M. T. Brandl, E. Belausov and S. Sela. (2009). Interactions of *Salmonella enterica* with lettuce leaves. J. Appl. Microbiol. J. Appl. Microbiol. 106: 1876–1885.

Kumar, C. G. and S. K. Anand. (1998). Significance of microbial biofilms in food industry: A review. Int. J. Food Microbiol. 42: 9–27.

Kyere, E. O., G. Foong, J. Palmer, J. J. Wargent, G. C. Fletcher and S. Flint. (2019). Rapid attachment of *Listeria monocytogenes* to hydroponic and soil grown lettuce leaves. Food Control 101: 77–80.

Kyere, E. O., G. Foong, J. Palmer, J. J. Wargent, G. C. Fletcher and S. Flint. (2020). Biofilm formation of *Listeria monocytogenes* in hydroponic and soil grown lettuce leaf extracts on stainless steel coupons. LWT-Food Sci. Technol. 126: 109114. Doi: 10.1016/j.lwt.2020.109114.

Kyle, J. L., C. T. Parker, D. Goudeau and M. T. Brandl. (2010). Transcriptome analysis of *Escherichia coli* O157: H7 exposed to lysates of lettuce leaves. Appl. And Environ. Microbiol. 76: 1375–1387.

Langsrud, S., B. Moen, T. Møretrø, M. Løype and E. Heir. (2016). Microbial dynamics in mixed culture biofilms of bacteria surviving sanitation of conveyor belts in salmon-processing plants. J. Appl. Microbiol. 120: 366–378.

Lapidot, A., U. Romling and S. Yaron. (2006). Biofilm formation and the survival of *Salmonella typhimurium* on parsley. Int. J. Food Microbiol. 109: 229–233.

Latasa, C., C. Solano, J. R. Penadés and I. Lasa. (2006). Biofilm-associated proteins. C. R. Biol. 329: 849–857.

Lee, J. J., J. D. Eifert, S. Jung and L. -K. Strawn. (2018). Cavitation bubbles remove and inactivate *Listeria* and *Salmonella* on the surface of fresh roma tomatoes and cantaloupes. Frontiers Sustain. Food Systems 2: 61.

Lee, J. S., Y. M. Bae, S. Y. Lee and S. Y. Lee. (2015). Biofilm formation of *Staphylococcus aureus* on various surfaces and their resistance to chlorine sanitizer. J. Food Sci. 80: M2279–M2286.

Lee, K. W. K., S. Periasamy, M. Mukherjee, C. Xie, S. Kjelleberg and S. A. Rice. (2014). Biofilm development and enhanced stress resistance of a model, mixed-species community biofilm. The ISME J. 8: 894–907.

Leff, J. W. and N. Fierer. (2013). Bacterial communities associated with the surfaces of fresh fruits and vegetables. PloS One 8: e59310. Doi: 10.1371/journal.pone.0059310.

Lemon, K. P., Higgins, D. E. and R. Kolter. (2007). Flagellar motility is critical for *Listeria monocytogenes* biofilm formation. J. Bacteriol. 189: 4418–4424.

Lequette, Y., G. Boels, M. Clarisse and C. Faille. (2010). Using enzymes to remove biofilms of bacterial isolates sampled in the food industry. Biofouling 26: 421–431.

Lewis, V. G., M. P. Ween and C. A. McDevitt. (2012). The role of ATP-binding cassette transporters in bacterial pathogenicity. Protoplasma 249: 919–942.

Li, N. -W., G. -L. Liu and J. Liu. (2017). Inactivation of *Bacillus cereus* biofilms on stainless steel by acidic electrolyzed water. J. Food Process. Preservation. 41: e13304. Doi: 10.1111/jfpp.13304.

Li, R., W. Du, J. Yang, Z. Liu and A. E. Yousef. (2018). Control of *Listeria monocytogenes* biofilm by paenibacterin, a natural antimicrobial lipopeptide. Food Control 84: 529–535.

Lianou, A. and K. P. Koutsoumanis. (2012). Strain variability of the biofilm-forming ability of *Salmonella enterica* under various environmental conditions. Int. J. Food Microbiol. 160: 171–178.

Likotrafiti, E., M. Anagnou, P. Lampiri and J. Rhoades. (2014). Effect of storage temperature on the behaviour of *Escherichia coli* O157: H7 and *Salmonella enterica* serotype Typhimurium on salad vegetables. J. Food Res. 3: 1. Doi: 10.5539/jfr.v3n2p1.

Lim, Y., M. Jana, T. T. Luong and C. Y. Lee. 2004. Control of glucose-and NaCl-induced biofilm formation by rbf in *Staphylococcus aureus*. J. Bacteriol. 186: 722–729.

Liu, J., S. Yu, B. Han and J. Chen. (2017). Effects of benzalkonium chloride and ethanol on dual-species biofilms of *Serratia liquefaciens* S1 and *Shewanella putrefaciens* S4. Food Control 78: 196–202.

Liu, N. T., A. M. Lefcourt, X. Nou, D. R. Shelton, G. Zhang and Y. Lo. (2013). Native microflora in fresh-cut produce processing plants and their potentials for biofilm formation. J. Food Prot. 76: 827–832.

Liu, N. T., X. Nou, A. M. Lefcourt, D. R. Shelton and Y. M. Lo. (2014). Dual-species biofilm formation by *Escherichia coli* O157: H7 and environmental bacteria isolated from fresh-cut processing facilities. Int. J. Food Microbiol. 171: 15–20.

Liu, N. T., G. R. Bauchan, C. B. Francoeur, D. R. Shelton, Y. M. Lo and X. Nou. (2016a). *Ralstonia insidiosa* serves as bridges in biofilm formation by foodborne pathogens *Listeria monocytogenes*, *Salmonella enterica*, and Enterohemorrhagic *Escherichia coli*. Food Control 65: 14–20.

Liu, W., H. L. Røder, J. S. Madsen, T. Bjarnsholt, S. J. Sørensen and M. Burmølle. (2016b). Interspecific bacterial interactions are reflected in multispecies biofilm spatial organization. Front. Microbiol. 7: 1366. Doi: 10.3389/fmicb.2016.01366.

Liu, Y., J. Zhang and Y. Ji. (2020). Environmental factors modulate biofilm formation by *Staphylococcus aureus*. Sci. Prog. 103: 1–14.

Lohse, M. B., M. Gulati, A. D. Johnson and C. J. Nobile. (2018). Development and regulation of single- and multi-species *Candida albicans* biofilms. Nature Rev. Microbiol. 16: 19.

López-Gálvez, F., M. I. Gil, P. Truchado, M. V. Selma and A. Allende. (2010). Cross-contamination of fresh-cut lettuce after a short-term exposure during pre-washing cannot be controlled after subsequent washing with chlorine dioxide or sodium hypochlorite. Food Microbiol. 27: 199–204.

Lopez-Galvez, F., A. Allende, F. Pedrero-Salcedo, J. J. Alarcon and M. I. Gil. (2014). Safety assessment of greenhouse hydroponic tomatoes irrigated with reclaimed and surface water. Int. J. Food Microbiol. 191: 97–102.

Lorite, G. S., C. M. Rodrigues, A. A. De Souza, C. Kranz, B. Mizaikoff and M. A. Cotta. (2011). The role of conditioning film formation and surface chemical changes on Xylella fastidiosa adhesion and biofilm evolution. J. Colloid. Interface. Sci. 359: 289–295.

Macarisin, D., J. Patel, G. Bauchan, J. A. Giron and V. K. Sharma. (2012). Role of curli and cellulose expression in adherence of *Escherichia coli* O157: H7 to spinach leaves. Foodborne Pathog. Dis. 9: 160–167.

Macarisin, D., J. Patel, G. Bauchan, J. A. Giron and S. Ravishankar. (2013). Effect of spinach cultivar and bacterial adherence factors on survival of *Escherichia coli* O157: H7 on spinach leaves. J. Food Prot. 76: 1829–1837.

Macarisin, D., J. Patel and V. K.Sharma. (2014). Role of curli and plant cultivation conditions on *Escherichia coli* O157: H7 internalization into spinach grown on hydroponics and in soil. Int. J. Food Microbiol. 173: 48–53.

Madrid, C., C. Balsalobre, J. García and A. Juárez. (2007). The novel Hha/YmoA family of nucleoid-associated proteins: Use of structural mimicry to modulate the activity of the H-NS family of proteins. Mol. Microbiol. 63: 7–14.

Madurkay, M., V. Kadlicekova, J. Turna and H. Drahovska. (2019). Bacteriophage application for control of Cronobacter in liquid media and in biofilms. J. Food Nutr. Research 58: 85–91.

Mahaudin, N. A., N. I. H. Mat Daud, N. -K. M. Ab Rashid, B. J. Muhialdin, N. Saari and W. N. Noordin. (2018). Bacterial attachment and biofilm formation on stainless steel surface and their *in vitro* inhibition by marine fungal extracts. J. Food Safety 38: e12456 Doi: 10.1111/jfs.12456Citations.

Mahmoud, B. S. M. (2010). Effects of X-ray radiation on *Escherichia coli* O157: H7, *Listeria monocytogenes*, *Salmonella enterica* and Shigella flexneri inoculated on shredded iceberg lettuce. Food Microbiol. 27: 109–114.

Martínez-Vaz, B. M., R. C. Fink, F. Diez-Gonzalez and M. J. Sadowsky. (2014). Enteric pathogen-plant interactions: Molecular connections leading to colonization and growth and implications for food safety. Microbes Environ. ME13139.

Mazaheri, T., C. Ripolles-Avila, A. S. Hascoet and J. J. Rodriguez-Jerez. (2020). Effect of an enzymatic treatment on the removal of mature *Listeria monocytogenes* biofilms: A quantitative and qualitative study. Food Control 114: 107266 Doi: 10.1016/j.foodcont.2020.107266.

Medrano-Félix, J. A., C. Chaidez, K. D. Mena, M. del Socorro Soto-Galindo and N. Castro-del Campo. (2018). Characterization of biofilm formation by *Salmonella enterica* at the air-liquid interface in aquatic environments. Environ. Monit. Assess. 190: 221. Doi: 10.1007/s10661-018-6585-7.

Méric, G., E. K. Kemsley, D. Falush, E. J. Saggers and S. Lucchini. (2013). Phylogenetic distribution of traits associated with plant colonization in *Escherichia coli*. Environ. Microbiol. 15: 487–501.

Mirani, Z. A., M. N. Khan, M. Aziz, S. Naz and S. I. Khan. (2012). Effect of stress on biofilm formation by *icaA* positive and negative strains of methicillin resistant *Staphylococcus aureus*. J. Coll. Physicians Surg. Pak. 22: 10–14.

Mitra, R., E. Cuesta-Alonso, A. Wayadande, J. Talley, S. Gilliland and J. Fletcher. (2009). Effect of route of introduction and host cultivar on the colonization, internalization, and movement of the human pathogen *Escherichia coli* O157: H7 in spinach. J. Food Prot. 72: 1521–1530.

Montañez-Izquierdo, V. Y., D. I. Salas-Vázquez and J. J. Rodríguez-Jerez. (2012). Use of epifluorescence microscopy to assess the effectiveness of phage P100 in controlling *Listeria monocytogenes* biofilms on stainless steel surfaces. Food Control 23: 470–477.

Moradi, M. and H. Tajik. (2017). Biofilm removal potential of neutral electrolyzed water on pathogen and spoilage bacteria in dairy model systems. J. Appl. Microbiol. 123: 1429–1437.

Moraes, J. O., E. A. Cruz, Í Pinheiro, T. C. Oliveira, V. Alvarenga, A. S. Sant'Ana et al. (2019). An ordinal logistic regression approach to predict the variability on biofilm formation stages by five *Salmonella enterica* strains on polypropylene and glass surfaces as affected by pH, temperature and NaCl. Food Microbiol. 83: 95–103.

Møretrø, T., L. Hermansen, A. L. Holck, M. S. Sidhu, K. Rudi and S. Langsrud. (2003). Biofilm formation and the presence of the intercellular adhesion locus ica among staphylococci from food and food processing environments. Appl. Environ. Microbiol. 69: 5648–5655.

Muhsin, J., T. Ufaq, H. Tahr and A. Saadia. (2015). Bacterial biofilm: Its composition, formation and role in human infections. J. Microbiol. Biotechnol. 4: 1–14.

Nahar, S., A. J. -W. Ha, K. -H. Byun, M. I. Hussain, M. F. R. Mirza and S. -D. Ha. (2021). Efficacy of flavourzyme against *Salmonella typhimurium*, *Escherichia coli*, and *Pseudomonas aeruginosa* biofilms on food-contact surfaces. Int. J. Food Microbiol. 336: 108897. Doi: 10.1016/j.ijfoodmicro.2020.108897.

Nesse, L. L., C. Sekse, K. Berg, K. C. Johannesen, H. Solheim, L. K. Vestby et al. (2014). Potentially pathogenic *Escherichia coli* can form a biofilm under conditions relevant to the food production chain. Appl. Environ. Microbiol. 80: 2042–2049.

Nicola, S., J. Hoeberechts, D. Saglietti and E. Fontana. (2004). Nitrogen fertilization regime and lettuce romaine types influence seedling growth, root architecture and transplant quality. pp. 217–225. *In*: Cantliffe, D. J., P. J. Stoffella and N. Shaw (eds.). VII International Symposium on Protected Cultivation in Mild Winter Climates: Production, Pest Management and Global Competition. ISHS Acta Horticulturae 659, Belgium.

Nilsson, R. E., T. Ross and J. P. Bowman. (2011). Variability in biofilm production by *Listeria monocytogenes* correlated to strain origin and growth conditions. Int. J. Food Microbiol. 150: 14–24.

Norwood, D. E. and A. Gilmour. (2000). The growth and resistance to sodium hypochlorite of *Listeria monocytogenes* in a steady-state multispecies biofilm. J. Appl. Microbiol. 88: 512–520.

Noyce, J. O., H. Michels and C. W. Keevil. (2006). Use of copper cast alloys to control *Escherichia coli* O157 cross-contamination during food processing. Appl. Environ. Microbiol. 72: 4239–4244.

Ölmez, H. and S. D. Temur. (2010). Effects of different sanitizing treatments on biofilms and attachment of *Escherichia coli* and *Listeria monocytogenes* on green leaf lettuce. LWT-Food Sci. Technol. 43: 964–970.

Omac, B., R. C. Moreira and E. Castell-Perez. (2018). Quantifying growth of cold-adapted *Listeria monocytogenes* and *Listeria innocua* on fresh spinach leaves at refrigeration temperatures. J. Food Eng. 224: 17–26.

O'Neill, E., C. Pozzi, P. Houston, D. Smyth, H. Humphreys, D. A. Robinson et al. (2007). Association between methicillin susceptibility and biofilm regulation in *Staphylococcus aureus* isolates from device-related infections. J. Clin. Microbiol. 45: 1379–1388.

Ono, K., R. Oka, M. Toyofuku, A. Sakaguchi, M. Hamada, S. Yoshida et al. (2014). cAMP signaling affects irreversible attachment during biofilm formation by *Pseudomonas aeruginosa* PAO1. Microbes Environ. 29: 104–106.

Oulahal, N., W. Brice, A. Martial and P. Degraeve. (2008). Quantitative analysis of survival of *Staphylococcus aureus* or *Listeria innocua* on two types of surfaces: Polypropylene and stainless steel in contact with three different dairy products. Food Control 19: 178–185.

Pagedar, A., J. Singh and V. K. Batish. (2010). Surface hydrophobicity, nutritional contents affect *Staphylococcus aureus* biofilms and temperature influences its survival in preformed biofilms. J. Basic Microbiol. 50: S98–S106.

Palmer, J., S. Flint and J. Brooks. (2007). Bacterial cell attachment, the beginning of a biofilm. J. Ind. Microbiol. Biotechnol. 34: 577–588.

Pang, X. Y., Y. S. Yang and H. G. Yuk. (2017). Biofilm formation and disinfectant resistance of *Salmonella* sp. in mono-and dual-species with *Pseudomonas aeruginosa*. J. Appl. Microbiol. 123: 651–660.

Pang, X. and H. G. Yuk. (2018). Effect of *Pseudomonas aeruginosa* on the sanitizer sensitivity of *Salmonella enteritidis* biofilm cells in chicken juice. Food Control 86: 59–65.

Papaioannou, E., E. D. Giaouris, P. Berillis and I. S. Boziaris. (2018). Dynamics of biofilm formation by *Listeria monocytogenes* on stainless steel under mono-species and mixed-culture simulated fish processing conditions and chemical disinfection challenges. Int. J. Food Microbiol. 267: 9–19.

Parijs, I. and H. P. Steenackers. (2018). Competitive inter-species interactions underlie the increased antimicrobial tolerance in multispecies brewery biofilms. ISME J. 12: 2061–2075.

Park, J. W., J. S. An, W. H. Lim, B. S. Lim and S. J. Ahn. (2019). Microbial changes in biofilms on composite resins with different surface roughness: An *in vitro* study with a multispecies biofilm model. J. Prosthet. Dent. 122: 493.e1–493.e8.

Parasion, S., M. Kwiatek, R. Gryko, L. Mizak and A. Malm. (2014). Bacteriophages as an alternative strategy for fighting biofilm development. Pol. J. Microbiol. 63: 137–145.

Parkar, S. G., S. H. Flint and J. D. Brooks. (2004). Evaluation of the effect of cleaning regimes on biofilms of thermophilic bacilli on stainless steel. J. Appl. Microbiol. 96: 110–116.

Patange, A., D. Boehm, D. Ziuzina, P. J. Cullen, B. Gilmore and P. Bourke. (2019). High voltage atmospheric cold air plasma control of bacterial biofilms on fresh produce. Int. J. Food Microbiol. 293: 137–145.

Patel, J. and M. Sharma. (2010). Differences in attachment of *Salmonella enterica* serovars to cabbage and lettuce leaves. Int. J. Food Microbiol. 139: 41–47.

Patel, J., M. Sharma, P. Millner, T. Calaway and M. Singh. (2011a). Inactivation of *Escherichia coli* O157: H7 attached to spinach harvester blade using bacteriophage. Foodborne Pathog. Dis. 8: 541–546.

Patel, J., M. Sharma and S. Ravishakar. (2011b). Effect of curli expression and hydrophobicity of *Escherichia coli* O157: H7 on attachment to fresh produce surfaces. J. Appl. Microbiol. 110: 737–745.

Pérez-Rodríguez, F., A. Valero, E. Carrasco, R. M. García and G. Zurera. (2008). Understanding and modelling bacterial transfer to foods: A review. Trends Food Sci. Technol. 19: 131–144.

Pilchová, T., M. Hernould, H. Prévost, K. Demnerová, J. Pazlarová and O. Tresse. (2014). Influence of food processing environments on structure initiation of static biofilm of *Listeria monocytogenes*. Food Control 35: 366–372.

Pires, D. P., H. Oliveira, L. D. Melo, S. Sillankorva and J. Azeredo. (2016). Bacteriophage-encoded depolymerases: Their diversity and biotechnological applications. Appl. Microbiol. Biotechnol. 100: 2141–2151.

Poortinga, A. T., R. Bos and H. J. Busscher. (2001). Electrostatic interactions in the adhesion of an ion-penetrable and ion-impenetrable bacterial strain to glass. Colloids Surf. B 20: 105–117.

Pratt, L. A. and R. Kolter. (1998). Genetic analysis of *Escherichia coli* biofilm formation: Roles of flagella, motility, chemotaxis and type I pili. Mol. Microbiol. 30: 285–293.

Prokopovich, P. and S. Perni. (2009). An investigation of microbial adhesion to natural and synthetic polysaccharide-based films and its relationship with the surface energy components. J. Mater. Sci.: Mater. Med. 20: 195–202.

Puga, C. H., C. SanJose and B. Orgaz. (2014). Spatial distribution of *Listeria monocytogenes* and *Pseudomonas fluorescens* in mixed biofilms. pp. 115–132. *In*: Hambrick, E.C. (ed.). *Listeria monocytogenes*: Food Sources, Prevalence and Management Strategies. Nova Publishers, New York, USA.

Qin, Z., X. Yang, L. Yang, J. Jiang, Y. Ou, S. Molin et al. (2007). Formation and properties of *in vitro* biofilms of ica-negative *Staphylococcus epidermidis* clinical isolates. J. Med. Microbiol. 56: 83–93.

Quilliam, R. S., A. P. Williams and D. L. Jones. (2012). Lettuce cultivar mediates both phyllosphere and rhizosphere activity of *Escherichia coli* O157: H7. PLoS One 7: e33842. Doi: 10.1371/journal. pone.0033842.

Raffaella, C., L. Casettari, L. Fagioli, M. Cespi, G. Bonacucina and W. Baffone. (2017). Activity of essential oil-based microemulsions against Staphylococcus aureus developed on stainless steel surface in different culture media and growth conditions. Int. J. Food Microbiol. 241: 132–140.

Rainey, P. B. and M. Travisano. (1998). Adaptive radiation in a heterogeneous environment. Nature 394: 69–72.

Reisner, A., K. A. Krogfelt, B. M. Klein, E. L. Zechner and S. Molin. (2006). *In vitro* biofilm formation of commensal and pathogenic *Escherichia coli* strains: Impact of environmental and genetic factors. J. Bacteriol. 188: 3572–3581.

Rendueles, O. and J. M. Ghigo. (2012). Multi-species biofilms: how to avoid unfriendly neighbors. FEMS Microbiol. Rev. 36: 972–989.

Rieu, A., S. Weidmann, D. Garmyn, P. Piveteau and J. Guzzo. (2007). Agr system of *Listeria monocytogenes* EGD-e: Role in adherence and differential expression pattern. Appl. Environ. Microbiol. 73: 6125–6133.

Ripolles-Avila, C., A. S. Hascoët, A. E. Guerrero-Navarro and J. J. Rodríguez-Jerez. (2018). Establishment of incubation conditions to optimize the *in vitro* formation of mature *Listeria monocytogenes* biofilms on food-contact surfaces. Food Control 92: 240–248.

Rode, T. M., S. Langsrud, A. Holck and T. Møretrø. (2007). Different patterns of biofilm formation in *Staphylococcus aureus* under food-related stress conditions. Int. J. Food Microbiol. 116: 372–383.

Römling, U. and M. Rohde. (1999). Flagella modulate the multicellular behavior of *Salmonella typhimurium* on the community level. FEMS Microbiol. Lett. 180: 91–102.

Römling, U., M. Rohde, A. Olsén, S. Normark and J. Reinköster. (2000). AgfD, the checkpoint of multicellular and aggregative behaviour in *Salmonella typhimurium* regulates at least two independent pathways. Mol. Microbiol. 36: 10–23.

Ryan, M. P., J. T. Pembroke and C. C. Adley. (2011). Genotypic and phenotypic diversity of *Ralstonia pickettii* and *Ralstonia insidiosa* isolates from clinical and environmental sources including high-purity water. Diversity in *Ralstonia pickettii*. BMC Microbiol. 11: 194. Doi: 10.1186/1471–2180–11–194.

Ryu, J. H., H. Kim, J. F. Frank and L. R. Beuchat. (2004). Attachment and biofilm formation on stainless steel by *Escherichia coli* O157: H7 as affected by curli production. Lett. Appl. Microbiol. 39: 359–362.

Saini, R., P. A. Giri, S. Saini and S. R. Saini. (2015). Dental plaque: A complex biofilm. Pravara Med. Rev. 7: 9–14.

Salazar, J. K., K. Deng, M. L. Tortorello, M. T. Brandl, H. Wang and W. Zhang. (2013). Genes ycfR, *sirA* and *yigG* contribute to the surface attachment of *Salmonella enterica* Typhimurium and Saintpaul to fresh produce. PLoS One 8: e57272. Doi: 10.1371/journal.pone.0057272.

Saldaña, Z., J. Xicohtencatl-Cortes, F. Avellno, A. D. Phillips, J. B. Kaper, J. L. Puente et al. (2009). Synergistic role of curli and cellulose in cell adherence and biofilm formation of attaching and effacing Escherichia coli and identification of Fis as a negative regulator of curli. Envion. Microbiol. 11: 992–1006.

Saldaña, Z., E. Sánchez, J. Xicohtencatl-Cortes, J. L. Puente and J. A. Girón. (2011). Surface structures involved in plant stomata and leaf colonization by Shiga-toxigenic *Escherichia coli* O157: H7. Front. Microbiol. 2: 119. Doi: 10.3389/fmicb.2011.00119.

Sapers, G. M. and M. P. Doyle. (2014). Scope of the produce contamination problem. pp. 3–20. *In*: Matthews, K. R., G. M. Sapers and C. P. Gerba (eds.). The Produce Contamination Problem: Causes and Solutions. Second Edition. Elsevier, Amsterdam, Netherlands.

Sauer, K., M. C. Cullen, A. H. Rickard, L. A. H. Zeef, D. G. Davies and P. Gilbert. (2004). Characterization of nutrient-induced dispersion in *Pseudomonas aeruginosa* PAO1 biofilm. J. Bacteriol. 186: 7312–7326.

Schauder, S. and B. L. Bassler. (2001). The languages of bacteria. Genes Dev. 15: 1468–1480.

Schembri, M. A., K. Kjærgaard and P. Klemm. (2003). Global gene expression in *Escherichia coli* biofilms. Mol. Microbiol. 48: 253–267.

Scher, K., U. Romling and S. Yaron. (2005). Effect of heat, acidification, and chlorination on *Salmonella enterica* serovar Typhimurium cells in a biofilm formed at the air-liquid interface. Appl. Environ. Microbiol. 71: 1163–1168.

Sela, S., S. Frank, E. Belausov and R. Pinto. (2006). A mutation in the luxS gene influences *Listeria monocytogenes* biofilm formation. Appl. Environ. Microbiol. 72: 5653–5658.

Sharma, M., J. H. Ryu and L. R. Beuchat. (2005). Inactivation of *Escherichia coli* O157: H7 in biofilm on stainless steel by treatment with an alkaline cleaner and a bacteriophage. J. Appl. Microbiol. 99: 449–459.

Sharma, M., G. Dashiell, E. T. Handy, C. East, R. Reynnells, C. White et al. (2017). Survival of *Salmonella* Newport on whole and fresh-cut cucumbers treated with lytic bacteriophages. J. Food Prot. 80: 668–673.

Sharma, R. P., S. D. Raut, A. S. Kadam, R. M. Mulani and R. S. Mane. (2020). *In vitro* antibacterial and anti-biofilm efficiencies of chitosan-encapsulated zinc ferrite nanoparticles. Appl. Physics A: Materials Science and Processing 126: 824.

Sharma, V. K. and B. L. Bearson. (2013). Hha controls *Escherichia coli* O157: H7 biofilm formation by differential regulation of global transcriptional regulators of FlhDC and CsgD. Appl. Environ. Microbiol. 79: 2384–2396.

Sharma, V. K. and T. A. Casey. (2014). Determining the relative contribution and hierarchy of hha and qseBC in the regulation of flagellar motility of *Escherichia coli* O157: H7. PLOS One 9: e85866. Doi: 10.1371/journal.pone.0085866.

Shaw, R. K., C. N. Berger, B. Feys, S. Knutton, M. J. Pallen and G. Frankel. (2008). Enterohemorrhagic *Escherichia coli* exploits EspA filaments for attachment to salad leaves. Appl. Environ. Microbiol. 74: 2908–2914.

Shen, C., Y. Luo, X. Nou, G. Bauchan, B. Zhou, Q. Wang et al. (2012). Enhanced inactivation of *Salmonella* and *Pseudomonas* biofilms on stainless steel by use of T-128, a fresh produce washing aid, in chlorinated wash solutions. Appl. Environ. Microbiol. 78: 6789–6798.

Shi, X., A. Namvar, M. Kostrzynska, R. Hora and K. Warriner. (2007). Persistence and growth of different *Salmonella* serovars on pre-and postharvest tomatoes. J. Food Prot. 70: 2725–2731.

Shi, X. and X. Zhu. (2009). Biofilm formation and food safety in food industries. Trends Food Sci. Technol. 20: 407–413.

Simm, R., M. Morr, A. Kader, M. Nimtz and U. Römling. (2004). GGDEF and EAL domains inversely regulate cyclic di-GMP levels and transition from sessility to motility. Mol. Microbiol. 53: 1123–1134.

Simões, M., L. C. Simões and M. J. Vieira. (2010). A review of current and emergent biofilm control strategies. LWT-Food Sci. Technol. 43: 573–583.

Sinde, E. and J. Carballo. (2000). Attachment of *Salmonella* spp. and *Listeria monocytogenes* to stainless steel, rubber and polytetrafluorethylene: The influence of free energy and the effect of commercial sanitizers. Food Microbiol. 17: 439–447.

Sivapalasingam, S., C. R. Friedman, L. Cohen and R. V. Tauxe. (2004). Fresh produce: A growing cause of outbreaks of foodborne illness in the United States, 1973 through 1997. J. Food Prot. 67: 2342–2353.

Solano, C., B. García, J. Valle, C. Berasain, J. M. Ghigo, C. Gamazo et al. (2002). Genetic analysis of *Salmonella enteritidis* biofilm formation: Critical role of cellulose. Mol. Microbiol. 43: 793–808.

Solomon, E. B., S. Yaron and K. R. Matthews. (2002). Transmission of *Escherichia coli* O157: H7 from contaminated manure and irrigation water to lettuce plant tissue and its subsequent internalization. Appl. Environ. Microbiol. 68: 397–400.

Somers, E. B. and A. C. Lee Wong. (2004). Efficacy of two cleaning and sanitizing combinations on *Listeria monocytogenes* biofilms formed at low temperature on a variety of materials in the presence of ready-to-eat meat residue. J. Food Prot. 67: 2218–2229.

Someya, N., K. Tsuchiya, S. Sugisawa, M. T. Noguchi and T. Yoshida. (2008). Growth promotion of lettuce (*Lactuca sativa* L.) by a Rhizobacterium *Pseudomonas fluorescens* strain LRB3W1 under iron-limiting condition. Environ. Control Biol. 46: 139–146.

Song, Y. J., H. H. Yu, Y. J. Kim, N. -K. Lee and H. -D. Paik. (2020). The use of papain for the removal of biofilms formed by pathogenic Staphylococcus aureus and Campylobacter jejuni. LWT-Food Sci. Technol. 127: 109383. Doi: 10.1016/j.lwt.2020.109383.

Soni, K. A. and R. Nannapaneni. (2010). Removal of *Listeria monocytogenes* biofilms with bacteriophage P100. J. Food Prot. 73: 1519–1524.

Soni, K. A., A. Oladunjoye, R. Nannapaneni, M. W. Schilling, J. L. Silva, B. Mikel et al. (2013). Inhibition and inactivation of *Salmonella typhimurium* biofilms from polystyrene and stainless steel surfaces by essential oils and phenolic constituent carvacrol. J. Food Protect. 76: 205–212.

Speranza, B., N. Monacis, M. Sinigaglia and M. R. Corbo. (2017). Approaches to removal and killing of *salmonella* spp. biofilms. J. Food Process. Preservation. 41: e12758. Doi: 10.1111/jfpp.12758.

Spiers, A. J., J. Bohannon, S. M. Gehrig and P. B. Rainey. (2003). Biofilm formation at the air–liquid interface by the *Pseudomonas fluorescens* SBW25 wrinkly spreader requires an acetylated form of cellulose. Mol. Microbiol. 50: 15–27.

Spiers, A. J., S. G. Kahn, J. Bohannon, M. Travisano and P. B. Rainey. (2002). Adaptive divergence in experimental populations of *Pseudomonas fluorescens*. I. Genetic and phenotypic bases of wrinkly spreader fitness. Genetics 161: 33–46.

Stepanović, S., I. Ćirković, L. Ranin and M. Svabić-Vlahović. (2004). Biofilm formation by *Salmonella* spp. and *Listeria monocytogenes* on plastic surface. Lett. Appl. Microbiol. 38: 428–432.

Stewart, P. S. (2015). Antimicrobial tolerance in biofilms. Microb. Biofilms 13: 269–285.

Sutherland, I. W. (1999). Polysaccharases for microbial exopolysaccharides. Carbohydr. Polym. 38: 319–328.

Tang, H., T. Cao, A. Wang, X. Liang, S. O. Salley, J. P. McAllister et al. (2007). Effect of surface modification of siliconeon *Staphylococcus epidermidis* adhesion and colonization. J. Biomed. Mater. Res. 80: 885–894.

Taylor, C. M., M. Beresford, H. A. Epton, D. C. Sigee, G. Shama, P. W. Andrew et al. (2002). *Listeria monocytogenes* relA and hpt mutants are impaired in surface-attached growth and virulence. J. Bacteriol. 184: 621–628.

Teplitski, M., A. Al-Agely and B. M. Ahmer. (2006). Contribution of the *SirA* regulon to biofilm formation in *Salmonella enterica* serovar Typhimurium. Microbiol. 152: 3411–3424.

Teplitski, M., J. D. Barak and K. R. Schneider. (2009). Human enteric pathogens in produce: Un-answered ecological questions with direct implications for food safety. Curr. Opin. Biotechnol. 20: 166–171.

Teplitski, M., R. I. Goodier and B. M. Ahmer. (2003). Pathways leading from BarA/*SirA* to motility and virulence gene expression in *Salmonella*. J. Bacteriol. 185: 7257–7265.

Tilahun, A., S. Haddis, A. Teshale and T. Hadush. (2016). Review on biofilm and microbial adhesion. Int. J. Microbiol. Res. 7: 63–73.

Todhanakasem, T. and G. M. Young. (2008). Loss of flagellum-based motility by *Listeria monocytogenes* results in formation of hyperbiofilms. J. Bacteriol. 190: 6030–6034.

Tomičić, R. M., I. S. Čabarkapa, D. M. Vukmirović, J. D. Lević and Z. M. Tomičić. (2016). Influence of growth conditions on biofilm formation of *Listeria monocytogenes*. Food Feed Res. 43: 19–24.

Tremoulet, F., O. Duche, A. Namane, B. Martinie and European *Listeria* Genome Consortium, J.C. Labadie. (2002). Comparison of protein patterns of *Listeria monocytogenes* grown in biofilm or in planktonic mode by proteomic analysis. FEMS Microbiol. Lett. 210: 25–31.

Tresse, O., V. Lebret, D. Garmyn and O. Dussurget. (2009). The impact of growth history and flagellation on the adhesion of various *Listeria monocytogenes* strains to polystyrene. Can. J. Microbiol. 55: 189–196.

Vadillo-Rodríguez, V., A. I. Guerra-García-Mora, D. Perera-Costa, M. L. Gónzalez-Martín and M. C. Fernández-Calderón. (2018). Bacterial response to spatially organized microtopographic surface patterns with nanometer scale roughness. Colloids. Surf. B 169: 340–347.

Vatanyoopaisarn, S., A. Nazli, C. E. Dodd, C. E. Rees and W. M. Waites. (2000). Effect of flagella on initial attachment of *Listeria monocytogenes* to stainless steel. Appl. Environ. Microbiol. 66: 860–863.

Vázquez-Sánchez, D., O. Habimana and A. Holck. (2013). Impact of food-related environmental factors on the adherence and biofilm formation of natural *Staphylococcus aureus* isolates. Curr. Microbiol. 66: 110–121.

Wang, H. H., K. P. Ye, Q. Q. Zhang, Y. Dong, X. L. Xu and G. H. Zhou. (2013). Biofilm formation of meat-borne *Salmonella enterica* and inhibition by the cell-free supernatant from *Pseudomonas aeruginosa*. Food Control 32: 650–658.

Wang, R., Y. Zhou, N. Kalchayanand, D. M. Harhay and T. L. Wheeler. (2020). Effectiveness and functional mechanism of a multicomponent sanitizer against biofilms formed by *Escherichia coli* O157: H7 and five *Salmonella* serotypes prevalent in the meat industry. J. Food Protect. 83: 568–575.

Warning, A. and A. K. Datta. (2013). Interdisciplinary engineering approaches to study how pathogenic bacteria interact with fresh produce. J. Food Eng. 114: 426–448.

White, A. P., D. L. Gibson, W. Kim, W. W. Kay and M. G. Surette. (2006). Thin aggregative fimbriae and cellulose enhance long-term survival and persistence of *Salmonella*. J. Bacteriol. 188: 3219–3227.

Winkelströter, L. K., F. L. Tulini and E. C. De Martinis. (2015). Identification of the bacteriocin produced by cheese isolate *Lactobacillus paraplantarum* FT259 and its potential influence on *Listeria monocytogenes* biofilm formation. LWT-Food Sci. Technol. 64: 586–592.

Wirtanen, G., U. Husmark and T. Mattila-Sandholm. (1996). Microbial evaluation of the biotransfer potential from surfaces with Bacillus biofilms after rinsing and cleaning procedures in closed food-processing systems. J. Food Prot. 59: 727–733.

Wolfe, A. J., D. E. Chang, J. D. Walker, J. E. Seitz-Partridge, M. D. Vidaurri, C. F. Lange et al. (2003). Evidence that acetyl phosphate functions as a global signal during biofilm development. Mol. Microbiol. 48: 977–988.

Wong, C. W., S. Wang, R. C. Levesque, L. Goodridge and P. Delaquis. (2019). Fate of 43 *Salmonella* strains on lettuce and tomato seedlings. J. Food Prot. 82: 1045–1051.

Xicohtencatl-Cortes, J., E. S. Chacón, Z. Saldana, E. Freer and J. A. Girón. (2009). Interaction of *Escherichia coli* O157: H7 with leafy green produce. J. Food Protect. 72: 1531–1537.

Yamazaki, A., J. Li, W. C. Hutchins, L. Wang, J. Ma, A. M. Ibekwe et al. (2011). Commensal effect of pectate lyases secreted from *Dickeya dadantii* on proliferation of *Escherichia coli* O157: H7 EDL933 on lettuce leaves. Appl. Environ. Microbiol. 77: 156–162.

Yao, Y. and O. Habimana. (2019). Biofilm research within irrigation water distribution systems: Trends, knowledge gaps, and future perspectives. Sci. Total Environ. 673: 254–265.

Yaron, S. (2014). Microbial attachment and persistence on plants. pp. 21–58. *In*: Matthews, K. R. (ed.). The Produce Contamination Problem, 2nd edition. Elsevier, San Diego, CA, USA.

Yaron, S. and U. Römling. (2014_. Biofilm formation by enteric pathogens and its role in plant colonization and persistence. Microb. Biotechnol. 7: 496–516.

Yawata, Y., N. Nomura and H. Uchiyama. (2008). Development of a novel biofilm continuous culture method for simultaneous assessment of architecture and gaseous metabolite production. Appl. Environ. Microbiol. 74: 5429–5435.

Yildiz, F. H. and G. K. Schoolnik. (1999). *Vibrio cholerae* O1 El Tor: Identification of a gene cluster required for the rugose colony type, exopolysaccharide production, chlorine resistance, and biofilm formation. Proc. Natl. Acad. Sci. 96: 4028–4033.

Yin, B., L. Zhu, Y. Zhang, P. Dong, Y. Mao, R. Liang et al. (2018). The characterization of biofilm formation and detection of biofilm-related genes in *Salmonella* isolated from beef processing plants. Foodborne Pathog. Dis 15: 660–667.

Yin, H. B., A. Boomer, C. H. Chen and J. Patel. (2019). Antibiofilm efficacy of peptide 1018 against *Listeria monocytogenes* and Shiga Toxigenic *Escherichia coli* on equipment surfaces. J. Food Prot. 82: 1837–1843.

Yousefi, M., M. Rahimi-Nasrabadi, S. M. Pourmortazavi, M. Wysokowski, T. Jesionowski, H. Ehrlich et al. (2019). Supercritical fluid extraction of essential oils. Trends Analyt. Chem. 118: 182–193.

Yu, H., Y. Liu, L. Li, Y. Guo, Y. Xie, Y. Cheng et al. (2020). Ultrasound-involved emerging strategies for controlling foodborne microbial biofilms. Trends Food Sci. Technol. 96: 91–101.

Zhang, C., C. Li, M. A. Abdel-Samie, H. Cui and L. Lin. (2020). Unraveling the inhibitory mechanism of clove essential oil against *Listeria monocytogenes* biofilm and applying it to vegetable surfaces. LWT-Food Sci. Technol. 134: 110210. Doi: 10.1016/j.lwt.2020.110210.

Zhao, T., M. P. Doyle and P. Zhao. (2004). Control of *Listeria monocytogenes* in a biofilm by competitive-exclusion microorganisms. Appl. Environ. Microbiol. 70: 3996–4003.

Ziech, R. E., A. P. Perin, C. Lampugnani, M. J. Sereno, C. Viana, C. Viana et al. (2016). Biofilm-producing ability and tolerance to industrial sanitizers in *Salmonella* spp. isolated from Brazilian poultry processing plants. LWT-Food Sci. Technol. 68: 85–90.

Ziuzina, D., L. Han, P. J. Cullen and P. Bourke. (2015). Cold plasma inactivation of internalised bacteria and biofilms for *Salmonella enterica* serovar Typhimurium, *Listeria monocytogenes* and *Escherichia coli*. Int. J. Food Microbiol. 210: 53–61.

Zogaj, X., M. Nimtz, M. Rohde, W. Bokranz and U. Römling. (2001). The multicellular morphotypes of *Salmonella typhimurium* and *Escherichia coli* produce cellulose as the second component of the extracellular matrix. Mol. Microbiol. 39: 1452–1463.

Index

A

Abiotic surfaces 248, 258–260, 269
Acute lung injury 141, 146, 147
Artificial intelligence 1, 3–5, 14
Artificial neural networks 10, 23

B

Bacterial attachment 250, 255, 260, 261
Balantidium 48, 51, 58
Biofilm 247–265, 268–278
Blastocystis 46, 48, 54–57, 59, 60, 63, 66–68, 73, 78–80, 84

C

Chatbot 1, 3, 11, 13, 27–32, 34
COVID-19 143, 176, 177
Cryptosporidium 47, 49, 51, 55–72, 75, 76, 78–82, 84–87
Cyber-molecular assays 1, 25
Cyclospora 47, 49, 55, 57, 58, 60–64, 79, 82, 85
Cystoisospora 46, 63

D

Deep learning 3, 5, 8, 10, 12–15, 19–21, 23–26, 28, 34
Diagnosis 118, 122–126, 128–134, 226–228
Diagnostic chatbot 1
Diagnostics 1–3, 6–8, 13, 16–19, 22, 23, 25, 27, 30, 31, 34
Disease 209, 226, 228
Disease diagnosis 190

E

ELISA 119, 120, 126–130
Entamoeba 46, 49, 51, 54, 57, 59, 60, 62, 63, 67, 69, 70, 72–74, 82, 84, 86, 87

F

Filarial nematodes 118, 121, 122, 124, 129, 131–133
Filariasis 118, 119, 121, 122, 125–129, 133
Fingerprint 197
Fresh produce 247–250, 254, 255, 258, 261–272, 274, 277, 278

G

Gel-based PCR 111, 112
Gene deletion 111
Giardia 46, 50, 53, 57, 59, 60, 62, 63, 65–72, 75, 84–86

H

High-resolution dye 239

I

ICT 119, 120, 127–129
Internal amplification control 242

L

Laboratory diagnostics 1, 3, 6–8, 16, 25
LAMP 111, 113, 115, 119, 120, 123, 130, 132–134
Language models 7
LIPS 119, 120, 127, 128
Loiasis 122, 128, 134
Lung inflammation 171, 173, 176
Lymphatic filariasis 118, 119, 121, 122, 125–128, 133

M

Machine learning 1, 4, 5
Malaria 104–115
Mansonellosis 118, 120

Mass spectrometry 190, 197, 198, 210, 211, 217, 219

Microorganism 191–193, 197–199, 203, 210, 212, 215, 226, 227

Microscopy 104, 105, 107, 108, 110–115, 119, 120, 122, 124, 127

Microsporidia 50, 51, 53, 55–57, 59–66, 73, 74, 85

Molecular diagnostics 16–19, 21–23, 27, 34

N

Neutrophils 149, 151–155, 165, 168, 173–176

O

Onchocerciasis 118–122, 124–128, 130, 133

P

Pathogens 247–249, 254–258, 260–267, 269–275, 277, 278

PCR 119, 120, 123, 125, 126, 130–134

Persistence 247–249, 252–254, 256, 260, 264–268, 277, 278

Personalized medicine 6, 17, 18

pfhrp2 111

Plasmodium Falciparum 104

Proteome 209, 210, 214, 217, 224, 226

R

Ramp rate 244

RDT 104, 108, 109–111, 113–115, 119, 122, 127, 134

Reaction efficiency 240

Reactive oxygen species 152

Real-time PCR 112, 114

S

Saturating dye 239

T

Transcription factor 157, 164, 166

V

Vascular endothelium 156, 169

For Product Safety Concerns and Information please contact our EU
representative GPSR@taylorandfrancis.com
Taylor & Francis Verlag GmbH, Kaufingerstraße 24, 80331 München, Germany